Clinical Teaching Strategies in Nursing

FOURTH EDITION

KATHLEEN B. GABERSON, PhD, RN, CNOR, CNE, ANEF

MARILYN H. OERMANN, PhD, RN, ANEF, FAAN

TERESA SHELLENBARGER, PhD, RN, CNE, ANEF

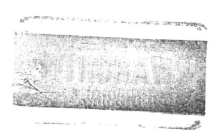

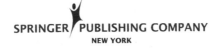

SPRINGER PUBLISHING COMPANY
NEW YORK

Springer Publishing Company, LLC
11 West 42nd Street
New York, NY 10036
www.springerpub.com

Acquisitions Editor: Margaret Zuccarini
Composition: diacriTech

ISBN: 978-0-8261-1961-2
e-book ISBN: 978-0-8261-1962-9
Instructors' Manual: 978-0-8261-2632-0
Instructors' PowerPoints: 978-0-8261-2633-7

Instructors' Materials: Instructors may request supplements by emailing textbook@springerpub.com

14 15 16 17 / 5 4 3 2 1

The author and the publisher of this Work have made every effort to use sources believed to be reliable to provide information that is accurate and compatible with the standards generally accepted at the time of publication. Because medical science is continually advancing, our knowledge base continues to expand. Therefore, as new information becomes available, changes in procedures become necessary. We recommend that the reader always consult current research and specific institutional policies before performing any clinical procedure. The author and publisher shall not be liable for any special, consequential, or exemplary damages resulting, in whole or in part, from the readers' use of, or reliance on, the information contained in this book. The publisher has no responsibility for the persistence or accuracy of URLs for external or third-party Internet websites referred to in this publication and does not guarantee that any content on such websites is, or will remain, accurate or appropriate.

Library of Congress Cataloging-in-Publication Data

Gaberson, Kathleen B., author.
  Clinical teaching strategies in nursing / Kathleen B. Gaberson, Marilyn H. Oermann, Teresa Shellenbarger.—Fourth edition.
    p. ; cm.
  Includes bibliographical references and index.
  ISBN 978-0-8261-1961-2—ISBN 978-0-8261-1962-9 (e-book)
  I. Oermann, Marilyn H., author. II. Shellenbarger, Teresa, author. III. Title.
  [DNLM: 1. Education, Nursing. 2. Teaching—methods. WY 18]
  RT73
  610.73071—dc23
                          2013047918

Special discounts on bulk quantities of our books are available to corporations, professional associations, pharmaceutical companies, health care organizations, and other qualifying groups. If you are interested in a custom book, including chapters from more than one of our titles, we can provide that service as well.

For details, please contact:
Special Sales Department, Springer Publishing Company, LLC
11 West 42nd Street, 15th Floor, New York, NY 10036-8002
Phone: 877-687-7476 or 212-431-4370; Fax: 212-941-7842
E-mail: sales@springerpub.com

Printed in the United States of America by McNaughton & Gunn, Inc.

Contents

Contributors to Previous Editions

Eric Bauman, PhD, RN

Suzanne Hetzel Campbell, PhD, WHNP-BC, IBCLC

Mickey Gilmore-Kahn, CNM, MN

Susan E. Stone, DNSc, CNM, FACNM

Diane M. Wink, EdD, FNP, ARNP

Contributor to the Fourth Edition

Debra Hagler, PhD, RN, ACNS-BC, CNE, CHSE, ANEF, FAAN
Clinical Professor
College of Nursing and Health Innovation
Arizona State University
Phoenix, Arizona

Preface

Teaching in clinical settings presents nurse educators with challenges that are different from those encountered in the classroom and in online environments. In nursing education, the classroom and clinical environments are linked because students must apply in clinical practice what they have learned in the classroom, online, and through other experiences. However, clinical settings require different approaches to teaching. The clinical environment is complex and rapidly changing, with a variety of new settings and roles in which nurses must be prepared to practice.

The fourth edition of *Clinical Teaching Strategies in Nursing* examines concepts of clinical teaching and provides a comprehensive framework for planning, guiding, and evaluating learning activities for undergraduate and graduate nursing students. It is a comprehensive source of information for full- and part-time faculty members whose responsibilities largely center on clinical teaching and for adjuncts and teachers whose sole responsibility is clinical teaching. Although the focus of the book is clinical teaching in nursing education, the content is applicable to teaching students in other health care fields.

The book describes clinical teaching strategies that are effective and practical in a rapidly changing health care environment. It presents a range of teaching strategies useful for courses in which the teacher is on site with students, in courses using preceptors and similar models, in simulation laboratories, and in distance education environments. The book also examines innovative uses of pedagogical technologies and nontraditional sites for clinical teaching.

A continuing feature in the fourth edition is an exhibit in each chapter that highlights sections of the Clinical Nurse Educator (CNE™) Examination Detailed Test Blueprint that relate to the chapter content; the entire test blueprint is reprinted as an appendix with permission of the

National League for Nursing. An instructor's manual with a course syllabus, learning activities for each chapter, suggestions for teaching this content, and PowerPoint presentations for each chapter are available to faculty members who adopt this textbook. **To obtain an electronic copy, contact Springer Publishing Company (textbook@springerpub.com)**.

The book is organized into three sections. The first section, "Foundations of Clinical Teaching," comprises six chapters that provide a background for clinical teaching and guide the teacher's planning for clinical learning activities. Chapter 1 discusses various elements of the context for clinical teaching, including the Synergy Model of Nursing Education, and presents a philosophy of clinical teaching that provides a framework for planning, guiding, and evaluating clinical learning activities. Chapter 2 discusses the intended and unintended results of clinical teaching; it emphasizes the importance of cognitive, psychomotor, and affective outcomes that guide clinical teaching and evaluation. Chapter 3 focuses on how to identify and develop appropriate clinical learning sites. It includes a discussion of how to effectively respond to increasing competition among nursing education programs for clinical sites. In Chapter 4, strategies for preparing clinical teachers, staff members, and students for clinical learning are discussed. This chapter includes suggestions for orienting faculty members and students to clinical agencies, how to prepare staff members for their role in assessing student performance, and the use of hand-held computing technology in student preparation for clinical learning activities. Chapter 5 discusses the process of clinical teaching, including identifying learning outcomes, assessing learning needs, planning learning activities, guiding students, and evaluating performance. Various clinical teaching models are described. This chapter also addresses important qualities of clinical teachers as identified in research on clinical teaching effectiveness and the stressful nature of clinical teaching and learning. Chapter 6 addresses ethical and legal issues inherent in clinical teaching, including the use of a service setting for learning activities, the effects of academic dishonesty in clinical learning, incivility between students and clinical teachers, and appropriate accommodations for students with disabilities.

The second section of the book focuses on effective clinical teaching strategies. One important responsibility of clinical teachers is the crafting of appropriate learning assignments. Chapter 7 discusses a variety of clinical learning assignments, in addition to traditional patient care activities, and suggests criteria for selecting appropriate assignments. Chapter 8 focuses on self-directed learning activities to achieve desired cognitive and affective learning outcomes. It reviews various approaches to meeting the individual needs of learners through the use of multimedia and computer-assisted instruction as well as the use of social media. In Chapter 9, the use of clinical simulation is discussed, including suggestions for designing and running simulation scenarios and debriefing students effectively. Suggestions for incorporating the use of electronic health records in clinical simulation are included. Chapter 10 is a new addition to the book; its focus is on the use of pedagogical technologies in clinical education. The chapter includes suggestions for selecting these technologies and the importance of matching the choice of technology to the intended type of learning. Strategies for acquiring new technologies and effectively using textbook publishers' supplementary materials are also presented. Chapter 11 discusses the use of case method, case study, and grand rounds as clinical teaching methods to guide the development of problem-solving and clinical judgment skills. In Chapter 12 the role of discussions in clinical learning and clinical conferences is explored. Effective ways to plan and conduct clinical conferences, questioning to encourage exchange of ideas and higher level thinking, and the roles of the teacher and learners in discussions and conferences are presented.

Chapter 13 describes effective strategies for using preceptors in clinical teaching. The selection, preparation, and evaluation of preceptors are discussed, and the advantages and disadvantages of using preceptors are explored. This chapter also discusses the use of learning contracts as a strategy for planning and implementing preceptorships.

The final section contains two chapters that focus on clinical evaluation and grading. Chapter 14 focuses on written assignments of various types, including short written assignments for critical thinking, journals, concept maps, and portfolios, among others. Suggestions are made for selecting and evaluating a variety of assignments related to important clinical outcomes. Chapter 15 is a succinct summary of three chapters in Oermann and Gaberson's *Evaluation and Testing in Nursing Education*, fourth edition (Springer Publishing Company, 2014). For a more extensive discussion of those topics, readers are referred to that companion book.

We would like to thank Debra Hagler, PhD, RN, ACNS-BC, CNE, CHSE, ANEF, FAAN, for writing Chapter 10 on pedagogical technologies and for contributing important content to Chapter 9 on clinical simulation. Dr. Hagler is clinical professor and coordinator, Teaching Excellence, at the College of Nursing and Health Innovation, Arizona State University.

Our thinking about and practice of clinical teaching has been shaped over many years by a number of teachers, mentors, and colleagues as well as through our own clinical teaching experience. It is impossible to acknowledge the specific contributions of each, but we hope that by the publication of this book, they will know how much they have influenced us as teachers. We also acknowledge Margaret Zuccarini, nursing publisher at Springer Publishing Company, for her patience, encouragement, and unfailing support.

Kathleen B. Gaberson
Marilyn H. Oermann
Teresa Shellenbarger

Foundations of Clinical Teaching

CHAPTER 1

Contextual Factors Affecting Clinical Teaching

Effective clinical teaching and learning is influenced by a number of factors. Clinical teaching is performed by a faculty within a curriculum that is planned and offered in response to professional, societal, environmental, and educational expectations and demands, using available human, intellectual, physical, and financial resources—the context of the curriculum.

However, considering that educational context is not enough for clinical teachers, they must also consider the health care context so that they are adequately preparing qualified nurses to be capable of responding to the needs and challenges of a rapidly changing health care environment. Curricula must be aligned with the practice setting (Veltri & Warner, 2012). Faculty members face a rapidly changing health care system burdened with financial pressures, consumption of services by patients with complex needs, delivery of care with expanding technology, and staff shortages. The context of the higher education environment is also a consideration for a nursing faculty. Within the educational environment nurse educators feel the pressures of tightening resources, increased workload demands, and changes in student characteristics.

Because the context is different for each nursing education program, each curriculum is somewhat unique (Iwasiw, Goldenberg, & Andrusyszyn, 2009, p. xi). Therefore, the practice of clinical teaching differs somewhat from program to program. It is not possible to recommend a set of clinical teaching strategies that will be equally effective in every nursing education program. Rather, the faculty must make decisions about clinical teaching that are congruent with the planned curriculum and relevant to its context (Iwasiw et al., 2009).

THE CURRICULUM PHILOSOPHY

In the sense that it is used most frequently in education, a philosophy is a system of enduring shared beliefs and values held by members of an academic or practice discipline. Philosophy as a comprehensive scientific discipline focuses on more than beliefs, but beliefs determine the direction of science and thus form a basis for examining knowledge in any science.

Philosophical statements serve as a guide for examining issues and determining the priorities of a discipline (Iwasiw et al., 2009, p. 172; Valiga, 2012, p. 108). Although a philosophy does not prescribe specific actions, it gives meaning and direction to practice, and it provides a basis for decision making and for determining whether one's behavior is consistent with one's beliefs. Without a philosophy to guide choices, a person is overly vulnerable to tradition, custom, and fad (Fitzpatrick, 2005; Tanner & Tanner, 2006).

A curriculum philosophy includes statements of belief about the goals of education, the nature of teaching and learning, and the roles of learners and teachers (Iwasiw et al., 2009, p. 172). It provides a framework for making curricular and instructional choices and decisions based on a variety of options. The values and beliefs included in a curriculum philosophy provide structure and coherence for a curriculum, but statements of philosophy are meaningless if they are contradicted by actual educational practice or incongruent with the parent institution (Iwasiw et al., 2009, pp. 172–173; Keating, 2011, p. 130; Valigia, 2012, p. 116). In nursing education, a curriculum philosophy directs the curriculum development process by providing a basis for selecting, sequencing, and using content and learning activities while aligning with the mission, vision, and values of the academic institution.

Although traditional views of curriculum development hold that a philosophy is essential as the foundation for building a curriculum, some nursing education leaders have suggested that a set of assumptions or one or more theories could be used instead (Boland, 2012; Iwasiw et al., 2009, p. 174). When used as a curriculum foundation, learning theories such as behaviorism, cognitive theories, and interpretive pedagogies reflect a faculty's beliefs about learning, teaching, student characteristics, and the educational environment. Nursing theories such as Rogers's Unitary Person

Model, Newman's Model of Health, and Watson's Theory of Human Caring may also serve as both theoretical and philosophical contexts for a curriculum (Iwasiw et al., 2009, pp. 173–174).

Contemporary nursing curriculum philosophies are often a blend of philosophy, nursing theory, and learning theory. Among others, these blended philosophical approaches include:

- Apprenticeship or cognitive apprenticeship
- Collaborative inquiry
- Constructivism
- Critical social theory
- Feminism
- Humanism
- Interpretive inquiry
- Phenomenology
- Pragmatism (Iwasiw et al., 2009, pp. 175–178)

While helpful in providing a guide for clinical education these philosophies do not always provide a focus on the learner, the nurse educator, and those they care for in clinical practice. Because nurse educators need to address health care needs of patients served, it might be wise to consider contemporary clinical practice models as a way of structuring curricula. One such model, the American Association of Critical-Care Nurses Synergy Model for Patient Care, provides a framework that guides nurses in providing optimal patient care by matching patient characteristics and needs with nursing characteristics (American Association of Critical-Care Nurses, 2013). The eight patient characteristics identified in the model are resiliency, vulnerability, stability, complexity, resource availability, participation in care and decision making, and predictability. Nurses drawing upon their knowledge, experience, and skills also bring eight nurse competencies to the nurse–patient interaction. These competencies include: clinical judgment, advocacy and moral agency, caring practices, collaboration, systems thinking, response to diversity, facilitation of learning, and clinical inquiry (American Association of Critical-Care Nurses, 2013). This Synergy Model, widely used in clinical practice with diverse patient populations, also has the potential to serve as a model to guide nursing staff education. It has been adapted and applied to staff development and preceptorship experiences. Drawing upon essential connections, it involves matching preceptor and preceptee characteristics and competencies to create synergy (Alspach, 2006; Kaplow, 2004). Green

(2006) also proposed applying the Synergy Model to academic nursing education. In this adaptation, learner needs are matched to educator competencies, thereby assisting in development of the learner and enhanced learning outcomes. The use of this Synergy Model of Nursing Education can be a helpful framework for faculty as they consider clinical teaching and their role in promoting learner development. Table 1.1 shows nurse educator competencies and learner characteristics.

This book provides a framework for planning, guiding, and evaluating the clinical learning activities of nursing students and health care providers based on the authors' philosophical approach to clinical teaching. That philosophical context for clinical teaching is discussed in the remainder of this chapter.

TABLE 1.1 Synergy Model of Nursing Education

Nurse educator competencies	Learner characteristics
Clinical judgment/clinical reasoning—clinical knowledge and experience used to develop learners	Resiliency—ability to adapt to different learning & teaching styles
Advocacy/moral agency—advocating for the learner's success	Readiness—preparedness & motivation to learn
Caring practices—responsive to the uniqueness of learners	Experiences—social and education influences that may affect learning
Collaboration—working with the learner and others to achieve goals	Vulnerability—susceptibility to actual or potential stressors
Systems thinking—recognizing and using resources to promote learning	Resource availability—extent of resources (personal, psychological, social, technical, fiscal) that learners bring to a situation
Response to diversity—sensitivity to incorporate individual differences in the learning plan	Participation in learning and decision making—extent to which one is engaged in the decision making and learning process
Clinical inquiry—questioning and evaluating practice	Predictability—a summative characteristic that leads to an expectation of the trajectory of learning
Facilitator of learning—use of self to facilitate learning	

Source: Green (2006, p. 279). © 2006 by Lippincott, Williams & Wilkins. Reprinted with permission.

A PHILOSOPHICAL CONTEXT FOR CLINICAL TEACHING

Every clinical teacher has a philosophical approach to clinical teaching, whether or not the teacher realizes it. That philosophical context determines the teacher's understanding of his or her role, approaches to clinical teaching, selection of teaching and learning activities, use of evaluation processes, and relationships with learners and others in the clinical environment. These beliefs serve as a guide to action, and they profoundly affect how clinical teachers practice, how students learn, and how learning outcomes are evaluated. Reflecting on the philosophical basis for one's clinical teaching may evoke anxiety about exposing oneself and one's practice to scrutiny, but this self-reflection is a meaningful basis for continued professional development as a nurse educator (O'Mara, Carpio, Mallette, Down, & Brown, 2000).

Readers may not agree with every element of the philosophical context discussed here, but they should be able to see congruence between what the authors believe about clinical teaching and the recommendations they make to guide effective clinical teaching. Readers are encouraged to articulate their own philosophies of nursing education in general and clinical teaching in particular to guide their clinical teaching practice.

A Lexicon of Clinical Teaching

Language has the power to shape thinking, and choice and use of words can affect the way a teacher thinks about and performs the role of clinical teacher. The following terms are defined so that the authors and readers will share a common frame of reference for the essential concepts in this philosophical approach to clinical teaching.

Clinical. This word is an adjective, derived from the noun *clinic.* *Clinical* means involving direct observation of the patient. Like any adjective, the word *clinical* must modify a noun. Nursing faculty members often are heard saying, "My students are in clinical today" or "I am not in clinical this week." Examples of correct use include "clinical practice," "clinical instruction," and "clinical evaluation."

Clinical teaching or *clinical instruction.* The central activity of the teacher in the clinical setting is clinical instruction or clinical teaching. The teacher does not supervise students. Supervision implies administrative functions such as overseeing, directing, and managing the work of others. Supervision is a function that is more appropriate for professional practice situations, not the learning environment.

The appropriate role of the teacher in the clinical setting is competent guidance. The teacher guides, supports, stimulates, and facilitates learning. The teacher facilitates learning by designing appropriate activities in appropriate settings and allows the student to experience that learning.

Clinical experience. Learning is an active, personal process. The student is the one who experiences the learning. Teachers cannot provide the experience; they can provide only the opportunity for the experience. The teacher's role is to plan and provide appropriate activities that will facilitate learning. However, each student will experience an activity in a different way. For example, a teacher can provide a guided observation of a surgical procedure for a group of students. Although all students may be present in the operating room at the same time and all are observing the same procedure, each student will experience something slightly different. One of the reasons teachers require students to do written assignments or to participate in clinical conferences is to allow the teacher a glimpse of what students have derived from the learning activities.

ELEMENTS OF A PHILOSOPHICAL CONTEXT FOR CLINICAL TEACHING

The philosophical context of clinical teaching that provides the framework for this book includes beliefs about the nature of professional practice, essential nurse educator competencies, the importance of clinical teaching, the role of the student as a learner, the need for learning time before evaluation, the climate for learning, the essential versus enrichment curricula, the espoused curriculum versus curriculum-in-use, and the importance of quality over quantity of clinical activities. Each of these elements serves as a guide to action for clinical teachers in nursing.

Clinical Education Should Reflect the Nature of Professional Practice

Nursing is a professional discipline. A professional is an individual who possesses expert knowledge and skill in a specific domain, acquired through formal education in institutions of higher learning and through experience, and who uses that knowledge and skill on behalf of society by serving specified clients. Professional disciplines are differentiated from academic disciplines by their practice component.

Clinical practice requires critical thinking and problem-solving abilities, specialized psychomotor and technological skills, and a professional value system. Practice in clinical settings exposes students to realities of professional practice that cannot be conveyed by a textbook or a simulation (Oermann & Gaberson, 2014). Schön (1987) represented professional practice as high, hard ground overlooking a swamp. On the high ground, practice problems can be solved by applying research-based theory and technique. The swampy lowland contains problems that are messy and confusing, that cannot easily be solved by technical skill. Nurses and nursing students must learn to solve both types of problems, but the problems that lie in the swampy lowlands tend to be those of greatest importance to society. Most professional practice situations are characterized by complexity, instability, uncertainty, uniqueness, and the presence of value conflicts. These are the problems that resist solution by the knowledge and skills of traditional expertise (Schön, 1983).

Because professional practice occurs within the context of society, it must respond to social and scientific demands and expectations. Therefore, the knowledge base and skill repertoire of a professional nurse cannot be static. Professional education must go beyond current knowledge and skills to prepare for practice in the future. Thus, clinical teaching must include skills such as identifying knowledge gaps, locating and using new information and technology, and initiating or managing change. Additionally, because health care professionals usually practice in interdisciplinary settings, nursing students must learn teamwork and collaboration skills to work effectively with others (Institute of Medicine, 2011; Oermann & Gaberson, 2014).

Thus, if clinical learning activities are to prepare nursing students for professional practice, they should reflect the realities of that practice. Clinical education should allow students to encounter real practice problems in the swampy lowland. Rather than focus exclusively on teacher-defined, well-structured problems for which answers are easily found in theory and research, clinical educators should expose students to ill-structured problems for which there are insufficient or conflicting data or multiple solutions (Oermann & Gaberson, 2014).

Clinical Teaching Is More Important Than Classroom Teaching

Because nursing is a professional practice discipline, what nurses and nursing students do in clinical practice is more important than what they can demonstrate in a classroom. Clinical learning activities provide real-life experiences and opportunities for transfer of knowledge to practical situations (Oermann & Gaberson, 2014). Some learners who perform well in the classroom cannot apply their knowledge successfully in the clinical area.

If clinical instruction is so important, why doesn't all nursing education take place in the clinical area? Clinical teaching is the most expensive element of any nursing curriculum. Lower student-to-teacher ratios in clinical settings usually require a larger number of clinical teachers than classroom teachers. Students and teachers spend numerous hours in the clinical laboratory; those contact hours typically exceed the number of credit hours for which students pay tuition. Even if the tuition structure compensates for that intensive use of resources, clinical instruction remains an expensive enterprise. Therefore, classroom instruction is used to prepare students for their clinical activities. Students learn prerequisite knowledge in the classroom and through independent learning activities that they later apply and test, first in the simulation laboratory and then in clinical practice.

The Nursing Student in the Clinical Setting Is a Learner, Not a Nurse

In preparation for professional practice, the clinical setting is the place where the student comes in contact with the patient or consumer for the purpose of testing theories and learning skills. In nursing education, clinical learning activities have historically been confused with caring for patients. In a classic study on the use of the clinical laboratory in nursing education, Infante (1985) observed that the typical activities of nursing students center on patient care. Learning is assumed to take place while caring. However, the central focus in clinical education should be on learning, not doing, as the student role. Thus, the role of the student in nursing education should be primarily that of learner, not nurse. For this reason, the term *nursing student* rather than *student nurse* is preferred, because in the former term, the noun *student* describes the role better.

Sufficient Learning Time Should Be Provided Before Performance Is Evaluated

If students enter the clinical area to learn, then it follows that students need to engage in activities that promote learning and to practice the skills that they are learning before their performance is evaluated to determine a grade. Many nursing students perceive that the main role of the clinical teacher is to evaluate, and many nursing faculty members perceive that they spend more time on evaluation activities than on teaching activities. Nursing faculty members seem to expect students to perform skills competently the first time they attempt them, and they often keep detailed records of students' failures and shortcomings, which are later consulted when determining grades.

However, skill acquisition is a complex process that involves making mistakes and learning how to correct and then prevent those mistakes. Because the clinical setting is a place where students can test theory and apply it to practice, some of those tests will be more successful than others. Faculty members should expect students to make mistakes and not hold perfection as the standard. Therefore, faculty members should allow plentiful learning time with ample opportunity for feedback before evaluating student performance summatively.

Clinical Teaching Is Supported by a Climate of Mutual Trust and Respect

Another element of this philosophy of clinical teaching is the importance of creating and maintaining a climate of mutual trust and respect that supports learning and student growth. Faculty members must respect students as learners and trust their motivation and commitment to the profession they seek to enter. Students must respect the faculty's commitment to both nursing education and society and trust that faculty members will treat them with fairness and, to the extent that it is possible, not allow students to make mistakes that would harm patients.

The responsibilities for maintaining this climate are mutual, but teachers have the ultimate responsibility to establish these expectations in the nursing program. In most cases, students enter a nursing education program with 12 or more years of school experiences in which teachers may have been viewed as enemies, out to get students, and eager to see students fail. Nurse educators need to state clearly, early, and often that they see nursing education as a shared enterprise, that they sincerely desire student success, and that they will be partners with students in achieving success. Before expecting students to trust them, teachers need to demonstrate their respect for students; faculty must first trust students and invite students to enter into a trusting relationship with the faculty. This takes time and energy, and sometimes faculty members will be disappointed when trust is betrayed. However, in the long run, clinical teaching is more effective when it takes place in a climate of mutual trust and respect, so it is worth the time and effort.

Clinical Teaching and Learning Should Focus on Essential Knowledge, Skills, and Attitudes

Most nurse educators believe that each nursing education program has a single curriculum. In fact, every nursing curriculum can be separated into knowledge, skills, and attitudes that are deemed to be essential to safe, competent practice and those that would be nice to have but are not critical. In other words, there is an essential curriculum and an enrichment curriculum. No nursing education program has the luxury of unlimited time for clinical teaching. Therefore, teaching and learning time is used to maximum advantage by focusing most of the time and effort on the most common practice problems that graduates and staff members are likely to face.

As health care and nursing knowledge grow, nursing curricula tend to change additively. That is, new content and skills are added to nursing curricula frequently, but faculty members are reluctant to delete anything. Neither students nor teachers are well served by this approach. Teachers may feel like they are drowning in content and unable to fit everything in; students resort to memorization and superficial, temporary learning, unable to discriminate between critical information and less important material. Faculty members must determine what content is critical and necessary and what information is nice to know but may not be necessary to include. Nurse educators in pre-licensure programs should focus on what knowledge is appropriate for the novice nurse, attend to the basic competencies, and ensure the provision of safe patient care while making the tough decisions about what content and clinical activities should remain and which can be removed (Dillard & Sitkberg, 2012).

Every nurse educator should be able to take a list of 10 clinical objectives or learning outcomes and reduce it to five essential objectives or learning outcomes by focusing on what is needed to produce safe, competent practitioners. To shorten the length of an orientation program for new staff members, the nurse educators in a hospital staff development department would first identify the knowledge, skills, and attitudes that were most essential for new employees in that environment to learn. If faculty members of a nursing education program wanted to design an accelerated program, they would have to decide what content to retain and what could be omitted without affecting the ability of their graduates to pass the licensure or certification examination and practice safely.

Making decisions like these is difficult, but what is often more difficult is getting a group of nurse educators to agree on the distinction between essential and enrichment content. Not surprisingly, these decisions are often made according to the clinical specialty backgrounds of the faculty; the specialties that are represented by the largest number of faculty members are usually deemed to hold the most essential content. These beliefs may explain why a group of nursing faculty members who teach medical-surgical or adult health nursing would suggest that a behavioral health clinical practice session should be cancelled so that all students may hear a guest speaker's presentation on arterial blood gases, or why many nursing faculty members advise students to practice for a year or two after graduation in a medical-surgical setting before transferring to the clinical setting in which students initially express an interest, such as behavioral health, community health, or perioperative settings.

This is not to suggest that the curriculum should consist solely of essential content. The enrichment curriculum is used to enhance learning, individualize activities, and motivate students. Students who meet essential clinical objectives can quickly select additional learning activities from the enrichment curriculum to satisfy needs for more depth and greater variety. Learners need to spend most of their time in the essential curriculum, but all students should have opportunities to participate in the enrichment curriculum as well.

The Espoused Curriculum May Not Be the Curriculum-in-Use

In a landmark guide to the reform of professional education, Argyris and Schön (1974) proposed that human behavior is guided by operational theories of action that operate at two levels. The first level, espoused theory (the "paper curriculum"), is what individuals say that they believe and do. Espoused theory is used to explain and justify action. The other level, theory-in-use (the "practice curriculum"), guides what individuals actually do in spontaneous behavior with others. Individuals are usually unable to describe their theories-in-use, but, when they reflect on their behavior, they often discover that it is incongruent with the espoused theory of action. Incongruity between espoused theory and theory-in-use can result in ineffective individual practice as well as discord within a faculty group.

Similarly, a nursing curriculum operates on two levels. The espoused curriculum is the one that is described in the self-study for accreditation or state approval and in course syllabi and clinical evaluation tools. This is the curriculum that is the subject of endless debate at faculty meetings. However, the curriculum-in-use is what actually happens. A faculty can agree to include or exclude certain learning activities, goals, or evaluation methods in the curriculum, but when clinical teachers are in their own clinical settings, they often do what seems right to them at the time, in the context of changing circumstances and resources. In fact, one of the competencies included on the National League for Nursing (NLN) Certified Nurse Educator (CNE™) Examination Detailed Test Blueprint is "Respond effectively to unexpected events that affect clinical . . . instruction" (NLN, 2012, p. 6). In other words, every teacher must interpret the espoused curriculum in view of circumstances and resources in the specific clinical setting and the individual needs of students and patients at the time. In reality, a faculty cannot prescribe to the last detail what teachers will teach (and when and how) and what learners will learn (and when and how) in clinical settings. Consequently, every student experiences the curriculum differently; hence the distinction between learning *activity* and learning *experience*.

When the notion of individualizing the curriculum is taken to extremes, an individual faculty member can become an "academic cowboy" (Saunders, 1999), ignoring the curriculum framework developed through consensus of the faculty in favor of his or her own "creative ideas and unconventional approaches to learning" (p. 30). Because a curriculum philosophy is designed to provide clear direction to the faculty for making decisions about teaching and learning, the integrity of the program of study may be compromised if the practice of an individual clinical teacher diverges widely from the collective values, beliefs, and ideals of the faculty. Academic freedom is universally valued in the educational community, but it is not a license to disregard the educational philosophy adopted by the faculty as a curriculum framework (Saunders, 1999). Thus, the exploration of incongruities between espoused curriculum and curriculum-in-use should engage the faculty as a whole on an ongoing basis while allowing enough freedom for individual faculty members to operationalize the curriculum in their own clinical teaching settings.

Quality Is More Important Than Quantity

Infante (1985) wrote, "The amount of time that students should spend in the clinical laboratory has been the subject of much debate among nurse educators" (p. 43). More than 25 years later, this statement still holds true for clinical teaching. Infante proposed that when teachers schedule a certain amount of time (4 or 8 hours) for clinical learning activities, it will be insufficient for some students and unnecessarily long for others to acquire a particular skill. The length of time spent in clinical activities is no guarantee of the amount or quality of learning that results. Both the activity and the amount of time need to be individualized.

Most nursing faculty members worry far too much about how many hours students spend in the clinical setting and too little about the quality of the learning that is taking place. A 2-hour activity that results in critical skill learning is far more valuable than an 8-hour activity that merely promotes repetition of skills and habit learning. Nurse educators often worry that there is not enough time to teach everything that should be taught, but, as noted in the previous section, a rapidly increasing knowledge base assures that there will never be enough time. There is no better reason to identify the critical outcomes of clinical teaching and focus most of the available teaching time on guiding student learning to achieve those outcomes.

USING A PHILOSOPHY OF CLINICAL TEACHING TO IMPROVE CLINICAL EDUCATION

In the following chapters, the philosophical context for clinical teaching articulated here will be applied to discussions of the role of the clinical teacher and the process of clinical teaching. Differences in philosophical approach can profoundly affect how individuals enact the role of clinical teacher. Every decision about teaching strategy, setting, outcome, and role behavior is grounded in the teacher's philosophical perspective.

The core values inherent in an educator's philosophy of clinical teaching can serve as the basis for useful discussions with colleagues and testing of new teaching strategies. Reflection on one's philosophy of clinical teaching may uncover the source of incongruities between an individual's espoused theory of clinical teaching and the theory-in-use. When the outcomes of such reflection are shared with other clinical teachers, they provide a basis for the continual improvement of clinical teaching.

Nurse educators are encouraged to continue to develop their philosophies of clinical teaching by reflecting on how they view the goals of clinical education and how they carry out teaching activities to meet those goals. A philosophical approach to clinical education will thus serve as a guide to more effective practice and a means of ongoing professional development (Valiga, 2012).

SUMMARY

The context in which clinical teaching occurs is a major determinant of its effectiveness. The context of the curriculum comprises internal and external influences, expectations, and demands that ground the curriculum and make it unique. The internal contextual factors include the faculty's shared beliefs about the goals of education, the nature of teaching and learning, and the roles of learners and teachers—the philosophical context of the curriculum.

Nursing education philosophies today are often a blend of philosophy, nursing theory, and learning theory. Recently, a widely used model of patient care has been adapted as the Synergy Model of Nursing Education. This model was proposed as a blueprint for aligning learner characteristics and needs and nurse educator competencies within the context of the health care system.

A philosophical context for clinical teaching influences one's understanding of the role of the clinical teacher and the process of teaching in clinical settings. This philosophy includes fundamental beliefs about the value of clinical education, roles and relationships of teachers and learners, and how to achieve desired outcomes. This philosophical approach to clinical teaching is operationalized in the remaining chapters of this book.

Terms related to clinical teaching were defined to serve as a common frame of reference. The adjective *clinical* means involving direct observation of the patient; its proper use is to modify nouns such as *laboratory, instruction, practice,* or *evaluation.* The teacher's central activity is *clinical instruction* or *clinical teaching* rather than supervision, which implies administrative activities such as overseeing, directing, and managing the work of others. Because learning is an active, personal process, the student is the one who experiences the learning. Therefore, teachers cannot provide *clinical experience,* but they can offer opportunities and activities that will facilitate learning. Each student will experience a learning activity in a different way.

The philosophical context of clinical teaching advocated in this book contains the following beliefs: Clinical education should reflect the nature of professional practice. Practice in clinical settings exposes students to realities of professional practice that cannot be conveyed by a textbook or a simulation. Most professional practice situations are complex, unstable, and unique. Therefore, clinical learning activities should expose students to problems that cannot be solved easily with existing knowledge and technical skills.

Another element of the philosophy of clinical teaching concerns the importance of clinical teaching. Because nursing is a professional practice discipline, the clinical practice of nurses and nursing students is more important than what they can demonstrate in a classroom. Clinical education provides opportunities for real-life experiences and transfer of knowledge to practical situations.

In the clinical setting, nursing students come in contact with patients for the purpose of applying knowledge, testing theories, and learning skills. Although typical activities of nursing students center on patient care, learning does not necessarily take place during caregiving. The central activity of the student in clinical education should be learning, not doing.

Sufficient learning time should be provided before performance is evaluated. Students need to engage in learning activities and practice skills before their performance is evaluated summatively. Skill acquisition is a complex process that involves making errors and learning how to correct and then prevent them. Teachers should allow plentiful learning time with ample opportunity for feedback before evaluating performance.

Another element of this philosophy of clinical teaching is the importance of a climate of mutual trust and respect that supports learning and student growth. Teachers and learners share the responsibility for maintaining this climate, but teachers are ultimately accountable for establishing expectations that faculty and students will be partners in achieving success.

Clinical teaching and learning should focus on essential knowledge, skills, and attitudes. Because every nursing education program has limited time for clinical teaching, this time is used to maximum advantage by focusing on the most common practice problems that learners are likely to face. Educators need to identify the knowledge, skills, and attitudes that are most essential for students to learn. Learners need to spend most of their time on this *essential curriculum.*

In clinical settings, the espoused curriculum may not be the curriculum-in-use. Although most faculty members would argue that there is one curriculum for a nursing education program, in reality, the espoused curriculum is interpreted somewhat differently by each clinical teacher. Consequently, every student experiences this curriculum-in-use differently. A faculty cannot prescribe every detail of what teachers will teach and what learners will learn in clinical settings. Instead, it is usually more effective to specify broader outcomes and allow teachers and learners to meet them in a variety of ways. Individual faculty members are cautioned not to take individualizing the curriculum as a license to ignore the shared philosophy that guides curriculum development and implementation.

Finally, the distinction between quality and quantity of clinical learning is important. The quality of a learner's experience is more important than the amount of time spent in clinical activities. Both the activity and the amount of time should be individualized.

Exhibit 1.1

CNE EXAMINATION TEST BLUEPRINT CORE COMPETENCIES

1. **Facilitate Learning**
   A. Implement a variety of teaching strategies appropriate to
      1. content
      2. setting
      3. learner needs
      4. learning style
      5. desired learner outcomes

   B. Use teaching strategies based on
      1. educational theory

   I. Create a positive learning environment that fosters a free exchange of ideas

(continued)

2. **Facilitate Learner Development and Socialization**

   D. Create learning environments that facilitate learners' self-reflection, personal goal setting, and socialization to the role of the nurse

4. **Participate in Curriculum Design and Evaluation of Program Outcomes**

   B. Actively participate in the design of the curriculum to reflect
   1. institutional philosophy and mission
   2. current nursing and health care trends
   3. community and societal needs
   5. educational principles, theory, and research

6. **Engage in Scholarship, Service, and Leadership**

   C. Function effectively within the organizational environment and the academic community
   1. Identify how social, economic, political, and institutional forces influence nursing and higher education.
   4. Consider the goals of the nursing program and the mission of the parent institution when proposing change or managing issues.

Note. This exhibit and the CNE Core Competency exhibits in subsequent chapters identify selected competencies that relate to content in each chapter. The lettering and numbering of competencies correspond to the structure of the Certified Nurse Educator (CNE™) Examination Detailed Test Blueprint.

Source: National League for Nursing. (2012). Copyright by National League for Nursing. Reprinted with permission.

REFERENCES

Alspach, G. (2006). Extending the Synergy Model to preceptorship. *Critical Care Nurse, 26*(2), 10, 12–13.

American Association of Critical-Care Nurses. (2013). *The AACN Synergy Model for patient care.* Retrieved from http://www.aacn.org/wd/certifications/content/synmodel.pcms?menu=certification

Argyris, C., & Schön, D. A. (1974). *Theory in practice: Increasing professional effectiveness.* San Francisco, CA: Jossey-Bass.

Boland, D. L. (2012). Developing curriculum: Frameworks, outcomes, and competencies. In D. M. Billings & J. A. Halstead (Eds.), *Teaching in nursing: A guide for faculty* (4th ed., pp. 138–149). St. Louis, MO: Elsevier Saunders.

Dillard, N., & Sitkberg, L. (2012). Curriculum development: An overview. In D. M. Billings & J. A. Halstead (Eds.), *Teaching in nursing: A guide for faculty* (4th ed., pp. 76–92). St. Louis, MO: Elsevier Saunders.

Fitzpatrick, J. J. (2005). Can we "escape fire" in nursing education? [Editorial]. *Nursing Education Perspectives, 26,* 205.

Green, D. A. (2006). A synergy model of nursing education. *Journal for Nurses in Staff Development, 22*, 277–285.

Infante, M. S. (1985). *The clinical laboratory in nursing education* (2nd ed.). New York, NY: Wiley.

Institute of Medicine. (2011). *The future of nursing: Leading change, advancing health.* Washington, DC: The National Academies Press.

Iwasiw, C. L., Goldenberg, D., & Andrusyszyn, M. (2009). *Curriculum development in nursing education* (2nd ed.). Sudbury, MA: Jones and Bartlett.

Kaplow, R. (2004). Applying the Synergy Model to nursing education. *Critical Care Nurse, 22*(3), 20, 22, 24–26.

Keating, S. B. (2011). *Curriculum development and evaluation in nursing.* New York, NY: Springer Publishing.

National League for Nursing. (2012). *Certified Nurse Educator (CNE) 2012–2013 Candidate Handbook.* Retrieved from http://www.nln.org/certification/handbook/cne.pdf

Oermann, M. H., & Gaberson, K. B. (2014). *Evaluation and testing in nursing education* (4th ed.). New York, NY: Springer Publishing.

O'Mara, L., Carpio, B., Mallette, C., Down, W., & Brown, B. (2000). Developing a teaching portfolio in nursing education: A reflection. *Nurse Educator, 25*, 125–130.

Saunders, R. B. (1999). Are you an academic cowboy? *Nursing Forum, 34*, 29–34.

Schön, D. A. (1983). *The reflective practitioner: How professionals think in action.* New York, NY: Basic Books.

Schön, D. A. (1987). *Educating the reflective practitioner.* San Francisco, CA: Jossey-Bass.

Tanner, D., & Tanner, L. (2006). *Curriculum development: Theory into practice* (4th ed.). Englewood Cliffs, NJ: Prentice Hall.

Valiga, T. M. (2012). Philosophical foundations of the curriculum. In D. M. Billings & J. A. Halstead (Eds.), *Teaching in nursing: A guide for faculty* (4th ed., pp. 107–118). St. Louis, MO: Elsevier Saunders.

Veltri, L., & Warner, J. (2012). Forces and issues influencing curriculum development. In D. M. Billings & J. A. Halstead (Eds.). *Teaching in nursing: A guide for faculty* (4th ed., pp. 92–106). St. Louis, MO: Elsevier Saunders.

CHAPTER 2

Outcomes of Clinical Teaching

In a study of the status of and proposed solutions for the global nursing faculty shortage, Nardi and Gyurko (2013) found that

> In many ways, nursing education appears to be stuck in the 19th and 20th centuries' apprentice model of a small group of nursing students following a clinical instructor around a hospital ward of inpatients for instruction and experience. In the real world of outpatient and nontraditional settings, quick and fragmented encounters, and high-tech delivery systems, this process is anachronistic and inefficient. It also makes nursing education, with its additional clinical practice component, a very expensive and time-consuming endeavor. (p. 320)

To justify the enormous expenditure of resources on clinical education in nursing, teachers must have clear, realistic expectations of the desired outcomes of clinical learning. What knowledge, skills, and values can be learned only in clinical practice and not in the classroom or through independent learning activities?

Nurse educators have traditionally focused on the *process* of clinical teaching. Many hours of discussion in faculty meetings have been devoted to how and where clinical learning takes place, which clinical activities should be required, and how many hours should be spent in the clinical area. However, current accreditation criteria for higher education in general and nursing in particular focus on evidence that the nursing education program is producing important intended outcomes of learning. Therefore, the effectiveness of clinical teaching should be judged on the extent to which it produces such outcomes.

This chapter discusses broad outcomes of nursing education programs that can be achieved through clinical teaching and learning. These outcomes may be operationally defined and stated as competencies and specific objectives in order to be useful in guiding teaching and evaluation. Competencies and specific objectives for clinical teaching are discussed in Chapter 5.

INTENDED OUTCOMES

Since the 1980s, accrediting bodies in higher education have placed greater emphasis on measuring the performance of students and graduates, holding faculty and institutions accountable for the outcomes of their educational programs (Dillard & Sitkberg, 2012). Outcomes are the products of educational efforts—the behaviors, characteristics, qualities, or attributes that learners display at the end of an educational program. Teachers are responsible for specifying outcomes of nursing education programs that are congruent with the current and future needs of society. Changes in health care delivery systems, demographic trends, technological advances, and developments in higher education influence the competencies needed for professional nursing practice (Boland, 2012). A nursing faculty must take these influences into account when designing a context-relevant curriculum (Iwasiw, Goldenberg, & Andrusyszyn, 2009).

In the curriculum development process, after the faculty agrees on the philosophical context for the nursing education program, it formulates curriculum outcome statements (Iwasiw et al., 2009). The desired outcomes for clinical teaching contribute to the achievement of the overall curriculum outcomes and therefore should be congruent with them.

In nursing education, a number of different terms are used to refer to professional abilities that learners are expected to demonstrate at program completion. *Outcomes* can be used to indicate the actual abilities demonstrated by program graduates or the intended or expected results of the education program. The latter connotation is more accurately referred to as *outcome statements*. Other terms used to denote such outcomes are *terminal objectives* (usually associated with a behaviorist philosophical approach) and *goals* (more broadly stated). Expectations of performance at the end of a curriculum level or course are often termed *competencies* (Iwasiw et al., 2009). In this book, we use the term *outcomes* to refer to the intended or expected results of clinical teaching.

The curriculum reform movement of the 1980s focused on the importance of outcomes rather than process in improving the quality of teaching and learning in nursing education. This approach suggests that an orderly curriculum design does not take into account each learner's individual needs, abilities, and learning style and that learners can reach the same goal by means of different paths. Development of an outcome-driven curriculum begins with specifying the desired ends and then selecting content and teaching strategies that will bring about those ends (Boland, 2012).

Thus, planning for clinical teaching should begin with identifying learning outcomes that are necessary for safe, competent nursing practice. These outcome statements are derived from the philosophical approach chosen to guide curriculum development and are related to the three domains of learning: cognitive (knowledge and intellectual skills), psychomotor (skills and technological abilities), and affective (professional attitude, values, and beliefs; Oermann & Gaberson, 2014). They also include outcomes that incorporate more than one of these domains.

Cognitive Domain Outcomes

Clinical learning activities enable students to transfer knowledge learned in the classroom and through independent learning activities to real-life situations. In clinical practice, theory and scientific evidence is translated into practice. By participating in clinical activities, students extend the knowledge that they acquired in the classroom, simulation lab, and in self-directed learning. To use resources effectively and efficiently, clinical learning activities should focus on the development of knowledge that cannot be obtained in the classroom or other settings.

As discussed in Chapter 1, new content is added to nursing curricula frequently, reflecting the growth of new knowledge in nursing and health care. If the faculty is not willing to delete content that is no longer current or essential, the potential exists for creating a congested, content-saturated curriculum in which both students and teachers lose focus on the essential knowledge outcomes. Nurse educators thus need to develop evidence-based teaching skills that will help them to critically evaluate the evidence for content additions and deletions and decide what knowledge is essential for students to acquire (Dillard & Sitkberg, 2012). For nursing education programs that prepare candidates for licensure or certification, consulting the licensure or certification examination test plans will help the faculty to focus attention on essential program content. The National Council of State Boards of Nursing (NCSBN) test plans for the National Council Licensing Examinations (NCLEX; NCSBN, 2013b) and the American Association of Colleges of Nursing (AACN) publications *The Essentials of Baccalaureate Education for Professional Nursing Practice* (AACN, 2008), *The Essentials of Master's Education for Advanced Practice Nursing* (AACN, 2011), and *The Essentials of Doctoral Education for Advanced*

Nursing Practice (AACN, 2006) are helpful resources for selecting and organizing essential content in undergraduate and graduate programs in nursing.

Knowing how to practice nursing involves high-level cognitive abilities such as problem solving, critical thinking, decision making, clinical reasoning, and clinical judgment. Traditional pedagogies that emphasize memorizing content and applying it in clinical practice are not sufficient for teaching the high-level thinking abilities necessary to ensure high-quality nursing care and patient safety in the complex environments of the contemporary health care system. Newer approaches such as narrative pedagogy promote teaching the process of thinking instead of content. Shifting emphasis away from covering content to engaging students in understanding the evolving context for nursing practice promotes development of thinking from multiple perspectives. When faculty members intend to teach high-level thinking, they should use approaches that engage students as participants in questioning, interpreting, and thinking about significant issues from multiple perspectives.

Problem Solving

Clinical learning activities provide rich sources of realistic practice problems to be solved. Some problems are related to patients and their health needs; some arise from the clinical environment. As discussed in Chapter 1, most clinical problems tend to be complex, unique, and ambiguous. The ability to solve clinical problems is thus an important outcome of clinical teaching and learning, and the nursing process itself is a problem-solving approach. Most nurses and nursing students have some experience in problem solving, but complex problems of clinical practice often require new methods of reasoning and problem-solving strategies. Nursing students may not be functioning on a cognitive level that permits them to problem solve effectively. To achieve this important outcome, clinical activities should expose the learner to realistic clinical problems of increasing complexity.

Many nurse educators and nursing students believe that problem solving is synonymous with critical thinking. However, the ability to solve clinical problems, while necessary, is insufficient for professional nursing practice, because it focuses on the solution or outcome instead of a more complete understanding of a situation in context. Problem solving involves identifying and defining the problem, collecting relevant data, proposing solutions, and implementing and evaluating their effectiveness. Students cannot solve problems for which they lack understanding and a relevant knowledge base. Only when students have a deep understanding of the problem in its context can they apply their knowledge and previous experience with similar patients as a framework for solving it (Oermann & Gaberson, 2014).

Critical Thinking

Critical thinking is an important outcome of nursing education. Early emphasis on developing critical thinking skills was stimulated by previous criteria for accreditation of prelicensure nursing education programs, but it is no longer an accreditation standard. However, current standards, competencies, and recommendations from the Institute of Medicine (2011), Quality and Safety Education for Nurses Institute (QSEN; 2013), AACN (2006, 2008, 2011), American Association of Colleges of Nursing QSEN Education Consortium (2012), and National League for Nursing (2008) address the importance of nurses who can think critically to promote patient safety and achieve cost-efficient, quality patient outcomes. The complexity of patient needs, the ever-expanding amount of health care information that nurses need to process in clinical settings, and multiple ethical issues faced by nurses require the ability to think critically to arrive at sound judgments about patient care (Oermann & Gaberson, 2014).

Because critical thinking is integral to the ability to practice professional nursing, most employers of new nursing graduates expect them to demonstrate this competency. However, it is important to remember that while critical thinking skills may be formed during the nursing education program, experience in nursing practice refines and strengthens them. Nurse educators face the challenge of developing true critical thinkers who will be comfortable practicing in the ever-changing health care environment of the future (Newton & Moore, 2013). This challenge suggests that clinical learning activities must focus intently on developing students' critical thinking skills and dispositions throughout the nursing education program, so that students can build on their experiences to begin to refine these skills before they enter the professional nursing workforce.

Many definitions of critical thinking exist, and the faculty must agree on a definition that is appropriate for a given program to provide direction for teaching and assessing this outcome as well as communicating the construct effectively to students. Critical thinking is a process used to determine a course of action involving collecting appropriate data, analyzing the validity and utility of the information, evaluating multiple lines of reasoning, and coming to valid conclusions. It is purposeful, outcome-directed, and evidence-based (Alfaro-LeFevre, 2013).

Students who think critically:

- ask questions and are curious and willing to search for answers,
- consider alternate perspectives and explanations,
- question current practices, and
- are open-minded. (Oermann & Gaberson, 2014)

Although most educators would classify critical thinking as a cognitive domain outcome, some definitions of critical thinking characterize it as a composite of attitudes, knowledge, and skills. It involves the ability to seek and analyze truth systematically and with an open mind as well as attitudinal dimensions of self-confidence, maturity, and inquisitiveness. Critical thinking is not restricted only to clinical situations. Professionals in every discipline use critical thinking, and this often results in uncertainty about how to measure and evaluate this important outcome. However, clinical learning activities help learners to develop discipline-specific critical thinking skills as they observe, participate in, and evaluate nursing care in an increasingly complex and uncertain health care environment.

Clinical Reasoning

Clinical reasoning is an essential feature of nursing competence, which is often demonstrated by experienced nursing (Banning, 2008). Clinical reasoning is critical thinking about patient care issues, for example, identifying, managing, and preventing patient problems. The result of clinical reasoning is *clinical judgment*, the inference or conclusion arrived at through clinical reasoning (Alfaro-LeFevre, 2013).

Clinical reasoning, therefore, is discipline-specific and applied in clinical settings. In nursing, clinical reasoning involves the process of evaluating the quantity, quality, and reliability of available evidence; analyzing and evaluating patient information; and making professional judgments about patient management (Banning, 2008). From this description, it is apparent that effective clinical reasoning, like the more general process of critical thinking, is dependent on a deep understanding of the context of a particular patient. Like critical thinking, clinical reasoning is a poorly defined construct that is therefore difficult to measure (Banning, 2008).

Decision Making

Professional nursing practice requires nurses to make decisions about patient care involving problems, possible solutions, and the best approach to use in a particular situation. Other decisions involve managing the clinical environment, care delivery, and other activities (Oermann & Gaberson, 2014). The decision-making process involves gathering, analyzing, weighing, and valuing information in order to choose the best course of action from among a number of alternatives. Selecting the best alternative in terms of its relative benefits and consequences is a rational decision. However, nurses rarely know all possible alternatives, benefits, and risks; thus, clinical decision making usually involves some degree of uncertainty. Decisions are also influenced by an individual's values and biases and by cultural norms, which affect the way the individual perceives and analyzes the situation. In nursing, decision making is mutual and participatory with patients and staff members so that the decisions are more likely to be accepted. Clinical learning activities should involve learners in many realistic decision-making opportunities to produce this outcome.

Psychomotor Domain Outcomes

Skills are another important outcome of clinical learning. Nurses must possess adequate psychomotor, communication, technological, and organizational skills to practice effectively in an increasingly complex health care environment. Skills often have cognitive and attitudinal dimensions, but the skill outcomes that must be produced by clinical teaching typically focus on the performance component.

Psychomotor Skills

Psychomotor skills are integral to nursing practice, and any deficiency in these skills among new graduates often leads to criticism of nursing education programs. Psychomotor skills enable nurses to perform effectively in action situations that require neuromuscular coordination. These skills are purposeful, complex, movement-oriented activities that involve an overt physical response. The term *skill* refers to the ability to carry out physical movements efficiently and effectively, with speed and accuracy. Therefore, psychomotor skill is more than the capability to perform; it includes the ability to perform proficiently, smoothly, and consistently under varying conditions and within appropriate time limits. Psychomotor skill learning requires practice with feedback in order to refine performance until the desired outcome is achieved. Thus, clinical learning activities should include plentiful opportunities for practice of psychomotor skills with knowledge of results to facilitate the skill-learning process.

However, psychomotor skill development involves more than technical proficiency. While performing technical skills, nursing students and staff members must also perform caring behaviors, critical thinking, clinical reasoning, problem solving, and decision making. However, the ability to integrate all of these competencies at once is not usually achieved until the technical skill component is so well developed that it no longer requires the nurse's or nursing student's conscious attention for successful performance. It is only at this point that the learner sees the whole picture and is able to focus on the patient as well as the technical skill performance.

Developing competence in using technology also involves psychomotor learning (Oermann & Gaberson, 2014). The growing use of electronic health records (EHRs) in various clinical settings requires students to have knowledge of this technology and at least a beginning ability to use EHRs to acquire patient information, use it to plan care, and document assessment findings and care given.

Interpersonal Skills

Interpersonal skills are used throughout the nursing process to assess patient and family needs, plan and implement care, evaluate the outcomes of care, and record and disseminate information. These skills include communication abilities, therapeutic use of self, and using the teaching process. Interpersonal skills involve knowledge of human behavior and social systems, but there is also a motor component largely comprising verbal behavior, such as speaking and writing, and nonverbal behavior, such as facial expression, body posture and movement, and touch. To encourage development of these outcomes, clinical learning activities should provide opportunities for students to form therapeutic relationships with patients; to develop collaborative relationships with health professionals; to document patient information, plans of care, care given, and evaluation results; and to teach patients, family members, and staff members individually and in groups.

Organizational Skills

Nurses need organization and time management skills to practice competently in a complex environment. In clinical practice, students learn how to set priorities, manage conflicting expectations, and sequence their work to perform efficiently.

One organizational skill that has become an important job expectation for professional nurses is delegation. In most health care settings, patient care is provided by a mix of licensed and unlicensed assistive personnel, and professional nurses must know how to delegate various aspects of patient care to others. "The importance of working with others and the abilities to delegate, assign, manage and supervise have never been as critical and challenging as in 21st century health care" (NCSBN, 2013a). Nurses need to know both the theory and skill of delegation—what to delegate, to whom, and under what circumstances—and to understand the legal aspects of empowering another person to carry out delegated tasks. However, students will not learn these skills unless they are given opportunities to practice them with faculty guidance. They need to learn to communicate clearly what is to be done; why, when, and how it should be done; and expectations for response or report back to the delegator. As discussed in Chapter 7, if clinical learning assignments focus exclusively on total patient care activities, students will not gain enough experience in carrying out this delegation responsibility to perform it competently as graduates.

Nursing faculty members, clinical teachers, and administrators and staff members in clinical facilities should provide opportunities for nursing students to understand delegation as a skill set that must be practiced to be performed competently. These skills may be initially developed in simulation activities. Debriefing after the simulation should focus not only on students' performance of delegation skills, but also on the clinical judgment process that resulted in the decision to delegate the work of others during the simulation and the effect that the simulated delegation would have had on clinical and financial outcomes (American Nurses Association and NCSBN, n.d.; Weydt, 2010).

Depending on the level of the learner (graduate or undergraduate student), clinical activities also provide opportunities to develop leadership and management skills. These skills include the ability to manage the care of a group of patients, to evaluate the performance of self and others, to allocate and coordinate resources, to work as part of a health care team, to ensure patient safety and quality of care, and to manage one's own career development. Clinical teachers may model these skills to students as well as encourage staff members in the clinical setting to do so. Examples of modeling opportunities include serving on a unit or institution-wide practice committee, demonstrating how to deal with a safety concern or health care error (Adelman-Mulally et al., 2012), and how to delegate effectively, as previously described. Because such activities are not always visible to nursing students in clinical settings, clinical teachers and staff members should discuss aloud the rationale for their decisions and actions with students, intentionally making the thinking process more apparent (Adelman-Mulally et al., 2012).

Affective Domain Outcomes

Clinical learning also produces important affective outcomes—beliefs, values, attitudes, and dispositions that are essential elements of professional nursing practice (Oermann & Gaberson, 2014). Affective outcomes represent the humanistic and ethical dimensions of nursing. Professional nurses are expected to hold and act on certain values with regard to patient care, such as respect for the patient's uniqueness, supporting patient autonomy and right to choose, and the confidentiality of patient information (Gardner & Suplee, 2010, p. 146). The values of professional nursing are expressed in the American Nurses Association *Code of Ethics for Nurses* (2005), and the nursing faculty should introduce the Code early in any nursing education program and reinforce its values by planning clinical learning activities that help students to develop them.

Additionally, professional nurses must be able to use the processes of moral reasoning, values clarification, and values inquiry. In an era of rapid knowledge and technology growth, nursing education programs must also produce graduates who are lifelong learners, committed to their own continued professional development.

Professional socialization is the process through which nurses and nursing students develop a sense of self as members of the profession, internalizing the norms and values of nursing in their own behavior. Professional socialization occurs at every level of nursing education: in initial preparation for nursing, when entering into the work setting as a new graduate, when returning to school for an advanced degree, and when changing roles within nursing.

Students are socialized into the role of professional nurse in the clinical setting, where accountability is demanded and the consequences of choices and actions are readily apparent. The clinical setting provides opportunities for students to develop, practice, and test these affective outcomes. Clinical education should expose students to strong role models, including nursing faculty members and practicing nurses who demonstrate a commitment to professional values, and it should provide value development opportunities that serve to socialize students to the profession.

Cultural Competence

Although in the previous discussion we attempted to classify outcomes according to cognitive, psychomotor, or affective domain, some intended outcomes of clinical learning are not easily categorized. One example is cultural competence, an outcome that includes elements of all three domains. Several related terms have been used to refer to different variations of this outcome. Kleiman, Frederickson, and Lundy (2004) defined these terms as follows:

- Cultural awareness: the recognition that people live within some cultural context, both inherited and experiential, that is particular to their group
- Cultural sensitivity: the belief that attention to the cultural contexts within patients' lives influences patient care and promotes beneficial patient outcomes
- Cultural competence: knowledge about an individual patient's cultural affiliations and the skill necessary to integrate them into the patient's care

The U.S. population is becoming increasingly multicultural. If current population trends continue, by the year 2050, the percentage of Americans of European descent will fall from the 69% reported in the 2004 census to 50%. The population of Americans of Asian and Hispanic descent is expected to triple, and African Americans are projected to double in number. To respond competently to these demographic changes, nursing students must be prepared to deal with diversity in all of its forms (Hines-Martin & Pack, 2009). The AACN Advisory Group on the Competencies for Cultural Competency in Baccalaureate Nursing Education's (2008) rationale for the integration of cultural competence in baccalaureate nursing education is to support the development of patient-centered care that identifies, respects, and addresses differences in patients' values, preferences, and expressed needs. This rationale includes a focus on eliminating health disparities, achieving social justice for vulnerable populations, and functioning in a global environment and in partnership with other health care disciplines.

Cultural competence has no specific end point; it can be described as an ongoing developmental process by which nurses understand, appreciate, and incorporate cultural expressions and worldviews into the care of patients and interactions with other health care providers (Campinha-Bacote, 2011; Warren, 2009). The development of this outcome begins with awareness of cultural diversity and specific knowledge about cultural values, beliefs, rules, and traditions of the nurse's own culture as well as the patient's, and progresses to appreciating the similarities and differences between the nurse's and patients' cultures. The culturally competent nurse is able to communicate with patients in ways that meet their needs and is knowledgeable about various cultures with regard to their health beliefs and behaviors (Hines-Martin & Pack, 2009). Three approaches can be used to deliver culturally competent care:

- *Cultural preservation:* supporting the use of scientifically valid cultural health practices, such as acupuncture for managing pain for an Asian American patient
- *Cultural accommodation:* supporting the use of cultural health practices that are known to be safe, such as placing a coin on the umbilicus of a newborn Hispanic infant
- *Cultural repatterning:* working with patients to help them change cultural health practices that are harmful, such as avoiding the use of herbs that interact adversely with anesthesia or prescribed medication (Huber, 2009)

Promoting culturally competent care is a priority in nursing and in nursing education. Therefore, clinical teachers should plan learning activities that will challenge learners to explore cultural differences and to develop culturally appropriate responses to patient needs.

UNINTENDED OUTCOMES

Although nurse educators usually have the intended outcomes in mind when they design clinical learning activities, those activities may produce positive or negative unintended outcomes as well. Positive unintended outcomes include career choices that students and new graduate nurses make when they have clinical experiences in various settings. Exposure to a wide variety of clinical specialties stimulates learners to evaluate their own desires and competence to practice in those areas and allows them to make realistic career choices. For example, nursing students who do not have clinical learning activities in an operating room are unlikely to choose perioperative nursing as a specialty. However, if students participate in clinical activities in the operating room, some will realize that they are well suited to practice nursing in this area, while others will decide that perioperative nursing is not for them. In either case, students will have a realistic basis for their career choices.

Clinical learning activities can produce negative unintended outcomes as well. Nurse educators often worry that students will learn bad practice habits from observing other nurses in the clinical environment. Often, students are taught to perform skills, document care, or organize their work according to practice standards or guidelines, the instructor's preferences, or school or agency policy. However, students may observe staff members in the clinical setting who adapt skills, documentation, and organization of work to fit the unique needs of patients or the environment. Students often imitate the behaviors they observe, including taking shortcuts and using work-arounds while performing skills, including omitting steps that the teacher may believe are important to produce safe, effective outcomes. The power of role models to influence students' behavior and attitudes should not be underestimated. However, the clinical teacher should be careful not to label the teacher's way as correct and all other ways as incorrect. Instead, the teacher should encourage learners to discuss the differences in practice habits that they have observed, evaluate them in terms of theory or principle, and identify more positive role models (Gardner & Suplee, 2010, pp. 9–10).

Another negative unintended outcome of clinical learning may be academic dishonesty. Academic dishonesty is intentional participation in deceptive practices such as lying, cheating, or false representation regarding one's academic work. Clinical teachers often try to instill the traditional health care cultural value that good nurses do not make errors. Even though the Institute of Medicine's report on health care errors (Kohn, Corrigan, & Donaldson, 2000) has caused growing concern about patient safety and the need to prevent errors, a standard of perfection is unrealistic for any practitioner, let alone nursing students and new staff members whose mistakes are an inherent part of learning new knowledge and skills. A teacher's emphasis on perfection in clinical practice may produce the unintended result of student dishonesty to avoid punishment for making mistakes. Punishment for mistakes, in the form of low grades or negative performance evaluations, is not effective in preventing future errors. The unintended result of punishment for mistakes may be that learners conceal errors or lack of knowledge or skill; bluffing their way through tasks or failure to report errors can have dangerous consequences for patients in clinical settings and also creates lost opportunities for learners to learn to correct and then prevent their mistakes (Kohn et al., 2000). If the instructor has established a learning climate of mutual trust and respect, acknowledges the possibility of errors, and assures students of respectful treatment when they admit their inadequacies, students will be less likely to behave dishonestly (Adelman-Mulally et al., 2012). Nursing faculty members and clinical teachers must also be exemplary role models of academic and professional integrity for students (Adelman-Mulally et al., 2012; Tippit et al., 2009).

SUMMARY

Outcomes of clinical teaching include abilities in cognitive, psychomotor, and affective domains that are acquired through clinical teaching and learning. Current nursing education program accreditation criteria focus on evidence that meaningful outcomes of learning have been produced. The effectiveness of clinical teaching can be judged on the extent to which it produces intended learning outcomes.

Clinical learning activities should focus on the development of *knowledge* that cannot be acquired in the classroom or other learning settings. In clinical practice, knowledge is applied to practice. In addition to understanding specific information, higher-level knowledge outcomes include cognitive skill in problem solving, critical thinking, decision making, and clinical reasoning. *Problem solving* ability is an important outcome of clinical teaching. Problems related to patients or the health care environment are typically unique, complex, and ambiguous and often require new methods of reasoning and problem-solving strategies. *Critical thinking* is a process used to determine a course of action after collecting appropriate data, analyzing the validity and utility of the information, evaluating multiple lines of reasoning, and coming to valid conclusions. Critical thinking is facilitated by attitudinal dimensions of self-confidence, maturity, and inquisitiveness. Clinical learning activities help learners to develop discipline-specific critical thinking and *clinical reasoning* skills as they observe, participate in, and evaluate nursing care. *Decision making* involves gathering, analyzing, weighing, and valuing information in order to choose the best course of action from among a number of alternatives. Because nurses rarely know all possible alternatives, benefits, and risks, clinical decision making usually involves some degree of uncertainty. Clinical education should involve learners in realistic situations that require them to make decisions about patients, staff members, and the clinical environment in order to produce this outcome.

Psychomotor skills are another important outcome of clinical learning. Many skills have cognitive and attitudinal dimensions, but clinical teaching typically focuses on the performance component. Psychomotor skill includes the ability to perform proficiently, smoothly, and consistently under varying conditions and within appropriate time limits. *Interpersonal skills* are used to assess client needs, plan and implement patient care, evaluate the outcomes of care, and record and disseminate information. These skills include communication, therapeutic use of self, and teaching patients and others. Interpersonal skills involve knowledge of human behavior and social systems, but there is also a motor component largely comprising verbal and nonverbal behavior. Nurses need *organizational skills* in order to set priorities, manage conflicting expectations, sequence their work to perform efficiently, and delegate nursing tasks to others appropriately. Clinical learning activities provide opportunities for learners to develop leadership and management skills.

Clinical learning also produces important affective outcomes that represent the humanistic and ethical dimensions of nursing. Professional nurses are expected to hold and act on certain values with regard to patient care and to use the processes of moral reasoning, values clarification, and values inquiry. These values are developed and internalized through the process of professional socialization. In an era of rapid knowledge and technological growth, nursing education programs must also produce graduates who are lifelong learners, committed to their own continued professional development.

One example of an outcome that encompasses all three domains is cultural competence. Cultural competence is the ability to provide care that fits the cultural beliefs and practices of patients. This outcome includes understanding and appreciating the similarities and differences between the nurse's and patients' cultures and incorporating cultural expressions and viewpoints into patient care.

Clinical learning activities also produce unintended positive and negative outcomes. Exposure to a wide variety of clinical specialties stimulates learners to evaluate their own desires and competence to practice in those areas and allows them to make realistic career choices. However, observing various role models in the clinical environment may result in students' learning bad practice habits. The unintended result of a teacher's unrealistic emphasis on perfection in clinical practice may be academically dishonest behavior among students, such as concealing lack of knowledge or skill or failing to report errors, both with potentially dangerous consequences.

Exhibit 2.1

CNE EXAMINATION TEST BLUEPRINT CORE COMPETENCIES

1. **Facilitate Learning**

   A. Implement a variety of teaching strategies appropriate to
      5. Desired learner outcomes

   G. Model reflective thinking practices, including critical thinking

   H. Create opportunities for learners to develop their own critical thinking skills

   (continued)

I. Create a positive learning environment that fosters a free exchange of ideas

J. Show enthusiasm for teaching, learning, and the nursing profession that inspires and motivates students

K. Demonstrate personal attributes that facilitate learning (e.g., caring, confidence, patience, integrity, respect, and flexibility)

P. Act as a role model in practice settings

2. **Facilitate Learner Development and Socialization**

D. Create learning environments that facilitate learners' self-reflection, personal goal setting, and socialization to the role of the nurse

E. Foster the development of learners in these areas
   1. cognitive domain
   2. psychomotor domain
   3. affective domain

G. Encourage professional development of learners

REFERENCES

Adelman-Mulally, T., Mulder, C. K., McCarter-Spalding, D. E., Hagler, D. A., Gaberson, K. B., Hanner, M. B., . . . Young, P. K. (2012). The clinical nurse educator as leader. *Nurse Education in Practice.* Retrieved from http://dx.doi.org/10.1016/j.nepr.2012.07.006

Alfaro-LeFevre, R. (2013). *Critical thinking clinical reasoning, and clinical judgment: A practical approach* (5th ed.). St. Louis, MO: Elsevier.

American Association of Colleges of Nursing (AACN). (2006). *The essentials of doctoral education for advanced nursing practice.* Washington, DC: Author. Retrieved from http://www.aacn.nche.edu/publications/position/DNPEssentials.pdf

American Association of Colleges of Nursing (AACN). (2008). *Essentials of baccalaureate education for professional nursing practice.* Retrieved from http://www.aacn.nche.edu/education-resources/BaccEssentials08.pdf

American Association of Colleges of Nursing (AACN). (2011). *Essentials of master's education in nursing.* Washington, DC: Author. Retrieved from: http://www.aacn.nche.edu/education-resources/MastersEssentials11.pdf

American Association of Colleges of Nursing Advisory Group on the Competencies for Cultural Competency in Baccalaureate Nursing Education. (2008). Cultural competency in baccalaureate nursing education. Retrieved from http://www.aacn.nche.edu/leading-initiatives/education-resources/competency.pdf

American Association of Colleges of Nursing QSEN Education Consortium. (2012). *Graduate-level QSEN competencies: Knowledge, skills, and attitudes.* Retrieved from http://www.aacn.nche.edu/faculty/qsen/competencies.pdf

American Nurses Association. (2005). *Code of ethics for nurses with interpretive statements.* Retrieved from http://nursingworld.org/MainMenuCategories/EthicsStandards/CodeofEthicsforNurses/Code-of-Ethics.pdf

American Nurses Association and National Council of State Boards of Nursing. (n.d.). *Joint statement on delegation*. Retrieved from https://www.ncsbn.org/Delegation_joint_statement_NCSBN-ANA.pdf

Banning, M. (2008). Clinical reasoning and its application to nursing: Concepts and research studies. *Nurse Education in Practice*, 8, 177–183. doi: 10.1016/j.nepr.2007.06.004

Boland, D. L. (2012). Developing curriculum: Frameworks, outcomes, and competencies. In D. M. Billings & J. A. Halstead (Eds.), *Teaching in nursing: A guide for faculty* (4th ed., pp. 138–159). St. Louis, MO: Elsevier Saunders.

Campinha-Bacote, J. (2011). Delivering patient-centered care in the midst of a cultural conflict: The role of cultural competence. *OJIN: The Online Journal of Issues in Nursing*, *16* (2), Manuscript 5. Retrieved from http://nursingworld.org/MainMenuCategories/ANAMarketplace/ANAPeriodicals/OJIN/TableofContents/Vol-16-2011/No2-May-2011/Delivering-Patient-Centered-Care-in-the-Midst-of-a-Cultural-Conflict.html

Dillard, N., & Sitkberg, L. (2012). Curriculum development: An overview. In D. M. Billings & J. A. Halstead (Eds.), *Teaching in nursing: A guide for faculty* (4th ed., pp. 76–92). St. Louis, MO: Elsevier Saunders.

Gardner, M. R., & Suplee, P. D. (2010). *Handbook of clinical teaching*. Sudbury, MA: Jones and Bartlett.

Hines-Martin, V. P., & Pack, A. H. (2009). INDE project: Developing a cultural curriculum within social and environmental contexts. In S. D. Bosher & M. D. Pharris (Eds.), *Transforming nursing education: The culturally inclusive environment*. New York, NY: Springer Publishing.

Huber, L. M. (2009). Making community health care culturally correct. *American Nurse Today*, 4(5), 13–15.

Institute of Medicine. (2011). *The future of nursing: Leading change, advancing health*. Washington, DC: The National Academies Press.

Iwasiw, C. L., Goldenberg, D., & Andrusyszyn, M. (2009). *Curriculum development in nursing education* (2nd ed.). Sudbury, MA: Jones and Bartlett.

Kleiman, S., Frederickson, K., & Lundy, T. (2004). Using an eclectic model to educate students about cultural influences on the nurse-patient relationship. *Nursing Education Perspectives*, 25, 249–253.

Kohn, L., Corrigan, J., & Donaldson, M. (2000). *To err is human: Building a safer health system*. Washington, DC: National Academy Press, Institute of Medicine.

Nardi, D., & Gyurko, C. C. (2013). The global nursing faculty shortage: Status and solutions for change. *Journal of Nursing Scholarship*, 45, 317–326.

National Council of State Boards of Nursing. (2013a). Delegation. Retrieved from https://www.ncsbn.org/1625.htm

National Council of State Boards of Nursing. (2013b). *Test plan for the National Council Licensure Examination for registered nurses*. Retrieved from https://www.ncsbn.org/2013_NCLEX_RN_Test_Plan.pdf

National League for Nursing. (2008). *NLN think tank on transforming clinical nursing education*. Retrieved from www.nln.org/facultydevelopment/pdf/think_tank.pdf

Newton, S. E., & Moore, G. (2013). Critical thinking skills of basic baccalaureate and accelerated second-degree nursing students. *Nursing Education Perspectives*, 34, 154–158.

Oermann, M. H., & Gaberson, K. B. (2014). *Evaluation and testing in nursing education* (4th ed.). New York, NY: Springer Publishing.

Quality and Safety Education for Nurses Institute. (2013). *Pre-licensure KSAs*. Retrieved from http://qsen.org/competencies/pre-licensure-ksas/

Tippit, M. P., Ard, N., Kline, J. R., Tilghman, B. C., Chamberlain, B., & Meagher, P. G. (2009). Creating environments that foster academic integrity. *Nursing Education Perspectives*, 30, 239–244.

Warren, B. J. (2009). Teaching the fluid process of cultural competence at the graduate level: A constructionist approach. In S. D. Bosher & M. D. Pharris (Eds.), *Transforming nursing education: The culturally inclusive environment.* New York, NY: Springer Publishing.

Weydt, A. (2010). Developing delegation skills. *The Online Journal of Issues in Nursing,* 15(2), Manuscript 1. Retrieved from http://nursingworld.org/MainMenuCategories/ANAMarketplace/ANAPeriodicals/OJIN/TableofContents/Vol152010/No2May2010/Delegation-Skills.aspx

CHAPTER 3

Developing Clinical Learning Sites

Nursing care occurs in diverse settings where there are patients (individuals, families, groups, and communities) who can benefit from the services of a professional nurse. Professional nurses assume multiple roles as they work with patients of all ages, races, ethnic groups, and cultures. These patients have the full scope of health promotion; health maintenance; and acute, chronic, and rehabilitation care needs.

In an ideal world, all nursing students would have clinical learning activities in all settings, with all patient populations, and in all professional nursing roles, and they would be prepared to adapt to rapid changes with patients, health issues, care locations, and approaches to care. Students would have opportunities to work with people from cultures other than their own and implement care that recognizes the global influences on both health and illness.

Nursing education does not exist in such an ideal world. All students cannot participate in every learning activity, nor can every student provide care for all these diverse groups during their nursing education. Faculty must make difficult choices about clinical education with the hope that the breadth and depth of students' clinical learning activities result in the development of the core competencies and skills needed for safe and effective nursing practice. For students who are already licensed nurses, their clinical experiences must help them grow as professionals as they move to more advanced levels of practice.

The traditional approach to clinical nursing education involves a faculty member working with a group of students (approximately 6–12, although this can vary from program to program), typically on an acute care unit in a hospital, for a portion of a clinical shift. This approach, while frequently used in nursing education, may provide an unpredictable and haphazard learning environment (Niederhauser, Schoessler, Gubrud-Howe, Magnussen, & Codier, 2012). Factors such as changing patient census, variable diagnoses and acuity of patients, diverse care needs, and staffing issues impact the learning opportunities during clinical practice. Because of the high patient acuity and complexity, many sites do not permit achievement of the full scope of clinical learning objectives. Collaboration with other disciplines, acting as a change agent, being a patient advocate, and the development of many key assessment and psychomotor skills can be difficult in a setting where all patients are critically ill. Because of the increasingly specialized nature of many acute care units (e.g., cardiovascular, orthopedic, endocrine), it is challenging for students to see a broad scope of patient problems when they have a finite number of clinical hours and a predetermined schedule. Additionally, due to decreasing length of inpatient stays and economic pressures to provide care in outpatient and community settings, limited (and, in some cases, decreased) numbers of clinical learning activities take place on hospital units that provide care for children, individuals with psychiatric illnesses, and women and families during pregnancy and childbirth. Even with these challenges, faculty respondents to a National League for Nursing (2008) survey about clinical nursing education indicated a belief that traditional rotations through medical specialty areas with specific numbers of clinical hours in those areas were important. However, they recognized the value of observation, learning in a wide variety of settings, and students being able to learn without faculty members being present.

Even when traditional acute care placements are appropriate, implementing clinical learning activities in such settings can be challenging. High demand for clinical placements from nursing education programs (often with rapidly increasing enrollments) and other health professional programs have overwhelmed many acute care agencies. Both staff members and patients can be asked to interact with students 24 hours a day, 7 days a week. As a result, acute care agencies often place limitations on the numbers of students per unit or the days and times that students can be present. In some cases, the mandated clinical group size is so limited that some students in a clinical group must be scheduled for observation activities elsewhere so that fewer students are present on the unit. In other cases, the group size has to be kept very small, a remedy that is usually neither economically feasible nor ideal for learning and meeting the educational goals of the course and the program. Engaging in these alternate clinical observation activities may decrease students' opportunity to actively participate in learning the professional nursing role and may also consume the time and resources of staff in these other areas. Faculty members must evaluate the appropriateness of these observation activities, address concerns about student guidance in the absence of a clinical instructor, and support staff members as they encounter different students arriving for observation activities each day.

The rapidly rising cost of health care in acute care settings and the demand for safe, quality care has led to the examination of health care delivery at a national level. The Institute of Medicine's (2011) report, *The Future of Nursing: Leading Change, Advancing Health* encourages the transformation of the health care system from acute care to community settings. The 2010 Affordable Care Act also represents a major overhaul to health care access that will ultimately affect nursing and nursing education. Lastly, Benner, Sutphen, Leonard, and Day (2009) reported that more than 50% of nurses work outside the hospital setting, yet a large portion of student learning still takes place in acute care clinical settings. They recommended increasing the variety of clinical settings to allow for a broader scope of experience for students. These widely referenced and respected sources are drawing national attention to nursing education and should encourage nursing faculty members to reexamine clinical nursing education and consider alternate settings for some portion of student clinical learning experiences.

As health care is increasingly delivered in nonacute care settings, clinical learning opportunities in these settings is also increased. Thus, while surgery was once performed almost exclusively in hospitals, many patients now have procedures in freestanding surgical centers. Patients once spent weeks recovering in hospitals after surgery or while recovering from trauma; they now recover at rehabilitation facilities or at home. No longer do patients who need long-term parenteral therapy or antibiotics stay in an inpatient facility. Full management of their care is carried out by nurses working in rehabilitation, long-term care, and home health settings.

Another driving force for the use of diverse settings for clinical learning is a call to increase the cultural competencies of graduates of nursing education programs. The American Association of Colleges of Nursing (AACN) proposed that, "Development of cultural competence in students and faculty occurs best in environments supportive of diversity and facilitated by guided experiences with diversity" (AACN, 2008, p. 2). Examples of these experiences include:

- Participation in a cultural immersion experience
- Participation in community projects involving community members—for example, health fairs, community forums and meetings, and the like—to understand concerns, values, and beliefs about health care
- Participation in or attendance at cultural celebrations or religious ceremonies

Clinical learning activities in diverse settings help to achieve these goals.

RE-IMAGINING CLINICAL LEARNING SETTINGS

Nursing care can be learned wherever students have contact with patients. Learning objectives do not prescribe a specific setting where the learning activities must take place. The core components of a clinical learning activity can be present in settings other than acute care hospital units and might include patient contact; opportunities for students to have an active role in assessment, goal setting, and then planning, implementing, and evaluating care; clinical reasoning and problem-solving opportunities; competent guidance (from the clinical teacher or someone designated to take on the teaching role in that site); and skill development (intellectual as well as psychomotor).

Benefits

Re-imagining and transforming clinical placements for nursing students has multiple benefits. These include preparing students to be a part of a health care system in which the acute care hospital is but one part. Not only will students learn about the varied settings in which health care is provided, but they will also have opportunities to develop skills that these settings are best able to provide. For example, development of a psychomotor skill such as initiation of intravenous therapy, including the clinical assessment and decision-making skills that go with this routine procedure, might be best learned in a perioperative setting. Development of therapeutic communication competencies might be best achieved in rehabilitation settings where it is possible to have sustained patient contact. The best opportunities to learn care planning, evaluation, and revision might be available in a home health setting where multidisciplinary care planning is fully integrated into patient services. The home health setting also lends itself to the development of collaboration skills as well as real-world knowledge about the impact of payer status and insurance reimbursement on the ability of the patient to pay for (and, in many cases, receive) needed care.

Clinical learning activities in community-based settings allow nursing students to work with patients where they live and work. Students see the challenges that patients face as they implement self-care for health promotion and maintenance, as well as see the impact on family members. Collaboration with other members of the health care team is a natural, necessary, and active part of care delivery in community-based settings.

Nursing students can participate in creatively designed, rigorous, high-quality clinical learning activities almost anywhere. This chapter discusses clinical learning opportunities in underused patient care sites, community-based sites, distant sites, and international settings. It also reviews various practical aspects of implementing clinical learning activities in these settings by addressing common agency, faculty, and student problems and suggesting solutions for such problems.

EXAMPLES OF DIVERSE CLINICAL LEARNING SETTINGS

Clinical learning activities in diverse settings include opportunities for students to meet specific learning objectives while caring for patients. Four categories will be used as examples of such activities. The first consists of patient care areas that are not used regularly as clinical learning sites. Some of these patient care sites (e.g., the operating room) have been virtually eliminated as clinical learning sites by nursing education programs, while others (e.g., outpatient clinics, nursing homes) are underused, despite the rich learning opportunities provided for students in these settings. The second category includes community-based sites where provision of health care may not be the prime focus of the site or agency but provide learning opportunities for clinical nursing students. Examples are schools, camps, and senior citizen programs and housing complexes. An example of learning activities in community-based sites is service learning. Chapter 7 provides more information on planning high-quality service learning activities. With the growth of technology and online nursing education, distance sites provide a third category of diverse clinical learning opportunities. The fourth category is the growing use of international clinical learning activities. Although these learning opportunities may be brief (often 1 week), students gain valuable experiences in diverse international settings while serving as part of a team providing health services.

There are other clinical learning activities not included in this discussion. One is an observation in which students' objectives are best achieved while they maintain a nonparticipant role in the clinical setting. Another is a special event held as part of a clinical rotation, (such as a trip to an art gallery or attending a play), designed to help students increase a specific skill, competency, or self-awareness. Also, clinical observations and interactions that are part of a didactic course are not included. Although potentially valuable as learning activities, riding in an ambulance with emergency medical service providers or visiting a hospital, clinic, or patient group as part of a course (whether at home or in another country) is not a clinical learning activity if there is no patient care in which the student participates.

CLINICAL LEARNING IN UNDERUSED PATIENT CARE SITES

With the diversity of clinical practice sites, there are many examples of clinical learning activities in underused patient care sites. Several examples will be used to illustrate how such sites can be optimized.

Outpatient Clinics

Outpatient settings such as primary care practices, specialty clinics, and rehabilitation programs are often difficult to use effectively as clinical learning sites because of the lack of registered nurse (RN) role models and the difficulty of placing large numbers of students at one site, which can make clinical teaching by the faculty difficult. This can be addressed through placement of students in a single large clinical facility. Major medical centers may have multiple specialty clinics and centers that allow students to participate in a multidisciplinary approach to patient care that may be focused on specific problems. For example, clinics that focus on pain management, wounds, gastroenterology, women's health, behavioral and mental health, diabetes, rehabilitation and sport medicine, and others may be appropriate for student learning. Students will have opportunities to engage in assessment, teaching, and delivery of focused care while interacting with a wide range of health care providers. Nursing staff members provide mentoring of the students while clinical teachers are available onsite and provide regular supervisory visits. Student–teacher conferencing activities allow for an assessment of student learning as well as an opportunity for students to ask questions. Group conferencing with several clinical nursing students can be used to share experiences with other students and enable them to make comparisons and contrasts between the learning settings, the care provided, and the patients seen.

Operating Room and Other Perioperative Settings

Most nursing education programs eliminated an operating room clinical rotation from their curricula many years ago, but in doing so, nursing faculties have overlooked many rich clinical learning opportunities. Many hospitalized patients for whom acute care nurses provide care pass though the operating room at some time during their hospitalization. Knowledge about patients' surgical experiences can greatly enhance the knowledge and skills of the nurse caring for the patients both before and after surgery. The Association of periOperative Registered Nurses (AORN) has encouraged nursing education programs to increase the use of perioperative settings for clinical nursing education. Perioperative environments are ideal settings for learning application of the nursing process, and perioperative clinical learning activities can contribute to the achievement of a wide variety of program outcomes. In addition to developing expected skills like aseptic technique, students see the use of the latest technology both in the surgical procedures and in the overall care of surgical patients. Possibly most important, students work with a team that demonstrates the interdisciplinary collaboration and communication essential for both safety and high-quality patient care in all settings (AORN, 2009). To help both perioperative staff members and clinical teachers implement such clinical learning activities, the AORN provides sample learning outcomes for perioperative experiences and relates these to overall program competencies such as those of the AACN. Objectives and a content outline for a model perioperative nursing course; objectives for a clinical rotation; and a document that relates objectives to content, activities, and competencies are all provided.

Nursing students can develop a wide array of psychomotor skills in perioperative settings, such as catheter care, insertion and maintenance of intravenous lines, pain management, skin and wound care, positioning, and care of unconscious patients. They also have opportunities to develop knowledge about evidence-based practice, leadership, quality improvement, and health care policy (Mott, 2012). Additionally, inclusion of perioperative learning activities in undergraduate nursing curricula will increase nurses' knowledge of patients' surgical experiences, and may also increase the number of nursing students who choose the perioperative specialty after graduation because "most graduate nurses seek employment in areas where they have had clinical experience" (Mott, 2012, p. 451).

Another way to include more perioperative clinical learning activities is with a practicum or capstone experience with preceptor guidance (Messina, Ianniciello, & Escallier, 2011; Mott, 2012). Such capstone courses allow students to apply knowledge and nursing principles learned from various courses throughout the program while being guided by an expert operating room (OR) clinician. Lastly, ambulatory surgery centers are another related and underused patient care site that may be appropriate for culminating clinical experiences for nursing students (Mathis, 2011).

Nursing Homes and Extended Care Facilities

Competency in the care of older adults, including frail elderly individuals, is a desired outcome of all nursing curricula. Given the growing aging population in the United States, almost all graduates will be caring for elderly patients, regardless of their future work setting. An underused clinical learning setting for gaining knowledge and competencies about care for the elderly is the nursing home or extended care facility.

Nursing homes provide an opportunity for students to practice multiple psychomotor skills and learn to provide long-term care to a single patient. In this setting, observation of changes over time is possible while caring for patients with complex needs. With a rich variety of patients, learning needs can be matched with clinical learning assignments as students provide holistic care while developing their health assessment, communication, leadership, and delegation skills with a wide range of residents (Lane & Hirst, 2012). Nursing homes provide many opportunities for students to practice implementing care that has a long-term impact. Bowel and urinary continence programs, programs to improve nutrition, and interventions to increase social interaction are a few examples of such activities.

Another benefit of student clinical learning in nursing homes is the opportunity to learn about the nursing role in improvement of care for the residents of the facility. Clinical teachers can serve as clinical experts and role models, and students have the time needed to implement and support programs that help patients achieve objectives that are hard to meet in today's rapidly changing acute health care environment. These settings also provide rich opportunities to learn and practice delegating nursing tasks to other licensed and unlicensed members of the care team.

There are some barriers to high-quality clinical learning experiences in nursing homes. One barrier is a negative attitude of some students toward elderly people, either preexisting or as a result of a previous nursing home experience. The clinical teacher's attitudes and approach to this situation can help prevent or address students' dislike of the experience (Mueller, Goering, Talley, & Zaccagnini, 2011). Another barrier facing clinical teachers in this setting is the lack of nursing role models. Clinical teachers can help overcome this concern by being positive role models themselves. Therefore, it is important to have clinical teachers who are committed to providing quality care for elderly residents, have knowledge about the special needs of aging residents, know regulations impacting nursing homes, and are enthusiastic about caring for this group of patients.

Faculty members need to carefully consider the agency selected for this clinical learning experience. Because there can be wide variability in quality of care provided to residents from facility to facility, it is critical for the faculty to assess indicators of quality in nursing homes and select appropriately. One measure that may provide insight into quality of care is the adequacy of staffing. Evaluating the patterns of staff turnover and retention rates may help determine if the number of RNs and other staff members present during clinical hours is adequate to meet resident needs and to assist students (Mueller et al., 2011). To provide information about other measures of nursing home quality, the Medicare website on nursing homes (www.medicare.gov/nursinghomecompare/search.html) presents reports about nursing home performance on indicators such as quality measures, staffing, and health inspections. This website supplies regular updates and overall ratings for over 15,000 Medicare- and Medicaid-certified nursing homes nationwide.

Once the quality of the nursing home is assessed, the teacher assigned to this clinical site should work on developing a partner relationship with the nursing home staff. This reciprocal relationship will help to build alliances and enable all staff members, teachers, and students to work collaboratively in delivering care, addressing patients' health care needs while providing relevant learning opportunities. Students can use this experience to improve collaboration skills as they work with a wide variety of staff members, including nursing assistants, licensed practical or vocational nurses, RNs, physical therapists, occupational therapists, dieticians, social workers, and administrators.

Hospice and Palliative Care

Competency in delivering end-of-life care is an expected student outcome of nursing education, yet many students may not have opportunities to develop skill in caring for these patients. It can be difficult to achieve these competencies in traditional cure-focused clinical settings where students have limited exposure and opportunity to interact with dying patients and their families. Clinical learning in hospice settings is an excellent way to expose students to the issues related to end-of-life care and to provide opportunities to develop many skills needed in all nursing roles and settings. Clinical teachers in community or mental health courses can work with hospice and palliative care providers to arrange for students to partner with hospice nurses and provide care to families receiving hospice services. Clinical teachers can use the End-of-Life Nursing Education Consortium (ELNEC) competencies to guide clinical educational experiences (AACN, 2013). Given the sensitive issues that arise during end-of-life care, it is important for clinical teachers to consider the emotional needs of students during these experiences and provide opportunities to discuss feelings. This can be accomplished through written reflective journals and conference activities. Faculty can structure clinical conferences similar to support group meetings and students can share their experiences, solve issues and problems, and discuss difficult topics (Hayes, 2005).

CLINICAL LEARNING IN COMMUNITY-BASED CLINICAL SITES

Almost all patients cared for by nurses in the acute care setting come from and return to the community. In addition, many issues, particularly those related to health promotion and maintenance and management of chronic disease, are best addressed in community settings. Community settings also offer many learning opportunities for development of key skills and competencies that are hard to meet in the acute care environment. For these reasons, inclusion of community-based clinical learning activities in nursing curricula is important. Community-based learning activities are often implemented under the umbrella of service learning. In service learning, students work collaboratively with community partners to meet both course and community objectives. Reflection on the experience and development of a sense of civic engagement are essential components. See Chapter 7 for an in-depth discussion of service learning.

Community-based experiences can occur in a wide variety of settings. These include health departments, schools, home health agencies, camps, shelters, day care centers for children or senior citizens, prisons, clinics, and nurse-managed wellness centers where students complete a wide variety of nursing interventions. The following section provides further details about some of these community-based clinical learning sites.

Childcare Settings

Because childcare-center–based care is provided to about 55% of U.S. children between the ages of 3 and 6 (Federal Interagency Forum on Child and Family Statistics, 2013), this is an opportune site for clinical learning for nursing students. Childcare and early education programs such as Head Start offer many opportunities for nursing students to develop observation, developmental assessment, physical assessment, and teaching skills. Children in these settings have more frequent respiratory illnesses, gastrointestinal illness, and otitis media, thereby providing nursing students with opportunities to learn more about these common childhood conditions and develop health promotion and teaching projects (Crowley, Cianciolo, Krajicek, & Hawkins-Walsh, 2012). Nursing students in these childcare settings can learn to provide a range of health care services that will benefit the children, their families, and even the childcare staff.

Schools

School-based clinical learning activities provide excellent opportunities for development of pediatric health assessment and promotion skills. This learning is enhanced if it takes place in the context of an ongoing program that demonstrates the principles of family-centered care and public health nursing rather than being a one-time event when the students drop into a school to take height and weight measurements or teach tooth-brushing. Schwartz and Laughlin (2008) described a program that is a long-term collaboration between a school of nursing and multiple K-12 schools. The students learn health assessment and promotion, disease prevention, and disease management in an environment where they see continuity of care. Through a program managed by a nursing coordinator, faculty members and students provide school nursing services that meet standards set by the state and the Association of School Nurses. These services include vision, height, weight, hearing, blood pressure, dental, and scoliosis screenings each year. Disease prevention and management are implemented as the students participate in immunization review and the design and implementation of plans of care for children with various health conditions and those who need medications while at school. Students also provide needed referrals based on outcomes of screenings (Schwartz & Laughlin, 2008).

Camps

Another community-based site that can meet many clinical learning objectives, particularly those related to the care of children with acute and chronic illnesses, is a camp. Clinical learning activities in summer camps for children provide a rich learning opportunity for nursing students to learn about growth and development, use physical assessment skills, and manage illnesses and emergencies. Camps that focus on specific health problems or chronic illnesses, such as diabetes, asthma, cancer, or developmental delays, allow nursing students to learn about these health problems during this immersion experience at the camp. Students also learn to manage campers' medications, manage infirmary issues, and deal with common camper issues like homesickness (Vogt, Chavez, & Schaffner, 2011). So that they are adequately prepared for the experiences, students may need appropriate clinical clearances (as discussed later in this chapter) and they should also be familiar with the camper's typical health problems and common medications administered. Since camp nurse responsibilities occur around the clock, students need to be prepared to deliver nursing care at all hours of the day and night, and ultimately deal with the camp living conditions and fatigue that may occur. Clinical teachers who guide these learning activities need to provide opportunities for student reflection on their experience and appropriate mentoring during the experience.

Senior Housing

The growing number of elderly people remaining in community settings provides multiple clinical learning opportunities for nursing students. One such setting involves senior housing. Davis, Beel-Bates, and Jensen (2008) described the Longitudinal Elder Initiative, during which undergraduate students made multiple visits to older adults living in the community. This promoted sustained meaningful interactions with residents with a variety of lifestyles, physical abilities, and interests and provided opportunities for nursing students to assess the comorbidities and differences among individuals in an aging population. Students developed relationships with the older adults as they met learning objectives. After practicing basic assessment skills in first-semester visits, the students examined the health care needs of patients and their unique risk factors based on physical and psychosocial factors such as chronic illnesses, finances, and cognitive status in the second semester. Common problems associated with aging were examined in the third semester's visits, and planning for aging-in-place was the culminating activity. To support these activities, multiple assessment tools from the Hartford Foundation and other sources were posted on the course website. Through this experience, students had an opportunity to view the older adult "in a context of change over time" (Davis et al., 2008, p. 181) and document their learning in a longitudinal portfolio that fostered reflection on factors resulting in positive and negative changes over time. On self-evaluation, students expressed increased confidence and competence in the areas of nutrition, depression and anxiety, financial aspects, sleep problems, polypharmacy, support systems, and community resources when compared with students who did not have the Longitudinal Elder Initiative experience (Davis et al., 2008).

Nurse-Managed Wellness Centers

Nurse-managed wellness centers offer a creative alternative to traditional clinical learning sites. These centers allow nurses to manage health services that focus on health promotion, disease prevention, health education, and wellness. Typically, these nurse-managed wellness centers are located in the community in places such as public housing, community or recreation centers, or homeless shelters where they serve vulnerable populations. Sometimes, clinical teachers serve as clinicians for the site and teach nursing students there as well (Aponte & Egues, 2010; Thompson & Bucher, 2013). In this dual role, clinical teachers serve as powerful nursing role models for students, and their first-hand knowledge of the community enriches the students' learning experiences as well as allows them to advocate for the populations served. However, when this model of nurse-managed wellness centers is used, nursing programs face the challenge of providing services during school breaks and holidays, and need to carefully plan programs and activities that are not disrupted by an interruption of services.

At these nurse-managed wellness centers, students have opportunities to address critical public health problems such as drug, nicotine, and alcohol addictions; stress and anxiety; and violence (National Nursing Centers Consortium, 2011). Students gain valuable experience assessing critical community issues and providing needed health services while establishing professional relationships. As with other clinical learning activities, students need the opportunity to reflect upon their experiences.

CLINICAL LEARNING AT DISTANT SITES

Distance education has become a respected and effective method of providing higher education in the United States. Jones and Wolf (2010) reported that 3.5 million students are learning online, with enrollments in online education growing at a substantially faster rate than overall higher education enrollments. The disciplines with the highest proportion of programs offered entirely online included health careers (Allen & Seaman, 2008). Nursing is following this trend. Students choose distance education programs for a variety of reasons, including issues related to distance from, and therefore access to, on-campus programs as well as the convenience of anytime, anyplace learning opportunities. Many distance learning programs operate asynchronously, allowing students to choose what time of the day or week they will participate. This makes distance learning programs especially attractive to adult learners who may be working or raising families or both while furthering their education (Johnson-Talbert, 2009).

But what about clinical education? Students enrolled in post-licensure undergraduate programs (RN-to-BSN) and graduate-level education may pursue distance education. The content in these programs depends heavily on acquiring not only the didactic knowledge base but also a set of necessary clinical skills. Ultimately, students must be able to demonstrate that they can apply clinical reasoning and function as safe, competent practitioners in a clinical environment. This is the segment of their education that cannot be completely taught or learned using computer technologies. Yet, the literature lacks information that can guide faculty members teaching in these programs, particularly in the clinical education component.

Faculty members in distance education programs need to carefully consider how students will acquire the necessary clinical skills and how these students will be evaluated. Available clinical sites and knowledgeable, skilled preceptors are needed. Typically, those preceptors working with online students are physically located in or near students' own communities, which may be hundreds of miles or more away from the nursing program. Although nurse educators have been able to provide didactic education to students who live almost anywhere using Internet technologies, schools traditionally have had affiliations only with clinical sites located geographically close to their campus, thus requiring development of new clinical sites for distance learners. The process of securing an appropriate clinical placement for students at distant locations involves a series of checks and balances to assure that students receive the education they need. The specific steps involved in selecting, preparing, evaluating, and rewarding preceptors are discussed in more detail in Chapter 13.

Evaluating students in the clinical setting is an ongoing challenge for preceptors and the nursing faculty, but can be particularly challenging with distance education. Goals of evaluation include identification of student strengths and problem areas as well as documentation of student progress. Faculty members must develop and maintain trusting work relationships with clinical preceptors who are at a distance. Contact between the nursing education program faculty member and the preceptor during a student's clinical experience needs to be timely and consistent. Preceptors need to know how to reach the designated faculty member with questions and concerns. At the same time, teaching and completing student evaluations can be time-consuming for the preceptor, and the nursing education program needs to avoid imposing unnecessary reporting burdens. When working at a distance, electronic communication using e-mail, Skype, or other synchronized audiovisual communication, such as Wimba, can be helpful to busy preceptors and faculty members alike.

Various tools have been developed by faculty members to assist in the evaluation process. Student self-evaluation is essential and includes regular written evaluation, reflection on clinical experiences, and plans for improvement. Involvement of the preceptor in written assessments provides documentation of the preceptor's observations of student performance that are necessary evidence for the faculty member's decision making. Self-identification of areas needing improvement can be stressful for students but is the basis for a mature practitioner's growth and should be fostered by the nursing education program.

Evaluation of clinical competence is more challenging when students are located in a distant setting. Some programs may require students to visit a campus for evaluation sessions and demonstration of essential clinical skills. Sometimes objective structured clinical exams (OSCEs) are used for this evaluation, particularly with nurse practitioner students. These exams assess student clinical competency with standardized patients portraying typical clinical problems. Students rotate through various stations and demonstrate skills such as history taking, assessments, or clinical procedures while a faculty evaluator uses a checklist or other rating tool to evaluate performance (Oranye, Ahmad, Ahmad, & Bakar, 2012; Robbins & Hoke, 2008). However, this type of evaluation may cause student stress and anxiety by creating a high-stakes testing environment. Additionally, concerns have been raised about the validity and reliability of this assessment method (Jones, Pegram, & Fordham-Clarke, 2010). One promising approach that addresses this concern uses video recordings of student performance with patients in the clinical setting (Strand, Fox-Young, Long & Bogossian, 2013). Although students in this pilot project had some difficulty with the technical aspect of video recording and uploading files, this method has the potential to provide feedback and assess student performance for distance education students. Other emerging possibilities include telehealth applications, virtual communities, and virtual clinical practicum experiences (Giddens & Walsh, 2010; Grady, 2011; Hawkins, 2012). Regardless of the method used, faculty need to plan for clinical learning at distance sites and carefully consider student guidance and evaluation.

CLINICAL LEARNING IN INTERNATIONAL SITES

Clinical placements in international sites can be rich opportunities to expand students' comfort and competence in the care of diverse patient populations, beyond that which can be gained in coursework focusing on such content. International learning experiences may increase cultural awareness and sensitivity while developing a better understanding of global issues. On a personal level, students may explore values, develop confidence, and learn or refine other skills. Learning activities that take place within the students' own cultures and familiar surroundings do not always help students meet goals related to becoming culturally sensitive, because the patients' world views do not predominate (Saenz & Holcomb, 2009). Nursing students whose clinical activities take place within other cultures, in both developed and developing countries, are challenged intellectually and emotionally to become more culturally aware. In an extensive review of the literature on international placements, Button, Green, Tengnah,

Johansson, and Baker (2005) found four benefits of such experiences: learning cultural differences, comparing health care systems, comparing nursing practice, and personal development.

Clinical experiences at international sites present unique challenges and require adequate preparation for both the student and the faculty member. Various factors must be considered as part of the planning process. The source institution for the nursing education program may have an international placement office that can assist with arrangements, offer travel suggestions, and facilitate the selection of appropriate sites. Establishing relationships with key personnel at the host location may enhance collaboration and facilitate planning. Once a site has been selected, preliminary and early travel arrangements should be completed because some preparation and planning time may be required. Students and faculty members must ensure that they are protected from developing health problems when traveling abroad. Participants will need to have updated immunizations and maintain current health and travel insurance. Depending upon the location of travel, they may also need to take preventative medications such as antimalarial drugs or get additional vaccinations. Most immunization series must be started well in advance of the planned trip. Students will need passports with an expiration date well beyond the end of the planned learning activity. Some trips, particularly those in developing countries, rural areas, or locations at significantly higher altitudes than students' city of origin, may also require physical conditioning. Students must also be informed of costs, which usually include tuition for the course, transportation, housing and food costs at the site, and cost of day-to-day expenses, including local travel. Completion of necessary paperwork usually includes a waiver of responsibility of the source educational institution and a separate application for the international activity.

Another important part of preparation involves understanding the practice environment, health care system, and nursing regulations at the destination site. Determine what students can legally do at the clinical site. Are there practice boundaries and restrictions on nursing care that they can provide? Students need to be prepared and understand that nursing practice, as well as the settings for that care, will be different. Make sure that students stay within regulated boundaries. Depending on the host location and type of site, verification of licensure of graduate nursing students and accompanying clinical teachers, and protocols to cover any nursing care to be delivered by students may be needed.

An understanding of the overall culture, customs, politics, economics, traditions, communication patterns, and values of the community and country in which they will be placed is also essential. This knowledge will be helpful and will ensure that students demonstrate respect and appreciation for the culture and challenges that the patients face. Practical aspects of life at the distant site must also be addressed. To prevent any misunderstandings while traveling, students need to consider the culture and their roles. Are there predetermined practices, customs, and expectations that they may need to follow? These include appropriate clothing for clinical activities. What does a nurse or volunteer health care provider wear in the host country? What equipment will the student need to provide? In some countries students may need to cover their heads and wear skirts (National League for Nursing, n.d.). Knowing these expectations prior to departing for the trip will facilitate appropriate planning and packing. If students are not fluent in the language spoken in the country, it is helpful to learn some basic language that will be used (e.g., thank you, goodbye) so they have some basic phrases they can use to communicate with others. If technology use is appropriate and available, consider using a mobile application for personal computing devices that assists with language translation. Preparation for day-to-day living conditions, including food and water safety, is essential. Housing should also be considered. Will the students be housed in a hotel, house, dormitory, or tent? Education related to personal safety, including both health and environmental risks, is essential. Lastly, encourage students to investigate common health and illnesses, causes of death, health beliefs, rituals, and practices, as this may facilitate preparation for health promotion and teaching at the clinical site.

Clinical teachers or preceptors must help students to understand that care may be different and that even the most generous care can result in harm. For example, use of antibiotics and provision of care and interventions that cannot be sustained after the team departs are not appropriate, however well-meaning (Crigger & Holcomb, 2007).

Emergency planning also is essential. Make sure that students know what to do if they become separated from the group. Have a frank discussion of what students and clinical teachers should do in case of a natural disaster or act of war or terrorism. Where should they go? When? Whom should they contact and how can that contact be completed? Monitor the U.S. Department of State website (www.travel.state.gov) for travel warnings for U.S. citizens and follow cautions and warnings.

Opportunities for reflection and sharing of experiences are critical because students may encounter emotional issues that need to be addressed. Even with adequate pretrip planning, students may not be prepared for the disparities and complex health issues they encounter, the limited resources available, the stereotypes they may experience, and their ethnocentric thinking (Kokko, 2011). Journaling (traditional or electronic format), development of a photolog, and sharing their experiences with classmates who did not participate provide opportunities for students to explore their feelings and reflect on their learning.

PRACTICAL ASPECTS OF CLINICAL PLACEMENTS IN DIVERSE SITES

When considering practical aspects of clinical placements in diverse sites, there are two major areas of concern. The first reflects the regulatory and accreditation requirements for clinical learning activities; the second involves preparation of the agency, clinical teachers, and students. All clinical learning activities must meet the requirements of state law and regulations (often set by the board of nursing) as well as the policies and requirements of accreditation agencies, the nursing education program (or its parent institution), and the site at which the clinical activities are to take place. Each nursing education program also has procedures in place that describe how contracts and similar formal communication with an agency are to be handled. While often clear from the school's perspective, this is not always the case from the agency's side. This a very important point for agencies that usually do not negotiate such contracts and for which there is no clearly identified contact person. Some agencies that appear to be freestanding may be part of larger agencies. Where the agency is part of a larger entity (e.g., a hospital system, local government program, state health department, school district, or federal agency such as the Veterans Administration), it can be both difficult and time-consuming to get the contract signed by all relevant parties. These agreements can dictate student and faculty requirements needed prior to entering the clinical agency for learning. These agreements are especially important when dealing with smaller agencies that may not have procedures in place related to orientation or placement of students in their facilities. Adhering to the agency guidelines is important to avoid conflicts, especially when multiple programs (nursing and other health professionals) are seeking placements for the same time period. Even if students are at one of the clinical entity's sites, the policy for the overall entity must be followed. Often, smaller and nontraditional sites (e.g., day care settings, church programs, food kitchens) and even some formal agencies that do not have large staffs (e.g., day treatment programs for substance abusers, nursing homes, assisted living facilities) do not require or have a formal orientation program. The clinical teacher should work with the staff to determine what preparation the students need to optimize their learning as well as protect and provide the best care for the patients they will encounter. On the other hand, a larger institution (e.g., a major hospital system) may be the parent organization of smaller community-based programs, and students may need to complete the full agency orientation to be placed in even a small, peripheral program. If these requirements become too onerous, expensive, or time-consuming, the value of clinical learning activities at these sites may be questioned by the nursing education program faculty and administration. Legal aspects of clinical learning experiences are more fully explored in Chapter 6, and a few aspects highly relevant to the use of diverse sites are presented in Exhibit 3.1.

Agency Preparation

As competition for clinical sites continues, clinical teachers seek creative ways to secure effectively and efficiently appropriate student learning opportunities. Clinical agency administrators and educators are also ready to embrace creative approaches that will decrease nursing program competition and rivalry in securing clinical sites while providing an equitable approach that will meet agency, nursing program, and student needs. Educational programs and health care providers must work together to meet common goals. One approach is the formation of a clinical placement consortium. In this model, school representatives, service agency liaisons, and clinical agency representatives meet to find appropriate learning opportunities for all. The use of web-based programs or course management systems is one way to manage and display clinical placement requests and facilitate open communication and negotiation among consortium members (Kline & Hodges, 2006).

Another approach to secure student clinical placements involves development of partnerships between health care organizations and nursing education programs. Academic service partnerships, also known as academic–community partnerships, are formal collaborative relationships between agencies that allow for sharing of knowledge, resources, clinical expertise, and opportunities with the intent of promoting both better patient care and nursing education. Formal partnerships generally allow for better access to clinical placements because the partners have clearly articulated a shared vision and mutually agreed upon goals, and have re-envisioned the roles of teacher and staff members. Partners work together to mobilize talents, leverage resources, and use assets effectively (Baiardi, Brush, & Lapides, 2010; Beal et al., 2012; Broussard, 2011).

Regardless of the type of relationship with the clinical agency or location of the clinical site, there are some basic considerations that will help to ensure a collegial work relationship with agency leaders and nursing staff. Details of the clinical learning activity (when will students be there, what

Exhibit 3.1

AREAS OF CONSIDERATION WHEN PLACING STUDENTS IN DIVERSE CLINICAL SITES

Legal and Regulatory Issues

- Does the placement meet requirements of relevant state laws and accompanying regulations related to approval, contract, faculty ratios, nature of faculty guidance, and student scope of practice?
- Must the clinical teacher be present for clinical learning activities for students to practice direct patient care?
- Can preceptors be used in the setting and in the manner planned?
- Can the clinical teacher delegate guidance and evaluation of students' learning to a registered nurse on staff at the agency if the clinical teacher is not present but in the building? What if the clinical teacher is not physically present?

Nursing Education Program Issues

- Is a contract required?
- Is travel reimbursement available?
- If the planned clinical learning activity will take place over more than the usual hours and day of a traditional clinical activity (e.g., on parts of most days of the week, during school breaks, on weekends), is this reflected in the clinical teacher's workload and compensation?
- Are there specific requirements of the education program's accreditation body that affect the planned clinical learning activity?

Agency Issues

- What are the agency's rules and policies related to nursing student clinical activities?
- Does the agency require a contract with the nursing education program? If so, who handles contracts with education programs?
- How are requests for clinical placements from multiple nursing education and other programs handled?
- What are the agency rules for student clearance (e.g., criminal background, child or elder abuse records, drug screening)?
- If screenings or background checks beyond the requirements of the nursing education program are required, who pays for them?
- Does the nursing education program need to document that students have demonstrated CPR or other competencies?
- What are the health requirements, such as tuberculosis testing or immunizations?
- Are there specific Health Information Portability and Accountability Act or patient privacy statements that must be completed?
- Does the agency need to keep a record of students for legal or regulatory purposes or to obtain future funding based on the value of student service to the organization? If yes, what is needed from the nursing education program?

(continued)

Student Issues

- What modes of transportation are available? Is there parking?
- What measures will help to ensure safety of students?
- What is the required orientation?

---

their learning goals are, what they are expected to do, and how they can participate) must be communicated with the staff. Settings that rarely host nursing students, as well as those that often do, can have problems getting this information to the staff members who will have the most contact with the students. Explore if there are methods to electronically share information with staff, such as through e-mail, so that it is disseminated in a convenient and efficient way. Misunderstandings about student activities and objectives do occur and can jeopardize the learning experience. Often course syllabi, clinical objectives, and guides to the clinical learning activity are provided to administrative staff of a clinical agency but may not be shared with the staff members who are directly working with the students and could benefit from access to this information. A meeting with the staff members who will work directly with the students, along with providing multiple copies of these written materials, will facilitate communication and ensure that the right people have the right information.

Including nursing staff in planning clinical learning activities can also prevent potential problems. Seeking input from staff nurses and understanding their workload demands can help clinical teachers plan effectively for student learning activities. Realizing the existing demands on staff members, such as precepting new nurses or supervising other staff members, will help clinical teachers form realistic expectations of the time available to assist students.

Clinical Teacher Preparation

Clinical teachers may need additional education, mentoring, and support as they implement clinical learning activities in new and diverse settings. A highly skilled clinical teacher who is at ease while teaching students to care for acutely ill patients in a critical care unit may not have the knowledge and skills needed to care for those patients in their homes a week after discharge. Like their students, clinical teachers may find that the fine points of adapting care to the home setting while respecting the family in their home and dealing with the virtual loss of the multiple support systems of the acute care setting will be new to them.

The organization and structure of clinical teaching outside of acute care settings will often be new to a faculty member. Some logistical issues will need to be addressed. If the students are not all in the same setting, how will faculty members conduct their clinical teaching activities at multiple sites? How will students and teachers communicate with each other? How will clinical conferences occur? What written assignments will be submitted to the faculty member and how and when will it be returned to students? Electronic technology can provide solutions for some of these issues. Course management platforms can be used to create forums for posting clinical updates and news, submission of course assignments, synchronous discussion boards, or even electronic discussion through Skype. Other electronic communication methods can be used to communicate with students during clinical practice. These methods include cellphones, although they are not always permitted at clinical sites. Short message service (SMS) or text messaging can be used to provide support and instant access between clinical teachers and students during clinical learning experiences activities. Use of this service is inexpensive and easy to use, and it allows for instant connectivity (Young et al., 2009).

Clinical teachers with nursing students in diverse sites, perhaps at different sites at the same time, have complex teaching obligations. Some sites, particularly those that are community-based or international, work beyond the days, times, or even weeks when traditional clinical learning activities occur, may need to maintain partnerships that work collaboratively to meet student and program needs.

Student Preparation

When students have clinical learning activities in unfamiliar sites or where the learning opportunities are not immediately clear to them, they report feeling confused, insecure, isolated, and unprepared for the experience (Leh, 2011). Provision of specific objectives, learning activities, preparation expectations, activity guides, and written expectations will greatly facilitate learning and make the expectations clear. This is especially true if the faculty member will not be present at the site at all times. See Exhibit 3.2 for an example of specific preparation, objectives, activities, and written expectations for a community-based experience. Orientation for the clinical experience is based on agency, site, and student needs. Regardless of the clinical setting, an overall orientation to the course expectations with a review of skills used frequently in the experiences and a discussion about preconceptions and expectations will provide students with essential preparation that will enable them to feel confident and prepared for the experience.

Student safety during the clinical learning experience will also need to be addressed. This is an issue in all clinical activities, but it is especially

Exhibit 3.2

EXAMPLE OF INSTRUCTIONS TO STUDENTS FOR COMMUNITY CLINICAL SITES

Preparation for All Community Clinical Learning Activities

- Review objectives and activities as listed for each assignment and do assigned reading before arriving at the site.
- Review key facts or existing guides (e.g., immunization schedules or classification of hypertension in adults) appropriate for the clinical area.
- Be at the site at the time indicated by your instructor.
- Wear your clean uniform (including identification) and follow the dress code. Dress appropriately for the weather.
- Bring a black pen, watch with a second hand, stethoscope, notebook, personal digital assistant, and pocket reference books, as appropriate, for the clinical learning activity.
- Check on transportation and directions to the site.
- Have contact information for your instructor (cell phone number, etc.) with you at all times.
- Share your schedule (where and when you are going) with your class partner.
- Bring a charged cell phone.
- Have the phone number and name of the site contact person.

Specific Preparation Before the Clinical Learning Activity Starts

- Read chapters XX, XX, and XX in the course text.
- Complete and submit the clinical preparation worksheet to your instructor.

General Clinical Activity Guidelines

- Work with the staff for an optimal learning experience.
- Your instructor will visit the site each day and be available by cell phone or text messaging.
- You should complete assessments, documentation, and teaching as described below. You may only administer medications under the direct observation of the registered nurse identified by your instructor.
- Review any unfamiliar medical diagnosis, medication, and care needed for patients you are seeing.
- Ask for help if something is unclear.

Clinical Activities

During this clinical learning activity, students will work with staff members to:
1. Follow agency policy for client intake for the visit, including completion of initial assessments and placement of clients and charts with appropriate provider.
2. Review patient's health record for history, diagnoses, medications, and lab test results.

(continued)

> 3. Follow patients through the physical exam to the end of the visit, if provider and patient agree.
> 4. Implement health teaching after review by the instructor.
> 5. Complete required clinical report.

important in situations where students may be in an unfamiliar area, making home visits, or going alone or in small groups to clinical sites at various times during the day or evening. Teachers must provide explicit guidelines for student safety during learning activities and document them in the course syllabus. Safety guidelines for home visits and going alone or in small groups to clinical sites should address proper methods of communication with faculty, agency, and patients. Ensure that students have the following information prior to the start of the clinical experience: clinical teacher and emergency contact information, clear travel directions, a reliable vehicle with adequate fuel, availability of a charged cell phone, and guidelines for appropriate dress and behavior while in a patient's home or at an agency or facility without an instructor present. The students must also be prepared for appropriate actions they may need to take if they find themselves in a dangerous situation, be it at an agency, out in the community, or at a patient's home (Dalton, Aber, & Fawcett, 2009).

Regular brief visits by the clinical teacher to each clinical site will help prevent problems and address issues that may arise from staff and students during the experience. Individual and group conferences with students will allow for sharing of experiences and provide additional time to assess learning and growth.

SUMMARY

Nursing care occurs anywhere there are clients who need the services of a professional nurse, and nursing students can learn to provide care wherever they have contact with clients. Traditionally, much of clinical nursing education has occurred in acute care settings because of long-held assumptions about how nurses must be prepared to practice. However, decreasing length of inpatient stays, high patient acuity, economic pressures to provide care in outpatient and community settings, and increasing competition with other educational programs for the same clinical sites have limited clinical learning opportunities located in traditional acute care settings. Using diverse sites for clinical learning activities can prepare nursing students for the challenges of contemporary nursing practice as clients, health needs, care locations, and approaches to care.

This chapter discussed options for planning and providing clinical learning opportunities for undergraduate and graduate nursing students in a wide variety of clinical sites. Examples of clinical learning opportunities in four categories were presented. The first category included patient care areas that are not used regularly as clinical learning sites (e.g., the operating room, outpatient clinics, nursing homes, and extended care facilities) despite the rich learning opportunities for students in these settings. The second category included sites where provision of health care is not the prime focus of the site or agency, such as schools, camps, and housing complexes. The third category is the use of distant clinical sites for online nursing students. The final category is the growing use of international clinical learning opportunities.

Practical aspects of clinical placements in diverse sites were also discussed. Two main areas of concern are the need to meet regulatory and accreditation requirements and the need for adequate preparation of agency staff members, clinical teachers, and students. Examples of methods and tools used for preparation of agency staff members, clinical teachers making the transition from traditional acute care sites, and nursing students were provided.

Exhibit 3.3

CNE EXAMINATION TEST BLUEPRINT CORE COMPETENCIES

1. **Facilitate Learning**
   A. Implement a variety of teaching strategies appropriate to
      2. setting
      3. learner needs
      5. desired learner outcomes
   C. Modify teaching strategies and learning experiences based on consideration of learners'
      1. cultural background
      2. past clinical experiences
   D. Use information technologies to support the teaching–learning process
   E. Practice skilled oral and written (including electronic) communication that reflects an awareness of self and relationships with learners (e.g., evaluation, mentorship, and supervision)
   F. Communicate effectively orally and in writing with an ability to convey ideas in a variety of contexts
   H. Create opportunities for learners to develop their own critical thinking skills

(continued)

> **M.** Develop collegial working relationships with clinical agency personnel to promote positive learning environments
> **O.** Demonstrate the ability to teach clinical skills
> **P.** Act as a role model in practice settings
> **Q.** Foster a safe learning environment
>
> 2. **Facilitate Learner Development and Socialization**
>
>   **D.** Create learning environments that facilitate learners' self-reflection, personal goal setting, and socialization to the role of the nurse
>   **E.** Foster the development of learners in these areas:
>   1. cognitive domain
>   2. psychomotor domain
>   3. affective domain
>
>   **F.** Assist learners to engage in thoughtful and constructive self and peer evaluation
>
> 3. **Use Assessment and Evaluation Strategies**
>
>   **C.** Use a variety of strategies to assess and evaluate learning in these domains:
>   1. cognitive
>   2. psychomotor
>   3. affective
>
>   **H.** Implement evaluation strategies that are appropriate to the learner and learning outcomes
>   **L.** Provide timely, constructive, and thoughtful feedback to learners
>
> 4. **Participate in Curriculum Design and Evaluation of Program Outcomes**
>
>   **H.** Collaborate with community and clinical partnerships to support educational goals
>
> 6. **Engage in Scholarship, Service, and Leadership**
>
>   **A.** Function as a change agent and leader
>   1. Model cultural sensitivity when advocating for change
>   7. Adapt to changes created by external factors

REFERENCES

Allen, E., & Seaman, J. (2008). Staying the course: Online education in the United States. *Sloan Consortium 2008*. Retrieved from www.sloan.org/publications/survey/pdf/staying_the_course.pdf

American Association of Colleges of Nursing. (2008). *Cultural competence in baccalaureate nursing education*. Retrieved from www.aacn.nche.edu/leading-initiatives/education-resources/competency.pdf

American Association of Colleges of Nursing. (2013). *ELNEC fact sheet*. Retrieved from www.aacn.nche.edu/elnec/about/fact-sheet

AORN, the Association of periOperative Registered Nurses. (2009). *Primer for undergraduate perioperative education: Didactic and clinical activities for the perioperative setting.* Retrieved from http://www.aorn.org/periopprimer

Aponte, J., & Egues, A. L. (2010). A school of nursing-wellness center partnership: Creating collaborative practice experiences for undergraduate US senior nursing students. *Holistic Nursing Practice, 24*, 158–168.

Baiardi, J. M., Brush, B. L., & Lapides, S. (2010). Common issues, different approaches: Strategies for community-academic partnership development. *Nursing Inquiry, 17*, 289–296.

Beal, J. A., Alt-White, A., Erickson, J., Everett, L. Q., Fleshner, I., Karshmer, J., ... Gale, S. (2012). Academic practice partnerships: A national dialogue. *Journal of Professional Nursing, 28*, 327–332.

Benner, P., Sutphen, M., Leonard, V., & Day, L. (2009). *Educating nurses: A call for radical transformation.* Sudbury, MA: Jossey-Bass.

Broussard, B. B. (2011). The bucket list: A service-learning approach to community engagement to enhance community health nursing clinical learning. *Journal of Nursing Education, 50*, 40–43.

Button, L., Green, B., Tengnah, C., Johansson, I., & Baker, C. (2005). The impact of international placements on nurses' personal and professional lives: Literature review. *Journal of Advanced Nursing, 50*, 315–324.

Crigger, N. J., & Holcomb, L. (2007). Practical strategies for providing culturally sensitive, ethical care in developing nations. *Journal of Transcultural Nursing, 18*, 70–76.

Crowley, A. A., Cianciolo, S., Krajicek, M. J., & Hawkins-Walsh, E. (2012). Childcare health and health consultation curriculum: Trends and future directions in nursing education. *Journal for Specialists in Pediatric Nursing, 17*, 129–135.

Dalton, J. M., Aber, C., & Fawcett, J. (2009). Students' perceptions of home visiting. *Home Healthcare Nurse, 27*, 253–261.

Davis, R., Beel-Bates, C., & Jensen, S. (2008). The longitudinal elder initiative: Helping students learn to care for older adults. *Journal of Nursing Education, 47*, 179–182.

Federal Interagency Forum on Child and Family Statistics. (2013). *America's children: Key national indicators of well-being.* Washington, DC: U. S. Government Printing Office. Retrieved from www.childsttats.gov/americaschildren/famsoc3.asp

Giddens, J. F., & Walsh, M. (2010). Collaborating across the pond: The diffusion of virtual communities for nursing education. *Journal of Nursing Education, 49*, 449–454.

Grady, J. L. (2011). The virtual clinical practicum: An innovative telehealth model for clinical nursing education. *Nursing Education Perspectives, 32*, 189–194.

Hawkins, S. Y. (2012). Telehealth nurse practitioner student clinical experiences: An essential educational component for today's health care setting. *Nurse Education Today, 32*, 842–845.

Hayes, A. (2005). A mental health nursing clinical experience with hospice patients. *Nurse Educator, 30*, 85–88.

Institute of Medicine. (2011). *The future of nursing: Leading change, advancing health.* Washington, DC: The National Academies Press.

Johnson-Talbert, J. J. (2009). Distance education: One solution to the nursing shortage? *Clinical Journal of Oncology Nursing, 13*, 269–270.

Jones, A., Pegram, A., & Fordham-Clarke, C. (2010), Developing and examining an objective structured clinical examination. *Nurse Education Today, 30*, 137–141.

Jones, D. P., & Wolf, D. M. (2010). Shaping the future of nursing education today using distant education and technology. *The ABNF Journal, 21*(2), 44–47.

Kline, K. S., & Hodges, J. (2006). A rational approach to solving the problem of competition for undergraduate clinical sites. *Nursing Education Perspectives, 27,* 80–83.

Kokko, R. (2011). Future nurses' cultural competencies: What are their learning experiences during exchange and studies abroad? A systematic literature review. *Journal of Nursing Management, 19,* 673–682.

Lane, A. M., & Hirst, S. P. (2012). Placement of undergraduate students in nursing homes: Careful considerations versus convenience. *Journal of Nursing Education, 51,* 145–149.

Leh, S. K. (2011). Nursing students' preconceptions of the community health clinical experience: Implications for nursing education. *Journal of Nursing Education, 50,* 620–627.

Mathis, D. S. H. (2011). Ambulatory surgery centers as clinical practice sites. *AORN Journal, 94,* 184.

Messina, B. A. M., Ianniciello, J. M., & Escallier, L. A. (2011). Opening the doors to the OR: Providing students with perioperative clinical experiences, *AORN Journal, 94,* 180–183, 185–188.

Mott, J. (2012). Implementation of an intraoperative clinical experience for senior level baccalaureate nursing students. *AORN Journal, 95,* 445–452. doi:10.1016/j.aorn.2011.05.024

Mueller, C., Goering, M., Talley, K., & Zaccagnini, M. (2011). Taking on the challenge of clinical teaching in nursing homes. *Journal of Gerontological Nursing, 37*(4), 32–38.

National League for Nursing. (n.d.). *Faculty preparation for global experiences toolkit.* Retrieved from www.nln.org/facultyprograms/facultyresources/toolkit_facprepglobexp.pdf

National League for Nursing. (2008). Summary of the survey on clinical education in nursing. *Nursing Education Perspectives, 29,* 238–245.

National Nursing Centers Consortium. (2011). *About nurse-managed care.* Retrieved from www.nncc.us/site/index.php/about-nurse-managed-care

Niederhauser, V., Schoessler, M., Gubrud-Howe, P. M., Magnussen, L., & Codier, E. (2012). Creating innovation models of clinical nursing education. *Journal of Nursing Education, 51,* 603–608.

Oranye, N. O., Ahmad, C., Ahmad, N., & Bakar, R. A. (2012). Assessing nursing clinical skills competence through objective structured clinical examination (OSCE) for open distance learning students in Open University Malaysia. *Contemporary Nurse, 41,* 233–241.

Robbins, L. K., & Hoke, M. M. (2008). Using objective structured clinical examinations to meet clinical competence evaluation challenges with distance education students. *Perspectives in Psychiatric Care, 44,* 81–88.

Saenz, K., & Holcomb, L. (2009). Essential tools for a study abroad nursing course. *Nurse Educator, 34,* 172–175.

Schwartz, M., & Laughlin, A. (2008). Partnering with schools: A win-win experience. *Journal of Nursing Education, 47,* 279–282.

Strand, H., Fox-Young, S., Long, P., & Bogossian, F. (2013). A pilot project in distance education: Nurse practitioner students' experience of personal video capture technology as an assessment method of clinical skills. *Nurse Education Today, 33,* 253–257.

Thompson, C. W., & Bucher, J. A. (2013). Meeting baccalaureate public/community health nursing education competencies in nurse-managed wellness centers. *Journal of Professional Nursing, 29,* 155–162.

Vogt, M. A., Chavez, R., & Schaffner, B. (2011). Baccalaureate nursing student experiences at a camp for children with diabetes: The impact of a service-learning model. *Pediatric Nursing, 37*, 69–73.

Young, P., Moore, E., Griffiths, G., Raine, R., Stewart, R., Cownie, M., & Frutos-Perez, M. (2009). Help is just a text away: The use of short message service texting to provide an additional means of support for health care students during practice placements. *Nurse Education Today, 30*, 118–123.

CHAPTER 4

Preparing for Clinical Learning Activities

Nurse educators should consider a number of factors in preparing for clinical learning activities. Equipping students to enter the clinical setting must be balanced with preparing staff members for the presence of learners in a service setting while also respecting the needs of patients. This chapter describes the roles and responsibilities of faculty members, staff members, and others involved in clinical teaching and suggests methods of preparing students and staff members for clinical learning activities. Strategies for selecting clinical learning activities will be discussed in Chapter 7.

UNDERSTANDING THE CONTEXT FOR CLINICAL LEARNING ACTIVITIES

To begin preparations for clinical teaching and learning, nurse educators should reflect on the context in which these activities take place. Teachers and learners use an established health care or community setting for a learning environment, thus becoming guests within that setting. What are the implications for clinical teaching and learning effectiveness under these conditions?

Over the last century, basic preparation for professional nursing has moved from service-based training and apprenticeship to academic educational programs in institutions of higher learning. As a result of this service-education separation, the clinical teacher and students who enter a clinical setting for learning activities are often regarded as guests of the health care agency or community site. They participate in the activities of the established system and attempt to follow the norms of its culture, but they are not a constant presence (MacIntyre, Murray, Teel, & Karshmer, 2009; Paton, 2007).

Traditionally, clinical teachers and students in an academic nursing education program comprise a temporary system within the permanent culture of the clinical setting. Similarly, a staff development instructor and orientees may represent a temporary system. A temporary system is a set of individuals who work together on a complex task over a limited period of time. Although clinical teachers are professional colleagues to nursing staff members and are viewed as nurses by patients, their primary role is that of educator. Even if they are employed by the agency as a staff member on a casual or part-time basis in addition to their academic positions, faculty members enact a different role in that agency when they are guiding the clinical learning activities of students, and role confusion is often inevitable (Paton, 2007).

Being a good guest involves knowing and adhering to the established routines, policies, and practices of the clinical setting. Clinical teachers negotiate with staff members for access to learning opportunities and resources while simultaneously protecting students from criticism and preventing errors. Often, students point out discrepancies between nursing staff practice and the standards or procedures that the students were taught. The teacher needs to explain such differences in terms of choice of approach to solving a clinical problem, when appropriate, rather than offering a value judgment. When possible, the clinical teacher should point out staff members who are positive role models of clinical excellence and professionalism.

At times, a clinical teacher's desire for positive relationships with staff members, reluctance to delay or slow patient care, and concern for patient and student safety result in minimizing students' risk taking in an effort to prevent errors. For example, teachers may select assignments for students that allow them to demonstrate previously developed competencies rather than choose learning activities that will challenge students to deepen their understanding and develop higher skill levels. If the teacher expects that a student will not be able to complete patient care activities in a timely manner, the instructor may forego a rich opportunity for the student to learn to prioritize, organize, and complete a complex set of tasks for the patient and to work collaboratively with other health care team members to do so efficiently. Excessive gatekeeping actions of this kind do not allow students to exhibit clinical problem solving, organize care activities, and learn to take appropriate, calculated risks.

Although clinical teachers and nursing students are seen as guests in the health care environment, they are also a vital resource to a health care agency. Nursing students represent potential future employees of that organization, and many health care administrators and managers view the presence of nursing students in the facility as a recruitment opportunity (Mullenbach, 2010). Positive clinical learning experiences may encourage nursing students to consider future employment in that agency, and nursing staff members who nurture the development of students can have a powerful influence on such a choice (Rebeschi & Aronson, 2009).

Many staff members, however, are unaware of or misinterpret these standards; they expect nursing students to participate fully in all unit activities, assume responsibility for patient care, take the same kinds of patient assignments, and complete the same patient care tasks as do staff members. They may recall their own clinical education as being more rigorous than the contemporary clinical activities that they witness; communicating those perceptions to nursing students can produce self-doubt, discouragement, and dissatisfaction among the novices. The teacher as culture broker must allow students to experience the real world of clinical nursing and, at the same time, communicate to staff members that trends and current issues in nursing education mean that "it's not your mother's nursing school." Keeping clinical agency staff members, managers, and administrators informed about the nature of contemporary nursing education and keeping students updated on current challenges and priorities in the health care environment will help to integrate students more effectively into the real world of clinical nursing.

SELECTING CLINICAL SETTINGS

Clinical teachers may have sole responsibility for selecting the settings in which clinical learning activities occur, or their input may be sought by those who make these decisions. In either case, selection of clinical sites should be based on important criteria such as compatibility of school and agency philosophy, availability of opportunities to meet learning objectives, geographical location, agency licensure or accreditation, availability of positive role models, complexity of patients, level of student, purpose and type of course, and physical resources (Gardner & Suplee, 2010, p. 18; O'Connor, 2006, pp. 26–27). In some areas, selection of appropriate clinical settings may be difficult because of competition among several nursing programs, and nursing programs must typically contract with a variety of agencies to provide adequate learning opportunities for students. Additionally, as nursing programs increase enrollments they face the challenge of securing adequate clinical placements, particularly in specialty areas such as pediatrics. Programs may be forced to use numerous clinical sites, which increases the time and energy required for teachers to develop relationships with staff, to obtain necessary information about agencies, and to develop and maintain competence to practice in diverse settings. It also creates an administrative burden to manage clinical agency approval, track student health requirement compliance, and coordinate clinical activities.

Selection Criteria

Nurse educators should conduct a careful assessment of potential clinical sites before selecting those that will be used. Faculty members who are also employed in clinical agencies may provide some of the necessary information, and teachers who have instructed students in an agency can provide ongoing input into its continued suitability as a practice site. State boards of nursing may have specific reporting requirements or forms that need to be completed as part of the selection and approval process for clinical sites. Nursing education programs may need to provide additional information for board of nursing review. For an example of an agency data form see www.portal.state .pa.us/portal/server.pt/community/state_board_of_nursing/12515/ licensure_information/572048#forms. Assessment of potential clinical agencies should address the following criteria (Stokes & Kost, 2012):

- *Opportunity to achieve learning outcomes.* Are sufficient opportunities available to allow learners to achieve learning objectives? For example, if planning, implementing, and evaluating preoperative teaching is an important course objective, the average preoperative patient census must be sufficient to permit learners to practice these skills. If the objectives require learners to practice direct patient care, does the agency allow this, or will learners only be permitted to observe? Will learners from other educational programs be present in the clinical environment at the same time? If so, how much competition for the same learning opportunities is anticipated? Will there be adequate patient census to ensure that appropriate learning opportunities are available?
- *Level of the learner.* If the learners are undergraduate students at the beginning level of the curriculum, the agency must provide ample opportunity to practice basic skills. Graduate students need learning activities that will allow them to develop advanced practice skills. Does the clinical agency permit graduate students to practice independently or under the guidance of a preceptor, without an on-site instructor? Are undergraduate students in a capstone

course permitted to participate in clinical learning activities under the guidance of an appropriate staff member as preceptor, without the physical presence of a faculty member?

■ *Degree of control by faculty.* Does the agency staff recognize the authority of the clinical teacher to plan appropriate learning activities for students, or do agency policies limit or prescribe the kinds and timing of student activities? Do staff members restrict the types of learning activities available? Do agency personnel view learners as additions to the staff and expect them to provide service to patients, or do they acknowledge the role of students as learners?

■ *Availability of role models for students.* As previously discussed, students often imitate the behaviors they observe in nursing staff members. Are the agency staff members positive role models for students and new staff nurses? If learners are graduate students who are learning advanced practice roles, are strong, positive role models available to serve as preceptors and mentors, Do they have the educational and experiential qualifications to guide students appropriately? Is staffing adequate to permit staff members to interact with students and participate in their learning, or are they overburdened? Are staff dismissive, exclusionary, and rude, or are they cooperative, inclusive, supportive, and welcoming of students?

■ *Geographical location.* Although geographical location of the clinical agency is not usually the most important selection criterion, it can be a crucial factor when a large number of clinical agencies must be used. Travel time between the campus and clinical settings for faculty and students must be considered, especially if learning activities are scheduled in both settings on the same day. Is travel to the agency via public transportation possible and safe, especially if faculty and students must travel in the evening or at night? Are public transportation schedules convenient; do they allow students and faculty to arrive at the agency in time for the scheduled start of activities, and do they permit a return trip to campus or home without excessive wait times? Does the value of available learning opportunities at the agency outweigh the disadvantages of travel time and cost?

■ *Physical facilities.* Are physical facilities such as conference space, locker rooms, cafeteria or other dining facility, library, and parking available for use by clinical teachers and students?

■ *Staff relationships with teachers and learners.* Do staff members respond positively to the presence of students, engage in effective communications with faculty and students, and welcome appropriate questions from them? Will the staff members cooperate with teachers in selecting appropriate learning activities, participate in orientation activities for faculty and students, and provide useful guidance and feedback about student performance?

■ *Orientation needs.* Some clinical agencies require faculty members to attend scheduled orientation sessions before they take students into the clinical setting. The time required for such orientation must be considered when selecting clinical agencies. If faculty members are also employed in the agency as casual or per diem staff, this orientation requirement may be waived. Can any parts of the orientation be completed without being present in the agency, such as online or via self-study? Is the clinical teacher who is new to a clinical setting permitted to work in the staff nurse role for several days prior to bringing students to the agency, to become familiar with the unit routines and to begin to form collaborative relationships with staff members? Are technology initiatives occurring that require faculty and student orientation, password clearances, and access to computer systems? If so, are there mechanisms in place for training and to allow clinical teachers and students to use these systems as part of the clinical learning activities?

■ *Opportunity for interdisciplinary activities.* As interprofessional skill development emerges as a critical component of nursing education, consider if there are opportunities for learners to practice as members of an interdisciplinary health care team. Will learners have contact with other health care practitioners, such as physical therapists, pharmacists, nutritionists, respiratory therapists, social workers, infection control personnel, and physicians?

■ *Agency requirements.* Unless the educational program and the clinical facility are parts of the same organization, a legal contract or agreement usually must be negotiated to permit students and faculty to use the agency as a clinical teaching site. Such contracts or agreements typically specify requirements such as school and individual liability insurance; competence in cardiopulmonary resuscitation; professional licensure for clinical teachers, graduate students, and RN-to-BSN students; immunization and other health requirements; dress code; use of name tags or identification badges; requirements for student drug testing; and requirements for criminal background checks for students and clinical teachers.

Health care agencies are mandating these requirements to ensure patient safety and comply with various regulations. Currently, the Centers for Disease Control and the Advisory Committee on Immunization Practices (ACIP) recommend that health professions students receive measles, mumps, rubella, hepatitis B, varicella, influenza, and pertussis vaccines (Lindley et al., 2011). Students may need to demonstrate compliance by showing evidence of immunizations or immunity, or they may require booster immunizations. Additional clinical requirements such as mandatory drug testing may also be specified by health care facilities (Cotter & Glasgow, 2012). Institutions may require testing for a specific panel of drugs or drug classifications. Typically students have a narrow window of time for completion of the drug testing at the start of a clinical practicum and must follow a specific protocol for this testing. Depending upon state regulations, students may also need to complete a variety of background checks to screen for offenses and criminal arrest records. These background checks may include child abuse, elder abuse, and criminal history checks. Some agencies require that students meet the same requirements that their staff members must meet, which may include financial background checks. As the Fair Credit Reporting Act requires, students should be notified about the purpose of these background checks and must provide written consent (Philipsen et al., 2012). All of these requirements should be communicated to students in print and, for ease of retrieval, in an online electronic format. Clear communication with students about these requirements will help to ensure that students understand them and have sufficient time to gather evidence of completion by the specified deadlines.

The list of clinical requirements may be quite lengthy and may require significant time and financial investment for students to comply; however, they must be completed before a student can begin clinical activities at a clinical site and risk violating the nursing education program's contract with the agency and jeopardize future access to that clinical site. Another concern for the educational institution involves managing these records. When gathering personal information about students, nursing education program personnel need to protect student privacy and prevent inappropriate disclosure of personal information obtained for clinical requirements. Some programs contract with agencies that conduct the background checks and provide reports to the administrator. Student consent is essential when releasing personally identifiable information to such outside agencies to ensure compliance with the Family Education Rights and Privacy Act (FERPA; Jones & Weninger, 2007; Shellenbarger & Stearns, 2010). Thus, nursing education programs should have guidelines for disclosure and a method of keeping this private information separate from students' academic records (Jones & Weninger, 2007).

Sufficient time must be allowed before the anticipated start of clinical activities to negotiate the contract and for clinical teachers and students to meet the requirements. Clinical teachers must usually have current unencumbered professional nursing licenses for each state in which they instruct in the clinical area, unless the clinical agencies are located in states that have adopted the Nurse Licensure Compact (National Council of State Boards of Nursing, n.d.) and the clinical teacher is also licensed in one of those states.

- *Agency licensure and accreditation.* Accreditation requirements for educational programs may specify that clinical learning activities take place in accredited health care organizations. If the agency must be licensed to provide certain health services, it is appropriate to verify current licensure before selecting that agency as a clinical site.
- *Costs.* In addition to travel expenses, there may be other costs associated with use of an agency for clinical learning activities. Any fees charged to schools for use of the agency or other anticipated expense to the educational program and to individual clinical teachers and students should be assessed.
- *Regulatory Board approvals.* State boards of nursing often require review and approval of clinical sites before a new site can be used for clinical nursing education. Faculty members or administrators may need to provide information about the health care institution, including bed capacity and average daily patient census, a list of other nursing education programs using the facility, number of students who will use the facility, and specific scheduling information.

PREPARATION OF FACULTY MEMBERS

When selection of the clinical site or sites is complete, the nurse educator must prepare for the teaching and learning activities that will take place there. Areas of preparation that must be addressed include clinical competence, familiarity with the clinical environment, and orientation to the agency or setting.

Clinical Competence

Clinical competence has been documented as an essential characteristic of effective clinical teachers. Clinical competence includes theoretical knowledge, expert clinical skills, and judgment in the practice area in which teaching occurs (Oermann & Gaberson, 2014).

Standards for accreditation and state approval of nursing education programs may require nurse faculty members to have advanced clinical preparation in graduate nursing programs in the clinical specialty area in which they are assigned to teach. In addition, faculty members should have sufficient clinical experience in the specialty area in which they teach. This is particularly important for faculty members who will provide direct, on-site guidance of students in the clinical area; the combination of academic preparation and professional work experience supports the teacher's credibility and confidence. Students often identify the ability to demonstrate nursing care in the clinical setting as an essential skill of an effective clinical instructor (Gardner & Suplee, 2010; Girija, 2012; Huo, Zhu, & Zheng, 2010; Kelly, 2007).

Clinical teachers should maintain current clinical knowledge through participation in continuing education and practice experience. Nurse educators who have a concurrent faculty practice or joint appointment in a clinical agency, or who work part time in a clinical role in addition to their academic assignment, are able to maintain their clinical competence by this means, especially if they practice in the same specialty area and clinical agency in which they teach.

Familiarity With the Clinical Environment

If the clinical teacher is entering a new clinical area, he or she may ask to work with the staff for a few days prior to returning to the site with students. This enables the teacher to practice using equipment and technology that may be unfamiliar and to become familiar with the agency environment, policies, and procedures. If this is not possible, the teacher should at least observe activities or shadow a nursing staff member in the clinical area to discern the characteristics of the patient population, the usual schedule and pace of activities, the types of learning opportunities available to develop desired outcomes, the diversity of health care professionals in the agency, and the presence of other learners (Di Leonardi & Oermann, 2010; O'Connor, 2006, pp. 31–33).

As previously mentioned, a clinical agency may require faculty members whose students use the facility to attend an orientation program. Orientation sessions vary in length, from several hours to a day or more, and typically include introductions to administrators, managers, and staff development instructors; clarification of policies such as whether students may administer intravenous medications; review of documentation procedures; and safety procedures. Faculty members may be asked to demonstrate competent operation of equipment, such as infusion pumps, that their students will be using or to submit evidence that they have met the same competency standards that are required of nursing staff members.

PREPARATION OF CLINICAL AGENCY STAFF

Preparation of the clinical agency staff usually begins with the nursing education program's initial contact with the agency when negotiating an agreement or contract between the program and the agency. Establishing an effective working relationship with the nursing staff is an important responsibility of the clinical teacher. Ideally, nursing staff members would be eager to work with the faculty member to help students meet their learning goals. Indeed, in academic health centers and other teaching institutions, participation in education of learners from many health care disciplines is a normal job expectation. Serving as a preceptor or working with students may be used for clinical ladder or magnet status designation evaluation criteria (Pierson, Liggett, & Moore, 2010). Regardless of the reasons for working with students, some staff members will enjoy working with students more than others. Because teachers cannot usually choose which staff members will be involved with students, it is important for the teacher to communicate the following information to all staff members.

Clarification of Roles

Staff members often expect the instructor to be responsible for the care of patients with whom students are assigned to work. Many clinical teachers remark that if they have 10 students and each student is assigned 2 patients, the instructor is responsible for 30 individuals. These role expectations are both unrealistic and unfair to all involved parties.

Although the clinical teacher is ultimately responsible for student learning, students have much to gain from close working relationships with staff members. Staff members can serve as useful role models of nursing practice in the real world; students can observe how staff members must adapt their practice to fit the demands of a complex, ever-changing clinical environment. At the same time, staff members are often stimulated and motivated by students' questions and the current information that they can share. The presence of students in the clinical environment often reinforces staff members' competence and expertise, and many nurses enjoy sharing their knowledge and skill with novices. Clinical teachers should therefore encourage staff members to participate in the instruction of learners within guidelines that teachers and staff members develop jointly. Students should be encouraged to use selected staff members as resources for their learning, especially when they have questions that relate to specific patients for whom the staff members are responsible.

An important point of role clarification is that the responsibility for patient care remains with staff members of the clinical agency, as mentioned earlier. If a student is assigned learning activities related to care of a specific patient, a staff member, often called the primary nurse, is assigned the overall responsibility for that patient's care. Students are accountable for their own actions, but the primary nurse and student should collaborate to ensure that patient needs are met. Staff members may give reports about patient status and needs to students who are assigned to work with those patients; students should be encouraged to ask questions of staff members about specific patient care requirements; to share ideas about patient care; and to report changes in patient condition, problems, tasks that they will not be able to complete, and the need for assistance with tasks (Di Leonardi & Oermann, 2010; O'Connor, 2006, p. 29).

Role expectation guidelines such as these should be discussed with staff members and managers. When mutual understanding is achieved, the guidelines may be written and posted or distributed to relevant personnel and students.

Level of Learners

Staff members can have reasonable expectations of learner performance if they are informed of the students' levels of education and experience. Beginning students and novice staff members will need more guidance; staff members working with these learners should expect frequent questions and requests for assistance. More experienced learners may need less assistance with tasks but more guidance on problem solving and clinical decision making. Sharing this information with staff members allows them to plan their time accordingly and to anticipate student needs.

It is especially important for faculty members to tell agency personnel what specific tasks or activities learners are permitted and not permitted to do. This decision may be guided by educational program or agency policy, the curriculum sequence, or by the specific focus of the learning activities on any given day. For example, during one scheduled clinical session, an instructor may want students to practice therapeutic use of self through interviewing and active listening, without relying on physical care tasks. The instructor should share this information with the staff and ask them to avoid involving students in physical care on that day.

Learning Outcomes

The overall purpose and desired outcomes of the clinical learning activities should be communicated to staff members. As demonstrated in the previous example, knowledge of the specific objectives for a clinical session permits staff members to collaborate with the teacher in facilitating learning. If students have the specific learning objective of administering intramuscular injections, staff members can be asked to notify the teacher if any patient needs an injection that day so that the student can take advantage of that learning opportunity.

Knowledge of the learning objectives allows staff members to suggest appropriate learning activities, even if the teacher is unable to anticipate the need. For example, an elderly patient who is confused may be admitted to the nursing unit; the staff nurse who is aware that students are focusing on nursing interventions to achieve patient safety might suggest that a student be assigned to work with this patient.

Need for Positive Role Modeling

The need for staff members to be positive role models for learners is a sensitive but important issue. As previously discussed, teachers often worry that students will learn bad practice habits from experienced nurses who may take shortcuts when giving care. When discussing this issue with staff members, instructors should avoid implying that the only right way to perform skills is the teacher's way. Instead, the teacher might ask staff members to point out when they are omitting steps from procedures and to discuss with learners the rationale for those actions. In this way, staff nurses can model how to think like a nurse, a valuable learning opportunity for nursing students.

Asking staff nurses to be aware of the behaviors that they model for students and seeking their collaboration in fostering students' professional role development is an important aspect of preparing agency staff to work with learners. To accomplish this goal, instructors need to establish mutually respectful, trusting relationships with staff members and to sustain dialogue about role modeling over a period of time.

The Role of Staff Members in Evaluation

Agency staff members have important roles in evaluating learner performance. The clinical performance of learners must be evaluated formatively and summatively. Formative evaluation takes the form of feedback to the student during the learning process; its purpose is to provide information to be used by the learner to improve performance. Summative evaluation occurs at the end of the learning process; its outcome is a judgment about the worth or value of the learning outcomes (Oermann & Gaberson, 2014). Summative evaluations usually result in academic grades or personnel decisions such as promotions or merit pay increases.

Teachers should explain carefully their expectations about the desired involvement of staff members in evaluating student performance. Agency personnel have an important role in formative evaluation by communicating with teachers and learners about student performance. Because staff members are often in close contact with students during clinical activities, their observations of student performance are valuable, but the teacher should keep in mind that staff members may have different expectations for student performance than the instructor does (Di Leonardi & Oermann, 2010). Staff members should be encouraged to report to the teacher any concerns that they may have about student performance as well as observations of exemplary performance; clinical instructors should accept this input and then validate the report by their own observations. Staff members should also feel free to praise students, point out any errors they may have made, or make suggestions for improving performance. Immediate, descriptive feedback is necessary for learners to improve their performance, and often staff members are better able than teachers to provide this information to students.

However, it is the teacher's responsibility to make summative evaluation decisions. Staff members should know that they are an important source of data on student performance and that their input is valued, but that it is the clinical teacher who ultimately certifies competence or assigns a grade.

PREPARING THE LEARNERS

Students need cognitive, psychomotor, and affective preparation for clinical learning activities. It is the clinical teacher's responsibility to assist students with such preparation as well as to assess its adequacy before students enter the clinical area.

Cognitive Preparation

General prerequisite knowledge for clinical learning includes information about the learning outcomes; the clinical agency; and the roles of teacher, student, and staff member. Additionally, in some nursing education programs, students are able and expected to prepare ahead of time for each clinical learning session. This preparation may include one or more of the following tasks: gathering information from patient records; interviewing patients and family members; assessing patient needs; performing physical assessment; reviewing relevant pathophysiology, nursing, nutrition, and pharmacology textbooks; and completing written assignments such as a patient assessment, plan of care, concept map, or instructor-designed preparation sheet. In some programs, students complete these types of learning activities during and following their clinical learning activities.

Teachers should ensure that the expected cognitive preparations for clinical learning do not carry more importance than the clinical learning activities themselves. That is, learning should be expected to occur during the clinical learning activities as well as during preclinical preparation. If students receive their learning assignments in advance of the scheduled clinical activity, they can be reasonably expected to review relevant textbook information and to anticipate potential patient problems and needs. If circumstances permit a planning visit to the clinical agency, the student may meet and interview the patient and review the patient's health record. However, requiring extensive written assignments to be completed before the actual clinical activity implies that learning takes place only before the student enters the clinical area. Students cannot be expected to formulate a realistic plan of care before assessing the patient's physical, psychosocial, and cultural needs; this assessment may begin before the actual clinical activity, but it usually comprises a major part of the student's activity in the clinical setting. Thus, preclinical planning should focus on preparations for the learning that will take place in clinical practice. For example, the teacher may require students to formulate a tentative nursing diagnosis from available patient information, formulate a plan for collecting additional data to support or refute this diagnosis, and plan tentative nursing interventions based on the diagnosis. A more extensive written assignment submitted after the clinical activity may require students to evaluate the appropriateness of the diagnosis and the effectiveness of the nursing interventions.

Additionally, because students often copy information from textbooks (or, regrettably, from other students) to complete such requirements, written assignments submitted before the clinical learning activity may not show evidence of clinical reasoning and problem solving, let alone comprehension and retention of the information. For example, some teachers require students to complete drug cards for each medication prescribed for a patient. Students often copy published pharmacologic information without attempting to retain this information and to think critically about why the medication was prescribed or how a particular patient might respond to it. A better approach is to ask students to reflect on the pharmacologic actions of prescribed drugs and to be prepared to discuss relevant nursing care implications, either individually with the instructor or in a group conference. If it is not possible for students to determine in advance which drugs are being used to treat patients whose care they will be participating in, the clinical instructor may ask students to study particular drug classifications and their prototype drugs and to be prepared to seek and use appropriate information resources when the student obtains the drug list. For example, if students are studying nursing care of patients who are at risk of a cerebral vascular accident, they should be familiar with several classifications of antihypertensive drugs and understand the common desired, side, and adverse effects. Students can then formulate a tentative plan of care for these patients and then modify and individualize the plan when they are able to assess specific patients.

Nursing students should learn to use a variety of reference materials both to prepare for clinical practice and as resources during clinical learning activities. Handheld devices such as personal digital assistants (PDAs) and smartphones are growing in popularity as resources that can be used to access reference materials (Robb & Shellenbarger, 2012). There is a growing body of information about PDA use by nursing students at various levels (Glasgow & Cornelius, 2005), but research-based evidence for its effectiveness is still limited (George & Davidson, 2005). In one survey of nursing education programs, 68% required students to purchase their own handheld devices (Smith & Pattrillo, 2006). Among nursing students who use electronic resources for clinical preparation, pharmacology books, medical dictionaries, and nursing diagnosis programs are most frequently used (Doran et al., 2010; Kuiper, 2010; Williams & Dittmer, 2009).

A quasi-experimental study of student preference for and use of e-books in one BSN program found that students used PDAs for both preclinical preparation and during clinical learning activities (Williams & Dittmer, 2009). Preference for e-book use as a resource over print resources grew among students in the experimental groups during the study, except for students in their first clinical nursing course, suggesting that beginning students need more guided learning activities with new technology tools. Students perceived that use of e-books on PDAs decreased the amount of time needed for preclinical preparation. Based on these results, Williams and Dittmer (2009) proposed that clinical teachers may need to view students' preclinical preparation differently: Should nursing students be allowed or even encouraged to search for information as needed throughout a clinical learning activity instead of completing a written preparation assignment? PDA and smart phone technology offers the convenience of fast, accessible, up-to-date information and possibly even increased productivity. Faculty members should consider the cost, connectivity issues, privacy and confidentiality concerns, available software, and student comfort with use if requiring these devices. Strategies to effectively implement this technology into clinical nursing education include: early introduction, opportunities for training and practice, technology support for problems, and clinical teacher role modeling (Cibulka & Crane-Wider, 2011; Kuiper, 2010; Zurmehly, 2010).

We recommend that students be expected to complete some cognitive preparation before clinical practice, but extensive, detailed written preparation assignments are unrealistic and often shift focus away from learning *during* clinical activities. Encouraging students' identification and use of appropriate, available information resources during clinical practice facilitates development of clinical reasoning and problem-solving abilities and increases students' self-confidence (Williams & Dittmer, 2009).

Meeting with students during a preclinical conference, either in a group or individually, also allows for assessment of student preparation. Clinical teachers can use questioning techniques to determine if students have adequate knowledge to care for patients. It also provides an opportunity for clarification about anticipated nursing care. Clinical teachers can assess student preparation and feel assured that students have an appropriate plan for care. Exhibit 4.1 provides sample questions that clinical teachers might use for preclinical conferences with students.

Exhibit 4.1

SAMPLE PRECLINICAL CONFERENCE QUESTIONING

- What are your priority nursing assessments?
- What is your plan of care for the day? What nursing care will you provide first?
- What lab or diagnostic tests were performed recently? What are the results? What are your nursing actions based upon these results?
- What medications are prescribed for your patient that will need to be administered? Why is the patient taking each medication? What are the actions, side effects, and nursing implications of these medications?

Psychomotor Preparation

Skill learning is an important outcome of clinical teaching. However, the length and number of clinical learning sessions are often limited in nursing education or new staff orientation programs. In a qualitative study completed by Killam and Heerschap (2013), students reported that lack of practice time and inadequate feedback about psychomotor skill performance were challenges to their learning in the clinical setting. As students develop into competent care providers they need to have adequate time to learn psychomotor skills in a practice setting and be given appropriate and informative feedback to enhance performance. When learning complex skills, it is more efficient for students to practice the parts first in an environment such as a simulation center or skills laboratory, free from the demands of the actual practice setting. In such a setting, students can investigate and discover alternative ways of performing skills, and they can make errors and learn to correct them without fear of harming patients. Thus, students should have ample skill practice time before they enter the clinical area so that they are not expected to perform a skill for the first time in a fast-paced, demanding environment. It is the clinical teacher's responsibility to assure that students have developed the desired level of skill before entering the clinical setting. The use of clinical simulation and technology in a nursing skills lab provides students with realistic learning opportunities to develop psychomotor skills in a controlled environment. Use of clinical simulation activities allows students to practice and refine psychomotor skills and incorporates cognitive and affective learning as well. A literature review of teaching psychomotor skills revealed that teaching methods that provide access to online instruction as part of psychomotor skills teaching was more effective than other approaches (McNett, 2012). Chapter 9 presents a comprehensive discussion of the use of clinical simulation.

Affective Preparation

Affective preparation of students includes strategies for managing their anxiety and for fostering confidence and positive attitudes about learning. Most students have some anxiety about clinical learning activities. Mild or moderate anxiety often serves to motivate students to learn, but excessive anxiety hinders concentration and interferes with information processing and learning and may undermine clinical performance (Cheung & Au, 2011). The role of the teacher in reducing the stress of clinical practice is discussed in more detail in Chapter 5. However, in preparation for clinical learning activities, teachers may employ strategies to identify students' fears and reduce their anxiety to a manageable level. A preclinical conference session might assess learners' specific concerns and assure students of the teacher's confidence in them, desire for their success, and availability for consultation and guidance during the clinical activities.

For example, during a preclinical conference on the first day of clinical practice in a course, the instructor may state that it is common for students to feel anxious before a clinical activity but that anxiety usually decreases during the experience. The teacher may encourage students to identify and name the specific source and nature of their anxieties; once these are identified, the teacher can help students to use a problem-solving approach to identify helpful responses. For instance, if students express concern that something may happen that they will not know how to handle, the teacher may help students to list all the potential adverse events and then brainstorm possible responses to them. Throughout such a discussion, teachers should reassure students of their availability to answer questions and assist them with clinical reasoning and problem solving during the clinical learning activities.

Orientation to the Clinical Agency

Like clinical teachers, students also need a thorough orientation to the clinical agency in which learning activities will take place. This orientation may take place before or on the first day of clinical activities. Staff members often assist the teacher in orienting students to the agency and helping them to feel welcome and comfortable in the new environment.

Orientation should include:

- The geographical location of the agency
- The physical setup of the specific unit where students will be placed
- Names, titles, and roles of personnel
- Location of areas such as rest rooms, dining facilities, conference room, locker rooms, public telephones, and library
- Information about transportation and parking
- Agency and unit policies
- Daily schedules and routines
- Emergency protocols (e.g., fire drill, rapid response codes, cardiac arrest procedures and equipment)
- Patient information documentation systems, including establishment of passwords and acquiring computer access to electronic health records and bedside medication administration systems

In addition, students need to have a telephone number at the clinical setting where they can be contacted in case of family emergency, know what procedures to follow in case of illness or other reason for absence on a clinical day, understand the uniform or dress requirements, and know what equipment to bring (e.g., stethoscope) and what to leave at home (e.g., personal valuables).

Given the growth of informatics in health care settings, faculty need to consider this for student orientation needs. Gone are the days of showing students hard-copy charts and explaining medication administration records and then moving quickly to delivering care. Instead, students need access codes for technology used at the clinical site. They will also need training for computer use, such as bar-coded bedside medication systems and electronic health records, before they can fully deliver care. Clinical teachers need to coordinate this technology training with nurse educators and health care information technology personnel. Of course, clinical teachers also need to ensure that they are up to date on this training so that they are prepared to guide student learning in the clinical setting.

Not all of this orientation information needs to be presented on site; some creative clinical teachers have developed electronic resources that provide a virtual tour of the facility. If the agency uses computer software to document patient information, the instructor may be able to acquire a copy of the software application and make it available in the school's computer facility. Or, the nursing program may purchase bar code scanning equipment that can be used to simulate medication administration in clinical practice labs. Learners can be expected to review these resources before coming to the clinical site. Because student and clinical teacher orientation to a clinical facility can be costly and time-intensive for staff development educators, some agencies are now using technology for orientation (Bowers et al., 2011; Brooks, & Erickson, 2012; Schumacher, 2010). Self-directed electronic learning modules can be delivered via a website or classroom management system that enables an efficient, flexible, and cost-effective delivery method for training. Mandatory education required by health care facilities, such as fire safety, Health Insurance Portibility and Accountability Act (HIPAA) training, infection control, or other topics can be delivered electronically. Clinical teachers and students can review needed training and complete appropriate evaluation materials. Spreadsheets or online systems can efficiently track compliance and completion of learning. Electronic delivery of clinical information can also be used throughout the year to share ongoing updates with clinical teachers and students in an efficient manner.

The First Day

Students almost always perceive the first day of clinical learning activities in a new setting as stressful; this is especially true of learners in their initial clinical nursing course. Students' first exposure to the clinical environment can either promote their independence as learners or foster dependence on the instructor due to fear. Clinical teachers should plan specific activities for the first day that will allow learners to become familiar with and comfortable in the clinical environment and at the same time alleviate their anxiety. These activities may include tours, conferences, games, and special assignments.

Even if learners have attended an agency orientation, it is helpful to take them on a tour of the specific areas they will use for learning activities, pointing out locations such as rest rooms, drinking fountains, fire alarms and extinguishers, emergency equipment, elevators, stairwells, and emergency exits. The instructor should introduce learners to staff members by name and title. If students need agency-specific identification badges, parking permits, or passwords for use of the computer system, the teacher may make the necessary arrangements ahead of time or accompany students to the appropriate locations where these items can be acquired. If an empty patient room is available, the instructor may demonstrate the use of equipment such as bed controls, call bell, oxygen delivery systems, and lighting controls.

Special assignments may include review and discussion of patient records, practice of computer documentation, and a scavenger hunt to help learners locate typical items needed for patient care. Exhibit 4.2 is an example of a scavenger hunt activity used in orienting students to a medical-surgical unit of a hospital. Learners may be asked to observe patient care for a specified period of time, interview a patient or family member, shadow a nurse, or complete a short written assignment focused on documenting an observation.

Exhibit 4.2

A SCAVENGER HUNT STRATEGY

Anywhere General Hospital
Unit 2C

Work in pairs to search for the location of the items or areas listed below. Check them off as you find them.

- Locker room
- Restrooms
- Oxygen shut-off valves
- Fire alarms
- Fire extinguishers
- Emergency exits
- Assignment board
- Patient health records
- Patient teaching materials
- Nurse manager's office
- Medication dispensing systems
- Linen carts

(continued)

- Kitchen
- Utility room
- Biohazardous waste containers
- Waterless hand sanitizer dispensers
- Reference materials
- Conference room
- Medical supply carts (IV bags, dressing change materials, gloves)
- Computer work stations

These activities may be followed by a short group conference, during which students are encouraged to discuss their impressions, experiences, and feelings. The teacher should review the roles of student, teacher, and staff members and should emphasize lines of communication. For example, students need to know who to ask for help and under what circumstances—that is, when to ask questions of staff members and when to seek assistance from the teacher. Handouts summarizing these expectations and requirements are useful because students can review them later when their anxiety is lower. If a dining facility is available in the clinical setting, pre- or postclinical conferences may take place in that location to allow students to relax with refreshments away from patient care areas. The conference may conclude by making plans for the next day of clinical practice, including selecting assignments and discussing how learners should prepare for their learning activities. Selection of clinical assignments is discussed in detail in Chapter 7.

SUMMARY

This chapter described the roles and responsibilities of faculty, staff members, and others involved in clinical teaching and suggested strategies for preparing students and staff members for clinical learning.

The teacher and learners comprise a temporary system within the permanent culture of the clinical setting. Negative consequences of this relationship can be avoided by establishing and maintaining regular communication between the instructor and staff members. Clinical teachers function as culture brokers and border spanners to help integrate students more fully into the real world of nursing practice.

Settings for clinical learning should be selected carefully, based on important criteria such as compatibility of school and agency philosophy, licensure and accreditation, availability of opportunities to meet learning objectives, geographical location, availability of positive role models, and physical resources. Selection of appropriate clinical settings may be complicated by competition among several nursing programs for a limited number of agencies. Specific criteria for assessing the suitability of potential clinical settings were discussed.

When clinical sites have been selected, educators must prepare for teaching and learning activities. Areas of preparation include clinical competence, familiarity with the clinical environment, and orientation to the agency. Clinical competence has been documented as an essential characteristic of effective clinical teachers and includes knowledge and expert skill and judgment in the clinical practice area in which teaching occurs. Teachers may maintain clinical competence through faculty practice, joint appointment in clinical agencies, part-time clinical employment, and continuing nursing education activities. The teacher may become familiar with a new clinical setting by working with or observing the staff for a few days prior to returning to the site with students. The clinical agency may require faculty members to attend an orientation program that includes introductions to agency staff, clarification of policies concerning student activities, and review of skills and procedures.

Preparation of the clinical agency staff usually begins with the teacher's initial contact with the agency. Roles of teacher, students, and staff members should be clarified so that staff members have guidelines for their participation in the instruction of learners. An important point of role clarification is that, although students are accountable for their own actions, the responsibility for patient care remains with staff members of the clinical agency. Staff members also need to be aware of specific learning objectives, the level of the learner, the need for positive role modeling, and expectations concerning their role in evaluating student performance. Although staff members' feedback is valuable in formative evaluation, the teacher is always responsible for summative evaluation of learner performance.

Students need cognitive, psychomotor, and affective preparation for clinical learning activities. Cognitive preparation includes information about the learning objectives; the clinical agency; and the roles of teacher, student, and staff member. Students may be expected to prepare for each clinical learning session through reading, interviewing patients, and completing written assignments. However, requirements for extensive written assignments to be completed before the actual clinical activity may imply that learning takes place only before the student enters the clinical area.

The instructor has a responsibility to assess that students have the desire level of skill development before entering the clinical setting. When learning complex skills, it is more efficient for students to practice the parts first in a simulated setting such as a skills laboratory, free from the demands of the actual practice setting. Students should have ample skill practice time before they enter the clinical area so that they are not expected to perform a skill for the first time in a fast-paced, demanding environment.

Affective preparation of students includes strategies for managing their anxiety and for fostering confidence and positive attitudes about learning. Most students have some anxiety about clinical learning activities. Mild or moderate anxiety often serves to motivate students to learn, but excessive anxiety hinders concentration and interferes with learning. In preparation for clinical learning activities, teachers may employ strategies such as a structured preclinical conference to identify students' fears and reduce their anxiety to a manageable level.

Students also need a thorough orientation to the clinical agency in which learning activities will take place. This orientation should include information about the location and physical setup of the agency, relevant agency personnel, agency policies, daily schedules and routines, and procedures for responding to emergencies and for documenting patient information.

Students almost always perceive the first day of clinical learning activities in a new setting as stressful. Clinical teachers should plan specific activities for the first day that will allow learners to become familiar with and comfortable in the clinical environment and at the same time alleviate their anxiety. These activities include tours, conferences, games, and special assignments.

Exhibit 4.3

CNE EXAMINATION TEST BLUEPRINT CORE COMPETENCIES

1. **Facilitate Learning**

   D. Use information technologies to support the teaching–learning process
   H. Create opportunities for learners to develop their own critical thinking skills
   I. Create a positive learning environment that fosters a free exchange of ideas
   K. Demonstrate personal attributes that facilitate learning (e.g., caring, confidence, patience, integrity, respect, and flexibility)
   M. Develop collegial working relationships with clinical agency personnel to promote positive learning environments
   O. Demonstrates ability to teach clinical skills
   P. Act as a role model in practice settings
   Q. Foster a safe learning environment

   (continued)

2. **Facilitate Learner Development and Socialization**

   D. Create learning environments that facilitate learners' self-reflection, personal goal setting, and socialization to the role of the nurse
   E. Foster the development of learners in these areas
      1. cognitive domain
      2. psychomotor domain
      3. affective domain

4. **Participate in Curriculum Design and Evaluation of Program Outcomes**

   A. Demonstrate knowledge of curriculum development including
      1. identifying program outcomes
      5. selecting appropriate clinical experiences

   H. Collaborate with community and clinical partnerships that support the educational goals

5. **Pursue Systematic Self-Evaluation and Improvement in the Academic Nurse Educator Role**

   A. Engage in activities that promote one's socialization to the role
   E. Participate in professional development opportunities that increase one's effectiveness in the role

6. **Engage in Scholarship, Service, and Leadership**

   C. Function effectively within the organizational environment and the academic community
      3. Integrate the values of respect, collegiality, professionalism, and caring to build an organizational climate that fosters the development of learners and colleagues

REFERENCES

Bowers, A. M., Kavanagh, J., Gregorich, T., Shumway, J., Campbell, Y., & Stafford, S. (2011). Student nurses and the electronic medical record. *CIN: Computers, Informatics, Nursing, 29*, 692–697. doi:10.1097/NCN.0b013e31822b8a8f

Brooks, C. L., & Erickson, L. K. (2012). What is the solution for clinical nurse educators and the electronic medical record? *Teaching and Learning in Nursing, 7*, 129–132. doi:10.1016/j.teln.2012.06.003

Cheung, R. Y., & Au, T. K. (2011). Nursing students' anxiety and clinical performance. *Journal of Nursing Education, 50*, 286–289. doi:10.3928/01484834–20110131–08

Cibulka, N. J., & Crane-Wider, L. (2011). Introducing personal digital assistants to enhance nursing education in undergraduate and graduate nursing programs. *Journal of Nursing Education, 50*, 115–118. doi:10.3928/01484834–20101230–07

Cotter, V. T., & Glasgow, M. E. S. (2012). Student drug testing in nursing education. *Journal of Professional Nursing, 28*, 186–189. doi:10.1016/j.profnurs.2011.11.017

Di Leonardi, B. C., & Oermann, M. H. (2010). Teaching in a clinical setting. In L. Caputi (Ed.), *Teaching nursing: The art and science* (pp. 82–141). Glen Ellyn, IL: College of DuPage Press.

Doran, D. M., Haynes, B., Kushniruk, A., Straus, S., Grimshaw, J. Hall, L. M., . . . Jedras, D. (2010). Supporting evidence-based practice for nurses through information technologies. *Worldviews on Evidence-Based Nursing, 7*(1), 4–15.

Gardner, M. R., & Suplee, P. D. (2010). *Handbook of clinical teaching.* Sudbury, MA: Jones and Bartlett.

George, L., & Davidson, L. (2005). PDA use in nursing education: Prepared for today, poised for tomorrow. *Online Journal of Nursing Informatics, 9*(2). Retrieved from http://ojni.org/9_2/george.htm

Girija, K. M. (2012). Effective clinical instructor: A step toward excellence in clinical teaching. *International Journal of Nursing Education, 4*(1), 25–27.

Glasgow, M. E., & Cornelius, F. (2005). Benefits and costs of integrating technology into undergraduate nursing programs. *Nursing Leadership Forum, 9,* 175–179.

Huo, X., Zhu, D., & Zheng, M. (2010). Clinical nursing faculty competence inventory – development and psychometric testing. *Journal of Advanced Nursing, 67,* 1109–1117. doi:10.1111/j.1365–2648.2010.05520.x

Jones, M. M., & Weninger, R. A. (2007). Student criminal background checks: Considerations for schools of nursing. *Journal of Nursing Law, 11,* 163–170.

Kelly, C. (2007). Students' perceptions of effective clinical teaching. *Nursing Education Today, 27,* 885–887.

Killam, L. A., & Heerschap, C. (2013). Challenges to student learning in the clinical setting: A qualitative descriptive study. *Nurse Education Today, 33,* 684–691. doi:10.1016/j.nedt.2012.10.008

Kuiper, R. (2010). Metacognitive factors that impact student nurse use of point of care technology in clinical settings. *International Journal of Nursing Education Scholarship, 7*(1), article 5. doi:10.2202/1548–923X.1866

Lindley, M. C., Lorick, S. A., Spinner, J. R., Krull, A. R., Mootrey, G. T., Ahmed, F., . . . Strikas, R. A. (2011). Student vaccination requirements of U.S. health professional schools: A survey. *Annals of Internal Medicine, 154,* 391–400. doi:10.7326/003–4819–154–6–201103150–00004

MacIntyre, R. C., Murray, T. A., Teel, C. S., & Karshmer, J. F. (2009). Five recommendations for prelicensure clinical nursing education. *Journal of Nursing Education, 48,* 447–453. doi:10.3928/01484834–20090717–03

McNett, S. (2012). Teaching nursing psychomotor skills in a fundamentals laboratory: A literature review. *Nursing Education Perspectives, 33,* 328–333. doi:10.5480/1536–5026–33.5.328

Mullenbach, K. F. (2010). Senior nursing students' perspectives on the recruitment and retention of medical-surgical nurses. *MEDSURG Nursing, 19,* 341–344.

National Council of State Boards of Nursing. (n.d.). *Nurse licensure compact.* Retrieved from https://www.ncsbn.org/nlc.htm

O'Connor, A. B. (2006). *Clinical instruction and evaluation: A teaching resource* (2nd ed.). Sudbury, MA: Jones and Bartlett.

Oermann, M. H., & Gaberson, K. B. (2014). *Evaluation and testing in nursing education* (4th ed.). New York, NY: Springer Publishing.

Paton, B. I. (2007). Knowing within: Practice wisdom of clinical nurse educators. *Journal of Nursing Education, 46,* 488–495.

Philipsen, N., Murray, T. L., Belgrave, L., Bell-Hawkins, A., Robinson, V., & Watties-Daniels, D. (2012). Criminal background checks in nursing: Safeguarding the public? *The Journal for Nurse Practitioners, 8,* 707–711. 10.1016/j.nurpra2012.07.033

Pierson, M. A., Liggett, C., & Moore, K. S. (2010). Twenty years of experience with a clinical ladder: A tool for professional growth, evidence-based practice, recruitment, and retention. *The Journal of Continuing Education in Nursing, 41*(1), 33–40. doi:10.3928/00220124–20091222–06

Rebeschi, L., & Aronson, B. (2009). Assessment of nursing student's learning outcomes and employment choice after the implementation of a senior capstone course. *International Journal of Nursing Education Scholarship, 6*(1), article 21. doi:10.2202/1548–923X.1775

Robb, M., & Shellenbarger, T. (2012). Using technology to promote mobile learning: Engaging students with cell phones in the classroom. *Nurse Educators, 37,* 258–261. doi:10.1097/NNC0b013e31826f27da

Schumacher, D. (2010). The electronic medical record and clinical nursing student instruction: Tips and tricks for success. *The Journal of Continuing Education in Nursing, 41,* 102–103. doi:10.3928/00220124–20100224–08

Shellenbarger, T., & Perez-Stearns, C. (2010). From the classroom to clinical: A Family Educational Rights and Privacy Act primer for the nurse educator. *Teaching and Learning in Nursing, 5,* 164–168.

Smith, C. M., & Pattrillo, R. E. (2006). PDAs in the nursing curriculum: Providing data for internal funding. *Nurse Educator, 31,* 101–102.

Stokes, L. G., & Kost, G. C. (2012). Teaching in the clinical setting. In D. Billings & J. Halstead (Eds.), *Teaching in nursing: A guide for faculty* (pp. 311–334). St. Louis, MO: Elsevier.

Williams, M. G., & Dittmer, A. (2009). Textbooks on tap: Using electronic books housed in handheld devices in nursing clinical courses. *Nursing Education Perspectives, 10,* 220–225.

Zurmehly, J. (2010). Personal digital assistants (PDAs): Review and evaluation. *Nursing Education Perspectives, 3,* 179–182. doi:10.1043/1536–5026–31.3.179

CHAPTER 5

Process of Clinical Teaching

Clinical teaching is a complex interaction between students and teachers. Influencing the clinical teaching process are characteristics of the teacher and learner; the clinical environment and nature of practice within that environment; patients, families, and others for whom students are caring; agency personnel and other health care providers; and the inherent nature of clinical practice with its uncertainties.

The process of clinical teaching is described in this chapter. The chapter provides a framework for the teacher to use in planning clinical activities appropriate for the learning outcomes and students, guiding students in the practice setting, and evaluating clinical performance. A framework assists clinical teachers to create an environment and opportunities for students to learn; the outcomes of those experiences, however, may vary considerably among students because of the many factors that influence the learning process. This chapter also describes characteristics of effective clinical teachers and models of clinical teaching, such as traditional, in which one teacher guides the learning of a small group of students; preceptor; and partnerships, including dedicated education units (DEUs).

TEACHING AND LEARNING

Teaching is a complex process intended to facilitate learning. While the goal of teaching is to lead students in discovering knowledge for themselves, the teacher encourages this discovery through deliberate teaching actions that lead in that direction. Self-discovery does not imply a lack of structure; instead, the teacher provides structure and learning activities for self-discovery by the student.

Clinical teaching is a series of deliberate actions on the part of the teacher to guide students in their learning. It involves a sharing and mutual experience on the part of both teacher and student and is carried out in an environment of support and trust. Teaching is not telling, it is not dispensing information, and it is not merely demonstrating skills. Instead, teaching is *involving* the student as an active participant in this learning. The teacher is a resource person with information to share for the purpose of facilitating learning and acquisition of new knowledge and skills.

Learning is a process through which people change as a result of their experiences. Some people view learning as an overt and measurable change in behavior resulting from an experience; however, this view negates a change in perception and insight as learning. In the clinical setting, new insights, ideas, and perspectives may be as critical to the student's learning and development as overt and measurable behaviors. Learning, therefore, may be a change in observable behavior or performance, or it may reflect a new perception and insight not manifested by an overt change in behavior.

The teaching–learning process is a complex interaction of these processes. The teacher is a facilitator of learning, and the student is an active participant. The need for students to be actively involved in their learning is critical in the teaching–learning process, particularly in the clinical setting. When students are actively involved in their learning and perceive a positive teacher–student relationship, they can be honest about their learning needs and how faculty can help them in developing their clinical competencies. Active learning may also foster students' higher level thinking as they reflect on patient problems and possible approaches. Studies on problem-based learning suggest that this method improves students' critical thinking (Kong, Qin, Zhou, Mou, & Gao, 2013).

Although teaching and learning are interrelated processes, each may occur without the other. Significant learning may result from the student's clinical activities without any teacher involvement. Similarly, the teacher's carefully planned assignments and activities for students may not lead to any new learning or development of competencies. The goal of clinical teaching is to create the environment and activities for learning, recognizing that each student will gain different insights and outcomes from them.

PROCESS OF CLINICAL TEACHING: FIVE COMPONENTS

The process of clinical teaching includes five steps:

1. Identifying the outcomes for learning
2. Assessing learning needs

3. Planning clinical learning activities
4. Guiding students
5. Evaluating clinical learning and performance

The process of clinical teaching is not linear; instead, each component influences others. For example, clinical evaluation provides data on further learning needs of students that in turn suggest new learning activities. Similarly, as the teacher works with students, observations of performance may alter the assessment and suggest different learning activities.

Identifying Outcomes for Learning

The first step in clinical teaching is to identify the goals and outcomes of clinical practice as discussed in Chapter 2. These intended learning goals and outcomes suggest areas for assessment, provide guidelines for teaching, and are the basis for evaluating learning. Nurse educators identify these outcomes in different ways. In some nursing programs, the outcomes of learning are stated as objectives to be achieved by students in the clinical course. In other programs, they are expressed in the form of clinical competencies to be demonstrated at the end of the course or for specific clinical activities. Clinical competencies often address 10 areas of learning. These areas are listed in Exhibit 5.1 with examples of competencies in each area.

In some clinical courses, students need to demonstrate learning and performance in all of these areas as well as others specific to the clinical specialty or setting. Other courses may focus on only a few of these areas of learning. Clinical competencies may be stated broadly, similar to most of the examples in Exhibit 5.1, or they can be more specific, such as, "administer intravenous injection of medications." In any clinical course, the competencies should be achievable by students, considering their prior knowledge, skills, and experiences; clinical learning opportunities available in the clinical setting, simulation, and through other learning experiences; and time allotted for clinical practice.

The clinical competencies should be communicated clearly to students, in written form, and understood by them. Similarly, the teacher has an important responsibility in *discussing* these outcomes and related clinical activities with agency personnel, not *telling* them. Agency personnel need input into decisions about the clinical activities and their match with the goals, philosophy, and care delivery system of the clinical setting. With this input, the teacher may need to alter intended clinical activities and plan simulations and other types of learning opportunities for students.

Exhibit 5.1

EXAMPLES OF CLINICAL COMPETENCIES

1. Concepts, theories, and other knowledge for clinical practice
   Analyzes the pathophysiological basis for the development of clinical manifestations in common patient conditions.
   Applies multicultural concepts of care to the community as client.

2. Use of research and other evidence in clinical practice
   Uses evidence on pain management interventions in planning care for patients.
   Evaluates research studies for applicability to long-term care of patients with dementia and their caregivers.

3. Assessment, diagnosis, plan, interventions, and evaluation of outcomes
   Collects data that are developmentally and age appropriate for healthy and ill children.
   Considers multiple nursing interventions for care of patients with complex health problems.

4. Psychomotor and technological skills, other types of interventions, and informatics competencies
   Demonstrates skill in conducting a physical examination.
   Uses informatics tools to retrieve and critically analyze information.

5. Values related to care of patients, families, and communities and other dimensions of health care
   Recognizes personal values that might conflict with professional nursing values.
   Accepts cultural, ethnic, and other differences of patients and communities.

6. Communication skills, ability to develop interpersonal relationships, and skill in collaboration with others
   Collaborates with other health providers in interdisciplinary care of children with disabilities.
   Communicates effectively with patients, families, staff, and others in the health care setting.

7. Development of knowledge, skills, and values essential for continuously improving the quality and safety of health care
   Identifies issues with quality of care in a clinical setting using relevant measures.
   Participates in analyzing system errors and designing unit-based improvements.

8. Management of care, leadership abilities, and role behaviors
   Manages care effectively for a small group of patients.
   Demonstrates the role and behaviors of a nurse as leader.

9. Accountability and responsibility of the learner
   Accepts responsibility for own actions and decisions.
   Values own role in preventing errors.

10. Self-development and continued learning
    Identifies own learning needs in clinical practice.
    Seeks learning opportunities to develop clinical competencies.

Students should also have input into the clinical competencies; there may be some already achieved by students and others to be added to meet their individual learning needs and goals. There should be some flexibility in the clinical course as long as students demonstrate the competencies and achieve the essential knowledge and skills for progressing through the nursing program.

It is important for all clinical teachers—full and part time, adjunct, and preceptors—to understand the clinical competencies of the course and prior courses that students have completed. The course leader is responsible for ensuring that all educators in a course, no matter what their role, use the outcomes and competencies to guide their selection of patients and other learning activities for students and to assess performance.

Assessing Learning Needs

Teaching begins at the level of the learner. The teacher's goal, therefore, is to assess the student's present level of knowledge and skill and other characteristics that may influence achieving the outcomes of the clinical practicum. The first area of assessment involves collecting data on whether the student has the prerequisite knowledge and skills for the clinical situation at hand and for completing the learning activities. For instance, if the learning activities focus on interventions for health promotion, students first need some understanding of health and behaviors for promoting health. Changing a sterile dressing requires an understanding of principles of asepsis. The teacher's role in assessment of the learner is important so that students engage in learning activities that build on their present knowledge and skills. When students lack the prerequisites, then the instruction can remedy these and more efficiently move students forward in their learning.

Not every student will enter the clinical course with the same prerequisite knowledge and skills, depending on past learning and clinical experiences. The teacher, therefore, should not expect the same entry competencies for all students. Assessment reveals the point at which the instruction should begin and does not imply poor performance for students, only that some learners may need different types of learning activities for the objectives. Assessment may also indicate that some students have already attained certain clinical competencies and can progress to new areas of learning.

The second area of assessment relates to individual characteristics of students that may influence their learning and clinical performance. Students and nurses today represent a diverse group of learners with varied cultural backgrounds, learning styles, ages, and other characteristics.

Students bring with them a wealth of life, work, and other experiences. In nursing programs, particularly second-degree programs, there is a wide range of ages of students, reflecting different generations and ways of thinking. Students in a nursing program may be baby boomers through the millennial/Net generation. There are different learning styles and expectations across these generations. Students who are gen Xers and millennials prefer experiential activities and being involved in decisions about their learning activities. Those students, in contrast to older students and most nursing faculty members, are part of the information age and grew up with the Internet, communicating with others electronically, and multitasking (Pardue & Morgan, 2008). Generational differences may affect how students approach their education. Nurse educators are challenged to design, implement, and evaluate innovative teaching–learning strategies to meet the needs of an increasingly diverse student and patient population (Bosher & Pharris, 2009; Jeffreys & Dogan, 2013).

In addition, many students combine their nursing education with other role responsibilities, such as family and work. Information about these characteristics, among others, gives the teacher a better understanding of the students and their responses to different learning situations. Faculty members need to accept individual differences among students and use this knowledge in planning the learning activities.

Planning Clinical Learning Activities

Following assessment of learner needs and characteristics, the teacher plans and then delivers the instruction. In planning the learning activities, the main considerations are the competencies to be developed in the clinical practicum, or outcomes to be met in the clinical component of the course, and individual learner needs. Other factors that influence decisions on clinical activities include evidence of the effectiveness of the clinical teaching method and learning activities being considered, characteristics of the clinical setting, and teacher availability to guide learners.

Clinical Competencies/Outcomes of Clinical Course

Clinical learning activities are selected to facilitate students' developing the essential competencies for clinical practice in that course or to meet the outcomes of the clinical practicum, depending on how these are stated by faculty members in the clinical course. The learning activities may include patient care assignment, but care of patients is not the only learning activity in which students engage in the practice setting. The specific competencies to be developed or outcomes to be achieved in that course should guide selection of learning activities. If the competencies focus on communication skills, then the learning activities may involve interviews with patients and families, papers analyzing those interactions, role play, and simulated patient–nurse interactions rather than providing direct care.

Learner Needs

While the clinical outcomes provide the framework for planning the learning activities, the other main consideration is the needs of the student. The activities should build on the student's present knowledge and skills and take into consideration other learner characteristics. Each student does not have to complete the same learning activities; the teacher is responsible for individualizing the clinical activities so that they best meet each student's needs while promoting achievement of the course outcomes.

Learning activities also build on one another. Planning includes organizing the activities to provide for the progressive development of knowledge and skills for each learner.

Evidence on Effectiveness of Clinical Teaching Method and Learner Activities

Decisions about the teaching methods to use and types of activities in which students will participate in the clinical setting should be based on evidence about what works best for promoting student learning. Nurse educators should review the literature to identify evidence to support the teaching methods they are planning and to get ideas about other strategies and activities for students that might be as or more effective. The evidence will also guide how a teaching method is implemented—for example, how to debrief after a simulation and the level of questions to ask to promote higher-level thinking. Evidence-based clinical nursing education involves four phases: (a) asking questions about best practices in teaching students in the clinical setting, (b) searching for research and other evidence to answer those questions, (c) evaluating the quality of the evidence and whether it is ready to be used in clinical teaching, and (d) deciding whether the findings are applicable to one's own clinical course, students, and setting (Oermann, 2007, 2009).

Characteristics of the Clinical Setting

The size of the agency, the patient population, the educational level and preparation of nurses and their availability and interest in working with students, other types of health care providers in the setting, and other characteristics of the clinical environment should be considered in planning the learning activities. These characteristics are considered in choosing an agency for use in a course, as discussed in Chapter 3, and they also guide the faculty in planning learning activities.

Teacher Availability

The teacher's availability to work with students in the clinical setting is an important consideration in planning the learning activities. Being available to students to guide their learning when needed is a characteristic of an effective clinical teacher (Kelly, 2007). The number and level of students in a clinical group, for instance, may influence the type of learning activities planned for a course. Beginning students and nurses new to a clinical practice area may require more time and guidance from the teacher than experienced students and nurses. This principle is also important in distance education and other courses using preceptors; the preceptor should be available to guide students' learning in clinical practice.

Guiding Learners in Clinical Practice

The next step in the process of clinical teaching is guiding learners to acquire the essential knowledge, technological and other skills, and values for practice. Guiding is a facilitative and supportive process that leads the student toward achievement of the outcomes. It is a process of coaching students in their learning. Guiding is not supervision; supervision is a process of overseeing. Effective clinical teaching requires that teachers guide students in their learning, not oversee their work.

This is the instructional phase in the clinical teaching process—the actual teaching of students in the clinical setting either on site or at a distance. For distance education courses, the instructional phase may be carried out by preceptors, advanced practice nurses (APNs) in the clinical setting, and other providers depending on the course outcomes. With some learning activities, the teacher has a direct instructional role—for instance, demonstrating an intervention to students and questioning them to expand their understanding of a clinical situation. Other teaching activities, though, may be indirect, such as giving feedback on papers and preparing preceptors for their role, among others.

Clinical teaching is more than guiding students in their learning. It also involves assisting them to integrate clinical information and assessment findings, helping them to make clinical judgments, and fostering a spirit of inquiry, among other outcomes (McNelis & Ironside, 2009). In clinical practice, students develop their clinical reasoning skills and learn to think like a nurse.

Clinical education provides the avenue for acquiring the knowledge and behaviors for practice in a particular role, whether it is a beginning professional nurse or new role such as APN. This process requires learning about the role as the initial step and observing and working with nurses in that role as the second step. In clinical instruction, the teacher guides the student in learning about the role and role behaviors of the nurse, and models important values and attributes of the professional in that role. Socialization comes from an integration of clinical and other experiences, not only from the guidance of the teacher. The experiences of students with preceptors, other nurses, and other health care providers contribute to this socialization process.

Skill in Observing Performance

In the process of guiding learners, the teacher needs to be skilled in: (a) observing clinical performance, arriving at sound judgments about that performance, and planning additional learning activities if needed and (b) questioning students to promote their thinking and clinical judgment. Observing students as they learn to care for patients and families and interact with others in the clinical environment allows the teacher to identify continued areas of learning and when assistance is needed from the teacher. This information, in turn, suggests new learning activities for clinical practice.

Observations of students may be influenced by the teacher's values and biases, which may affect *what they see* as they observe a student's performance and their *impressions* of the quality of that performance. All educators should know their own values and biases that might influence their observations of student performance in clinical practice and judgments about student performance of the competencies. Guidelines for observing students are summarized in Exhibit 5.2.

Skill in Questioning Students

The second skill needed by the teacher to effectively guide clinical learning activities is an ability to ask thought-provoking questions without students feeling that they are being interrogated. Open-ended questions about students' thinking and the rationale they used for arriving at clinical judgments foster development of critical thinking skills, an important outcome of clinical practice (Hoffman, 2008; Hsu, 2007; Oermann, 2008; Profetto-McGrath, Smith, Day, & Yonge, 2004). Rowles and Russo (2009) suggested that engaging students through use of questions promotes higher level problem solving, transfer of learning to clinical practice, use of

Exhibit 5.2

GUIDELINES FOR OBSERVING STUDENTS IN CLINICAL PRACTICE

- Examine your values and biases that may influence observations of students in clinical practice and judgments about clinical performance.
- Do not rely on first impressions for these might change significantly with further observations of the student.
- Make a series of observations before drawing conclusions about clinical performance.
- Share with students on a continual basis observations made of clinical performance and judgments about whether students are meeting the clinical competencies.
- Focus observations on the outcomes of the clinical course or competencies to be achieved.
- When the observations reveal other aspects of performance that need further development, share these with students and use the information as a way of providing feedback on performance.
- Discuss observations with students, obtain their perceptions of performance, and be willing to modify judgments when a different perspective is offered (Oermann & Gaberson, 2014).

evidence for solving problems, identification of underlying assumptions, and improved student–faculty interactions. Use of a questioning strategy also helps students begin to think like a nurse (Konradi, 2012).

Faculty members, however, tend to ask questions that focus on recall of facts rather than ones that foster critical thinking (Profetto-McGrath et al., 2004). When questioning students in clinical practice, the teacher should assess understanding of relevant concepts and theories and how they apply to patient care. Other questions can ask students about different approaches and decisions possible in a clinical situation, consequences of each decision, what they would do, and their rationale; possible problems, interventions, and their evidence base; and assumptions underlying their thinking. Questions should encourage learners to think beyond the obvious.

The way in which questions are asked is also significant. The purpose of questioning is to encourage students to consider other perspectives and possibilities, not to drill them and create added stress. In the beginning of a clinical course, and particularly in the beginning of the nursing program, the teacher should discuss the purpose of questioning and its relationship to developing thinking and clinical reasoning skills. The teacher can demonstrate the type of questions that will be asked in the course and emphasize that the goal is to help them learn and begin to think like a nurse.

Because questioning is for instructional purposes, students need to be comfortable that their responses will not influence their clinical grades. Instead, the questions asked and answers given are an essential part of the teaching process, to promote learning and development of critical thinking skills, not for grading purposes. Only with this framework will students be comfortable in responding to higher level questions and evaluating alternative perspectives, using the teacher as a resource.

Evaluating Clinical Learning and Performance

The remaining component of the clinical teaching process is evaluation. Clinical evaluation serves two purposes: formative and summative. Through formative evaluation, the teacher monitors student progress toward meeting the outcomes of the clinical course and demonstrating competency in clinical practice. Formative evaluation provides information about further learning needs of students and where additional clinical instruction is needed. Clinical evaluation that is formative is not intended for grading purposes; instead, it is designed to diagnose learning needs as a basis for further instruction.

Summative evaluation, in contrast, takes place at the end of the learning process to ascertain whether the course outcomes have been achieved and competencies developed (Oermann & Gaberson, 2014). Summative evaluation provides the basis for determining grades in clinical practice or certifying competency. It occurs at the completion of a course, an educational program, orientation, and other types of programs. This type of clinical evaluation determines what *has been* learned rather than what *can be* learned.

There are many clinical evaluation strategies that can be used in nursing courses. These are discussed and examples are provided in Chapter 15.

QUALITIES OF EFFECTIVE CLINICAL TEACHERS

Clinical teaching requires an educator who is knowledgeable about the clinical practice area, is clinically competent, knows how to teach, relates effectively to students, and is enthusiastic about clinical teaching. The teacher also serves as a role model for students or selects clinicians who will model important professional behaviors.

There has been much research in nursing education on characteristics and qualities of an effective clinical teacher. Every clinical teacher should be aware of behaviors that promote learning in the practice setting and ones that impede student learning.

Knowledge

Teachers in nursing, as in any field, need to have expertise in the subject they are teaching. In clinical teaching, this means that educators are knowledgeable about the types of patient problems in the clinical setting, how to manage them, new technologies in patient care, and related research (Beitz & Wieland, 2005; Hanson & Stenvig, 2008; Kelly, 2007; Tang, Chou, & Chiang, 2005). In a study by Kelly (2007), teacher knowledge was most important, followed by feedback and communication skills. Students identified the need for the teacher to be knowledgeable in four areas: as it relates to the clinical setting, curriculum, students, and pedagogy. Teachers must also be up-to-date in the area of clinical practice in which they are working with students. This is particularly true in the traditional model of clinical teaching, in which the teacher is responsible for planning and guiding student learning in practice.

In a study by Tang and colleagues (2005), having "sufficient professional knowledge" was one of the three highest ranked clinical teacher behaviors. In another study, Wolf and associates (2004) analyzed student evaluations of faculty performance. Strengths of the teacher included characteristics such as being knowledgeable, creating a positive learning environment, being professional and supportive of students, and displaying scholarly attributes.

Clinical Competence

Teachers cannot guide student learning in clinical practice without being competent themselves. Clinical competence is an important characteristic of effective clinical teaching in nursing (Tang et al., 2005). Teachers need to be experts in their clinical specialty, maintain their clinical skills, be able to explain and demonstrate nursing care in a real situation, and guide students in developing essential clinical competencies.

This quality of teaching may be problematic for faculty members who teach predominantly in the classroom or change practice settings frequently and do not keep current in their clinical specialty. In some nursing education programs, clinical faculty members are required to maintain a clinical practice certification, which encourages continued competency. For programs without such a requirement, it is up to the teacher to maintain clinical expertise and skills.

Skill in Clinical Teaching

Skill in clinical teaching includes the ability of the teacher to assess learning needs, plan instruction that meets those needs and fosters achievement of the outcomes of the clinical course, guide students in developing their clinical competencies, and evaluate learning fairly. These teaching skills are described more specifically in Exhibit 5.3.

The clinical teacher needs to know *how to teach*. While this seems obvious, in some settings, clinical teachers, preceptors, and others working with students are not prepared educationally for their roles. They have limited knowledge about how to guide students' learning in the clinical setting and assess their performance. Being an expert clinician is not enough. In a study by Wetherbee, Nordrum, and Giles (2008) with physical therapy clinical educators, there was a positive correlation between the number of years of clinical teaching experience and scores on the Nursing Clinical Teacher Effectiveness

---

Exhibit 5.3

CLINICAL TEACHING SKILLS

- Assesses learning needs of students, recognizing and accepting individual differences
- Plans assignments that help in transfer of learning to clinical practice, meet learning needs, and promote acquisition of knowledge and development of competencies
- Communicates clearly to students outcomes of learning and expectations of students in clinical practice
- Considers student goals and needs in planning the clinical activities
- Structures clinical assignments and activities in clinical practice so they build on one another
- Explains clearly concepts and theories applicable to patient care
- Demonstrates effectively clinical skills, procedures, and use of technology
- Provides opportunities for practice of clinical skills, procedures, and technology and recognizes differences among students in the amount of practice needed
- Is well prepared for clinical teaching
- Develops clinical teaching strategies that encourage students to problem solve, arrive at clinical decisions, and think critically in a clinical situation
- Asks higher level questions that assist students in thinking through complex clinical situations and cases requiring critical thinking
- Encourages students through teaching and assessment to think independently and beyond accepted practices and to try out new interventions
- Varies clinical teaching strategies and learning activities to stimulate student interest and meet individual needs of students
- Guides learning and students' use of resources for learning
- Is available to students in clinical practice when they need assistance
- Serves as a role model for students
- Provides specific, timely, and useful feedback on student progress
- Shares observations of clinical performance with students
- Encourages students to evaluate their own performance
- Corrects mistakes without belittling students
- Exhibits fairness in evaluation

Inventory. With experience, educators can refine their skills in clinical teaching and develop their expertise, using self-reflection and feedback from students.

In a study by Berg and Lindseth (2004), the instructional skills of the teacher were ranked second highest when students (n = 171) were asked to describe characteristics of an effective teacher in nursing. When those same students were asked about ineffective teachers, lack of teaching skill was ranked highest.

Skills in evaluating clinical performance both formatively, for feedback, and summatively, at the end of a period of time in the clinical course, are critical for effective teaching. Research has shown that effective teachers are fair in their evaluations of students, correct student errors without belittling students and diminishing their self-confidence, and give prompt feedback that promotes further learning and development.

Interpersonal Relationships With Students

The ability of the clinical teacher to interact with students, both on a one-to-one basis and as a clinical group, is another important teacher behavior. Qualities of an effective teacher in this area are showing confidence in students, respecting students, being honest and direct, supporting students and demonstrating caring behaviors, being approachable, and encouraging students to ask questions and seek guidance when needed. Considering the demands on students as they learn to care for patients, students need to view the teacher as someone who supports them in their learning. In a study by Hanson and Stenvig (2008), students identified three attributes of a good clinical nursing educator. These were knowledge, interpersonal relationships with students, and use of appropriate teaching strategies.

Personal Characteristics of the Clinical Teacher

Personal attributes of the teacher also influence teaching effectiveness. These attributes include enthusiasm, a sense of humor, willingness to admit limitations and mistakes honestly, patience, and flexibility when working with students in the clinical setting, among others (Berg & Lindseth, 2004; Tang et al., 2005). Students often describe effective teachers as ones who are friendly and provide an opportunity for them to share feelings and concerns about patients. Three other personal qualities important in teaching in any setting are integrity, perseverance, and courage (Glassick, Huber, & Maeroff, 1997). While these characteristics were originally used to describe the teacher as a scholar, they are just as important in carrying out the clinical teaching role. Integrity implies truthfulness with students and fairness in dealing with them in the process of learning and in clinical evaluation. The teacher develops an atmosphere of trust for students to engage in open discussions, examine alternatives, and discuss conflicting opinions with the faculty member. Fairness "involves the presentation of one's own interpretations and conclusions in ways that keep open an examination of alternatives" (Glassick et al., 1997, p. 64).

In clinical teaching, faculty members need to persevere in their efforts to improve their teaching competencies. They should be willing to reflect on their teaching and evaluation practices and consider better ways of designing clinical activities and guiding students in their learning. Good teachers, like good scholars, strive to perfect their teaching skills over time and avoid stagnation in their teaching approaches.

STRESSES OF STUDENTS IN CLINICAL PRACTICE

Clinical practice is inherently stressful. In the clinical setting, students face uncertainties and unique situations that they may not have encountered in their prior learning. For some students, clinical practice is stressful because they are unsure about approaches and interventions to use. Interacting with the teacher, other health care providers, the patient, and family members may also contribute to the stress that students experience in clinical practice.

Other stresses, from the students' perspective, relate to the changing nature of patient conditions, a lack of knowledge and skill to provide care to patients, excessive workload, unfamiliarity in the clinical setting, working with difficult patients, developing technological skills, and being observed and evaluated by the teacher (Gorostidi et al., 2007; Li, Wang, Lin, & Lee, 2011; Moscaritolo, 2009; Suresh, Matthews, & Coyne, 2013). In a study by Li, Wang, Lin, and Lee (2011), stress from lack of knowledge and skills for practice was ranked highest by students. Studies also document student stress in academic and personal situations, but students perceive clinical stresses more intensely (Jimenez, Navia-Osorio, & Diaz, 2010).

In many of these studies, the clinical teacher and behaviors of the teacher created the most stress for students. This finding reinforces the need for the faculty to develop supportive and trusting relationships with students in the clinical setting and be aware of the stressful nature of clinical learning activities. A climate that supports the process of learning in clinical practice is dependent on a caring relationship between teacher and student rather than an adversarial one. When students experience stress, they need clinical teachers who are sensitive to their concerns, demonstrate empathy, and provide clear guidance (Gibbons, Dempster, & Moutray, 2008).

Learning in clinical practice occurs in public under the watchful eye of the teacher, the patient, and others in the setting. By keeping the nature of clinical learning in mind and using supportive behaviors when interacting with students, the teacher can reduce some of the stress that students naturally feel in clinical practice.

STRESSFUL NATURE OF CLINICAL TEACHING

Clinical teaching can be stressful for the teacher. First, it is time consuming. A three-credit theory or online course usually requires 3 hours per week of instruction, one clock hour for each credit hour, not including preparation time. However, a three-credit clinical course may require 6 to 9 hours of clinical teaching a week, two to three clinical practice hours per credit hour, and even more in some nursing education programs. This time commitment for clinical teaching may create stress for faculty members who are also involved in research, scholarship, professional service, and clinical practice. In many nursing education programs, faculty members are responsible for writing grant proposals, conducting research, writing for publication, serving on committees, providing community service, and maintaining a clinical practice. With growth in enrollments in nursing programs, academic advisement of students may consume more faculty time. These multiple roles are demanding for clinical educators.

In addition to demands associated with the multiple roles of a nursing faculty member, other aspects of clinical teaching may be stressful. These include:

- Coping with the many expectations associated with clinical teaching
- Feeling exhausted and emotionally drained at the end of a clinical teaching experience with students
- Teaching interfering with activities of personal importance and requiring working outside of regular hours
- Too heavy a workload
- Pressure to maintain clinical competence or a clinical practice without time to do so
- Feeling unable to satisfy the demands of students, clinical agency personnel, patients, and others
- Teaching inadequately prepared students
- Lack of monetary compensation (Oermann, 1998; Whalen, 2009)

For some new clinical teachers, their stress relates to a lack of preparation for their role. While clinicians have expert knowledge and skills in their specialty area, they may have limited knowledge of how to teach. Reid et al. (2013) emphasized that preparation for the role of clinical teacher was essential to promote job satisfaction and reduce attrition. They prepared experienced clinicians as part-time clinical teachers using multiple teaching strategies (face-to-face and online instruction, simulations, and group mentoring sessions). As part of the preparation they also explored challenges faced by clinical teachers and provided mentoring for new faculty members.

Novice faculty members and teachers new to a nursing education program should find a mentor in the school who can support them as they learn the educator role in that setting. Mentoring is a strategy to promote the well-being of nursing faculty and facilitate the transition of new teachers into their role (Dunham-Taylor, Lynn, Moore, McDaniel, & Walker, 2008; Shirey, 2006; Weidman, 2013). Mentors can be good sources of guidance on how to balance clinical teaching with other faculty roles. Faculty members on the tenure track may need release time from clinical teaching responsibilities to work on research and scholarship; changes in workload should be negotiated early in one's career to allow adequate time for scholarly activities.

MODELS OF CLINICAL TEACHING

There are different models of clinical teaching: traditional, in which the teacher is directly responsible for guiding students in the clinical setting; preceptor; and clinical teaching partnership, including DEUs. In the preceptor and partnership models, preceptors and others in the clinical setting provide the clinical instruction, with the faculty member responsible for overall planning, coordinating the experience, grading clinical practice, and assuming other course-related responsibilities.

Traditional Model

In the traditional model of clinical teaching, the educator provides the instruction and evaluation for a small group of nursing students and is on site during the clinical experience. A benefit of this model is the opportunity to assist students in using the concepts and theories learned in class, through online instruction, in readings, and through other learning activities in patient care. The teacher can select clinical activities that best meet the students' needs and are consistent with course goals and objectives. Because the clinical teacher is involved to varying degrees with the nursing curriculum overall, the clinical activities may be more carefully selected to reflect the concepts and theories that students are learning in the course than when preceptors or partners provide the instruction. In addition, the faculty member may be more committed to implementing the philosophy of the nursing program than preceptors or clinicians hired only for clinical teaching, often on a short-term basis.

Disadvantages, though, are the large number of students for whom faculty members may be responsible; not being accessible to students when needed because of demands of other students in the group; teaching procedures, clinical skills, and use of technologies for which the faculty member may lack expertise; the time commitment of providing on-site clinical instruction for faculty members with multiple other roles; and high costs for the nursing program. Faculty members who are part time or adjunct may not be sufficiently familiar with the philosophy and goals of the program, overall curriculum, clinical competencies developed prior to and following the course in which they are teaching, and other program characteristics, which may affect their planning of clinical activities for students and their expectations of students in the course. It is critical for the full-time faculty to prepare and orient part-time and adjunct faculty members involved in clinical teaching so they are not only aware of their role and responsibilities but also understand how their course relates to the overall nursing curriculum.

In the traditional model, the clinical learning experiences are dependent on patients in the setting at the time when students are present. As patients' conditions change, students may lack the requisite knowledge and skills to care for them. Nielsen (2009) identified another disadvantage in that students in acute care settings may prepare for particular assignments, but when they arrive on the unit, the patient is discharged. In courses in which students provide total patient care, they have limited time for contact with other patients in the setting. Nielsen proposed a concept-based approach in which students focus their learning on concepts—for example, oxygenation—and clinical practice provides experiences in those concepts across different patients. Nielsen, Noone, Voss, and Mathews (2013) described their model of clinical teaching, which is based on the intentional planning of clinical learning activities based on course competencies rather than a focus on total patient care experiences.

Another disadvantage of the traditional model of clinical teaching is that the educator and students may not be part of the health care system in which students have clinical practice. They are outsiders to the clinical setting and may not understand the system of care in that setting and its culture. As such, faculty members must work closely with the managers and clinical nursing staff to ensure an effective clinical experience for students. It is up to the faculty member to develop a working relationship with the staff, which is essential to create an environment for learning and take advantage of experiences available in the setting. In the traditional model of clinical teaching, faculty members who are not also practicing in the clinical setting often invest extensive time in developing and maintaining these relationships.

The relationships that nursing faculty members develop in the clinical setting are not only with nursing staff but also involve other health care providers. With the emphasis on interprofessional care, nursing students need clinical learning activities in which they examine their own role in relationship to other providers, collaborate with other health professionals, and learn to work as a team. This learning can occur with simulations. Simulations that involve nursing, medical, pharmacy, and other students provide a way for students to learn to collaborate and gain an understanding of different perspectives to patient care. Interprofessional education with simulation is an effective strategy to teach students about collaborative models of care delivery and prepare future health professionals to work effectively within teams (Brock et al., 2013; King, Conrad, & Ahmed, 2013; Tullmann, Shilling, Goeke, Wright, & Littlewood, 2013).

Preceptor Model

In the preceptor model of clinical teaching, an expert nurse in the clinical setting works with the student on a one-to-one basis in the clinical setting. Preceptors are staff nurses and other nurses employed by the clinical agency who, in addition to their ongoing patient care responsibilities, provide on-site clinical instruction for students. In addition to one-to-one teaching, the preceptor guides and supports the learner and serves as a role model. Omansky (2010) defined the preceptor as someone who guides nursing students to apply classroom knowledge in the clinical setting, serves as a role model, teaches clinical skills, and models critical thinking. With a preceptor's guidance, students can transition into independent practice, become socialized into their professional role, and develop their clinical competencies (Blum, 2009; McClure & Black, 2013; Smedley & Penney, 2009). In addition to improving clinical skills, a preceptorship fosters development of perceived competence among nursing students and their self-confidence (Happell, 2009; King, Singh, & Harris, 2009).

In the preceptor model of clinical instruction, the faculty member from the nursing program serves as the course coordinator, liaison between the nursing education program and clinical setting, and resource person for the preceptor. The faculty member, however, is typically not on site during the clinical practicum. The preceptor model involves sharing clinical teaching responsibilities between nursing program faculty members and expert clinicians from the practice setting.

One strength of the preceptor model is the consistent one-to-one relationship of the student and preceptor, providing an opportunity for the student to work closely with a role model. This close relationship promotes professional socialization and enables students to gain an understanding of how to function in the role for which they are being prepared. Other advantages of preceptorships are that students are able to work closely with a clinical expert in the field, develop self-confidence, improve their critical thinking and decision-making skills, and learn new clinical skills under the guidance of the preceptor.

Potential disadvantages of the preceptor model are lack of integration of theory, research, and practice; lack of flexibility in reassigning students to other preceptors if needed; and time and other demands made on the preceptors. Preceptors must be well prepared for their roles. This preparation should include instruction on methods to facilitate adult learning, teaching methods, communication, evaluation, and conflict resolution consistent with the specific goals of the nursing program (McClure & Black, 2013). Although preceptors should be prepared educationally for this role, some preceptors may lack clinical teaching skills. The preceptor model is commonly used at upper levels of the prelicensure curriculum, often in the final clinical course; for graduate nursing students; and in distance education courses. However, preceptors can also be used with beginning nursing students, providing an opportunity for them to develop their clinical knowledge and skills guided by an expert in the role and gain a realistic view of clinical practice. In distance education courses, when students do not live locally, clinical settings can be established close to the students' homes with preceptors providing the clinical instruction.

Partnership Model

There are varied types of partnerships in nursing education. Some of these are the result of nursing program faculties and administrators searching for ways to increase student enrollment and cope with budgetary constraints, a nursing faculty shortage, and not enough clinical sites, and others are intended to address the gap in preparation for practice readiness (American Association of Colleges of Nursing, 2008; Beal, 2012; Frank, 2008; Wyte-Lake, Tran, Bowman, Needleman, & Dobalian, 2013). In partnerships, nursing education programs collaborate with clinical agencies and the community to respond to these issues as well as work together to meet the health care needs of the community (Beal, 2012; Campbell & Filer, 2008; Campbell & Jeffers, 2008; Francis-Baldesari & Williamson, 2008; Stolder, Rosemeyer, & Zorn, 2008).

Partnerships vary widely. In some programs, the partnership model is a collaborative relationship between a clinical agency and nursing program that involves sharing an APN or a clinician in another role and academic faculty member. The APN teaches students in the clinical setting, with the faculty member serving as course coordinator, and the faculty member in turn contributes to the clinical agency—for example, by conducting research and serving as a consultant. Expertise and services are shared between the partners. In this type of partnership, the APN may work with a graduate or prelicensure nursing student on an individualized basis or may teach a small group of prelicensure students, as in the traditional clinical teaching model. At both the undergraduate and graduate levels, the faculty member works closely with the clinicians and agency to ensure the selection of relevant clinical activities for students.

Another example of a partnership for clinical teaching is the clinical scholar model, which originated in 1984 as a joint initiative between the University of Colorado College of Nursing and University of Colorado Hospital in Denver. In this model, clinical nurse experts coordinate student placements and learning experiences, provide consistent instruction for nursing students, and contribute to the evaluation of students' clinical competencies. These clinical experts are master's prepared in nursing and have a minimum of 5 years of experience in a nursing specialty practice and 2 years of employment in the health care agency (Preheim, 2008; Preheim & Foss, 2015). This model gives students an opportunity to be taught by expert clinicians practicing in the setting. Other partnerships are community based, linking education, practice, and research.

Another type of partnership is the DEU. A DEU is a learning community in which agency clinical staff members teach prelicensure nursing students (Freundl et al., 2012). While there are varied DEU models in the United States and other countries, a common element is the active engagement of nursing and other staff in the education of students. In these models, nurse clinicians serve as clinical teachers with academic faculty members in the role as liaison, guiding the clinician to ensure a quality clinical experience and that course outcomes are met. The goal of this model is to better prepare nursing students for clinical practice and with fewer faculty members from the school of nursing (Dapremont & Lee, 2013; Moscato, Nishioka, & Coe, 2013). Rhodes and associates (2012) reported that students were highly satisfied with their clinical experience on DEUs, and they developed strong relationships with the staff nurses. Students also reported experiencing patient-centered care first hand. In addition, DEU nurses were satisfied with their involvement in the students' education. In a project by McKown, McKown, and Webb (2011), DEU students were able to achieve the Quality and Safety Education for Nurses (QSEN) competencies.

Selecting a Clinical Teaching Model

There is no one model that meets the needs of every nursing education program, clinical course, or group of students. The teacher should select a model considering these factors:

- Educational philosophy of the nursing program
- Philosophy of the faculty about clinical teaching
- Goals and intended outcomes of the clinical course and activities
- Level of nursing student
- Type of clinical setting
- Availability of preceptors, expert nurses, and other people in the practice setting who provide clinical instruction
- Willingness of clinical agency personnel and partners to participate in teaching students and other educational activities

SUMMARY

The process of clinical teaching begins with identification of the goals and outcomes for clinical learning and proceeds through assessing the learner, planning clinical learning activities, guiding students, and evaluating clinical learning and performance. The goals and outcomes suggest areas for assessment, provide guidelines for teaching, and are the basis for evaluating learning. They may be expressed in the form of clinical objectives, outcomes, or competencies and may be established for an entire course or for specific clinical activities. The outcomes of clinical practice should be communicated clearly to students, in written form, and understood by them. Similarly, the teacher has an important responsibility in discussing these outcomes and related clinical activities with agency personnel.

Teaching begins at the level of the learner. The teacher's goal, therefore, is to assess the student's present level of knowledge and skill and other characteristics that may influence developing the clinical competencies. This assessment is important so that students engage in learning activities that build on their present knowledge and skills. When students lack the prerequisites, then the instruction can remedy these deficiencies and more efficiently move students forward in their learning. The second area of assessment relates to individual characteristics of students that may influence their learning and clinical performance, such as age, learning style, and cultural background.

Following assessment of learner needs and characteristics, the teacher plans and then delivers the instruction. In planning the learning activities, the main considerations are the objectives and individual learner needs. The next step in the process of clinical teaching is that of guiding learners to acquire essential knowledge, skills, and values for practice. In this process of guiding learners, the teacher needs to be skilled in (a) observing clinical performance, arriving at sound judgments about that performance, and planning additional learning activities if needed and (b) questioning learners to encourage critical thinking but without interrogating them.

The last component of the clinical teaching process is evaluation. Clinical evaluation can be formative or summative. Through formative evaluation, the teacher monitors student progress in meeting the clinical outcomes and demonstrating competency in clinical practice. Summative evaluation, in contrast, takes place at the end of the learning period to ascertain whether the outcomes have been achieved and competencies developed. It occurs at the completion of a course, an educational program, orientation, and other types of programs. This type of clinical evaluation determines what *has been* learned rather than what *can be* learned.

Teaching in the clinical setting requires a faculty member who is knowledgeable, is clinically competent, knows how to teach, relates effectively to students, and is enthusiastic about clinical teaching. The research in nursing education over the years has substantiated that these qualities are important in clinical teaching.

Clinical practice is stressful for students. Students have identified dimensions of clinical learning that often produce anxiety, such as fear of making a mistake that would harm the patient; interacting with the patient, the teacher, and other health care providers; the changing nature of patient conditions; a lack of knowledge and skill to practice giving care to patients; and working with difficult patients, among others. In some research studies, students have reported that the teacher is a source of added stress for them. These findings highlight the need for faculty members to develop supportive and trusting relationships with students in the clinical setting and to be aware of the stressful nature of this learning experience. A climate that supports the process of learning in clinical practice is dependent on a caring relationship between teacher and student rather than an adversarial one.

The teacher chooses a model for clinical teaching: traditional, preceptor, or partnership, including the DEU model. In the traditional model of clinical teaching, the instruction and evaluation of a group of students are carried out by a faculty member. In the preceptor model of clinical teaching, an expert nurse in the clinical setting works with the student typically on a one-to-one basis. The preceptor also guides and supports the learner and serves as a role model. The faculty member is typically not on site during the clinical experience but has important responsibilities for the course, such as serving as course coordinator, providing the classroom instruction, serving as a liaison between the nursing education program and clinical setting, and being a resource person for the preceptor.

Partnerships were also described in this chapter. The partnership model varies with the academic institution but is generally a collaborative relationship between the nursing education program and a clinical agency or with the community. Partnerships emphasize collaboration among partners to meet the needs of the partners and community as a whole. Another type of partnership is the DEU, in which agency clinical staff members teach prelicensure nursing students. In these models, nurse clinicians serve as clinical teachers with academic faculty members in the role of liaison, guiding the clinician to ensure a quality clinical experience and that course outcomes are met.

Exhibit 5.4

CNE EXAMINATION TEST BLUEPRINT CORE COMPETENCIES

1. **Facilitate Learning**

   A. Implement a variety of teaching strategies appropriate to
      1. content
      2. setting (clinical)
      3. learner needs
      4. learning style
      5. desired learner outcomes
      6. method of delivery

   B. Use teaching strategies based on
      1. educational theory
      2. evidence-based practices related to education

   C. Modify teaching strategies and learning experiences based on consideration of
      1. cultural background
      2. past clinical experiences
      3. past educational and life experiences

   F. Communicate effectively orally and in writing with an ability to convey ideas in a variety of contexts
   G. Model reflective thinking practices, including critical thinking
   H. Create opportunities for learners to develop their own critical thinking skills
   I. Create a positive learning environment that fosters a free exchange of ideas
   J. Show enthusiasm for teaching, learning, and the nursing profession that inspires and motivates students

(continued)

    K. Demonstrate personal attributes that facilitate learning (e.g., caring, confidence, patience, integrity, respect, and flexibility)
    L. Respond effectively to unexpected events that affect instruction
    M. Develop collegial working relationships with clinical agency personnel to promote positive learning environments
    N. Use knowledge of evidence-based practice to instruct learners
    O. Demonstrate ability to teach clinical skills
    P. Act as a role model in practice settings
    Q. Foster a safe learning environment

2. Facilitate Learner Development and Socialization

    A. Identify individual learning styles and unique learning needs of learners
    B. Provide resources for diverse learners to meet their individual learning needs
    C. Advise learners in ways that help them meet their professional goals
    D. Create learning environments that facilitate learners' self-reflection, personal goal setting, and socialization to the role of the nurse
    E. Foster the development of learners in these areas
        1. cognitive domain
        2. psychomotor domain
        3. affective domain

    F. Assist learners to engage in thoughtful and constructive self and peer evaluation
    H. Encourage professional development of learners

5. Pursue Systematic Self-Evaluation and Improvement in the Academic Nurse Educator Role

    A. Engage in activities that promote one's socialization to the role
    D. Demonstrate a commitment to lifelong learning
    E. Participate in professional development opportunities that increase one's effectiveness in the role
    F. Manage the teaching, scholarship, and service demands as influenced by the requirements of the institutional setting

6. Engage in Scholarship, Service, and Leadership

    B. Engage in scholarship of teaching
        1. Exhibit a spirit of inquiry about teaching and learning, student development, and evaluation methods
        2. Use evidence-based resources to improve and support teaching

    C. Function effectively within the organizational environment and academic community
        3. Integrate the values of respect, collegiality, professionalism, and caring to build an organizational climate that fosters the development of learners and colleagues

REFERENCES

American Association of Colleges of Nursing. (2008). *Essentials of baccalaureate education for professional nursing.* Retrieved from http://www.aacn.nche.edu/education-resources/BaccEssentials08.pdf

Beal, J. A. (2012). Academic-service partnerships in nursing: An integrative review. *Nursing Research and Practice, 2012,* Article ID 501564. doi:10.1155/2012/501564

Beitz, J. M., & Wieland, D. (2005). Analyzing the teaching effectiveness of clinical nursing faculty of full- and part-time generic BSN, LPN-BSN, and RN-BSN nursing students. *Journal of Professional Nursing, 21,* 32–45.

Berg, C. L., & Lindseth, G. (2004). Research brief. Students' perspectives of effective and ineffective nursing instructors. *Journal of Nursing Education, 43,* 565–568.

Blum, C. (2009). Development of a clinical preceptor model. *Nurse Educator, 34,* 29–33.

Bosher, S. D., & Pharris, M. D. (2009). *Transforming nursing education: The culturally inclusive environment.* New York, NY: Springer.

Brock, D., Abu-Rish, E., Chia-Ru, C., Hammer, D., Wilson, S., Vorvick, L., . . . Zierler, B. (2013). Interprofessional education in team communication: Working together to improve patient safety. *BMJ Quality & Safety, 22,* 414–423. doi:10.1136/bmjqs-2012-000952

Campbell, S., & Filer, D. (2008). How can we continue to provide quality clinical education for increasing numbers of students with decreasing numbers of faculty? *Annual Review of Nursing Education, 6,* 45–63.

Campbell, S., & Jeffers, B. (2008). The sister model: A framework for academic and service partnerships in nursing home settings. *Journal of Gerontological Nursing, 34*(9), 18–24.

Dapremont, J., & Lee, S. (2013). Partnering to educate: Dedicated education units. *Nurse Education in Practice, 13,* 335–337. doi:10.1016/j.nepr.2013.02.015

Dunham-Taylor, J., Lynn, C., Moore, P., McDaniel, S., & Walker, J. (2008). What goes around comes around: Improving faculty retention through more effective mentoring. *Journal of Professional Nursing, 24,* 337–346.

Francis-Baldesari, C., & Williamson, D. (2008). Integration of nursing education, practice, and research through community partnerships: A case study. *Advances in Nursing Science, 31*(4), E1–E10. doi:10.1097/01.ANS.0000341416.11586.3a

Frank, B. (2008). Enhancing nursing education through effective academic-service partnerships. *Annual Review of Nursing Education, 6,* 25–43.

Freundl, M., Anthony, M., Johnson, B., Harmer, B., Carter, J., Boudiab, L., & Nelson, V. (2012). A dedicated education unit: VA Medical Centers and baccalaureate nursing programs partnership model. *Journal of Professional Nursing, 28,* 344–350. doi:10.1016/j.profnurs.2012.05.008

Gibbons, C., Dempster, M., & Moutray, M. (2008). Stress and eustress in nursing students. *Journal of Advanced Nursing, 61,* 282–290.

Glassick, C. E., Huber, M. T., & Maeroff, G. I. (1997). *Scholarship assessed.* San Francisco, CA: Jossey-Bass.

Gorostidi, X., Egilegor, X., Erice, M., Iturriotz, M., Garate, I., Lasa, M., & Cascante, X. (2007). Stress sources in nursing practice: Evolution during nursing training. *Nurse Education Today, 27,* 777–787.

Hanson, K. J., & Stenvig, T. E. (2008). The good clinical nursing educator and the baccalaureate nursing clinical experience: Attributes and praxis. *Journal of Nursing Education, 47,* 38–42.

Happell, B. (2009). A model of preceptorship in nursing: Reflecting the complex functions of the role. *Nursing Education Perspectives, 30,* 372–376.

Hoffman, J. (2008). Teaching strategies to facilitate nursing students' critical thinking. In M. Oermann (Ed.), *Annual review of nursing education: Clinical nursing education* (pp. 225–236). New York, NY: Springer.

Hsu, L-L. (2007). Conducting clinical post-conference in clinical teaching: A qualitative study. *Journal of Clinical Nursing, 16*, 1525–1533.

Jeffreys, M. R., & Dogan, E. (2013). Evaluating cultural competence in the clinical practicum. *Nursing Education Perspectives, 34*, 88–94.

Jimenez, C., Navia-Osorio, P. M., & Diaz, C. V. (2010). Stress and health in novice and experienced nursing students. *Journal of Advanced Nursing, 66*, 442–455. doi:10.1111/j.1365–2648.2009.05183.x

Kelly, C. (2007). Students' perceptions of effective clinical teaching revisited. *Nurse Education Today, 27*, 885–892. doi:10.1016/j.nedt.2006.12.005

King, A. E. A., Conrad, M., & Ahmed, R. A. (2013). Improving collaboration among medical, nursing and respiratory therapy students through interprofessional simulation. *Journal of Interprofessional Care, 27*, 269–271. doi:10.3109/13561820.2012.730076

King, M., Singh, M., & Harris, L. (2009). A critical care bridging program to prepare fourth-year baccalaureate students for specialty practice. *Dynamics, 20*(1), 12–17.

Kong, L. N., Qin, B., Zhou, Y. Q., Mou, S. Y., & Gao, H. M. (2013). The effectiveness of problem-based learning on development of nursing students' critical thinking: A systematic review and meta-analysis. *International Journal of Nursing Studies*. doi:10.1016/j.ijnurstu.2013.06.009; 10.1016/j.ijnurstu.2013.06.009

Konradi, D. B. (2012). Learning to think like a professional nurse: A critical questions strategy. *Journal of Nursing Education, 51*, 359–360. doi:10.3928/01484834-20120522-03

Li, H. C., Wang, L. S., Lin, Y. H., & Lee, I. (2011). The effect of a peer-mentoring strategy on student nurse stress reduction in clinical practice. *International Nursing Review, 58*, 203–110. doi: 10.1111/j.1466–7657.2010.00839.x

McClure, E., & Black, L. (2013). The role of the clinical preceptor: An integrative literature review. *Journal of Nursing Education, 52*, 335–341. doi:10.3928/01484834-20130430-02

McKown, T., McKown, L., & Webb, S. (2011). Using Quality and Safety Education for Nurses to guide clinical teaching on a new dedicated education unit. *Journal of Nursing Education, 50*, 706–710. doi:10.3928/01484834-20111017-03

McNelis, A., & Ironside, P. (2009). National survey on clinical education in prelicensure nursing education programs. In N. Ard & T. M. Valiga (Eds.), *Clinical nursing education: Current reflections* (pp. 29–38). New York, NY: National League for Nursing.

Moscaritolo, L. (2009). Interventional strategies to decrease nursing student anxiety in the clinical learning environment. *Journal of Nursing Education, 48*, 17–23.

Moscato, S. R., Nishioka, V. M., & Coe, M. T. (2013). Dedicated education unit: Implementing an innovation in replication sites. *Journal of Nursing Education, 52*, 259–267. doi:10.3928/01484834-20130328-01

Nielsen, A. (2009). Educational innovations. Concept-based learning activities using the clinical judgment model as a foundation for clinical learning. *Journal of Nursing Education, 48*, 350–354.

Nielsen, A. E., Noone, J., Voss, H., & Mathews, L. (2013). Preparing nursing students for the future: An innovative approach to clinical education. *Nurse Education In Practice, 13*, 301–309. doi:10.1016/j.nepr.2013.03.015

Oermann, M. H. (1998). Work-related stresses of clinical nursing faculty. *Journal of Nursing Education, 37*, 302–304.

Oermann, M. H. (2007). Approaches to gathering evidence for educational practices in nursing. *Journal of Continuing Education in Nursing, 38*, 250–257.

Oermann, M. H. (2008). Ideas for postclinical conferences. *Teaching and Learning in Nursing, 3,* 90–93.

Oermann, M. H. (2009). Evidence-based programs and teaching/evaluation methods: Needed to achieve excellence in nursing education. In M. Adams & T. Valiga (Eds.), *Achieving excellence in nursing education* (pp. 63–76). New York, NY: National League for Nursing.

Oermann, M. H., & Gaberson, K. B. (2014). *Evaluation and testing in nursing education* (4th ed.). New York, NY: Springer Publishing.

Omansky, G. L. (2010). Staff nurses' experiences as preceptors and mentors: An integrative review. *Journal of Nursing Management, 18,* 697–703. doi:10.1111/j.1365-2834.2010.01145.x

Pardue, K., & Morgan, P. (2008). Millennials considered: A new generation, new approaches, and implications for nursing education. *Nursing Education Perspectives, 29,* 74–79.

Preheim, G. (2008). The Clinical Scholar Model: Competency development within a caring curriculum. In M. Oermann (Ed.), *Annual review of nursing education: Clinical nursing education* (pp. 3–23). New York, NY: Springer.

Preheim, G., & Foss, K. (2015). Partnerships with clinical settings: Roles and responsibilities of nurse educators. In M. H. Oermann (Ed.), *Teaching in nursing and role of the educator: The complete guide to best practice in teaching, evaluation, and curriculum development* (pp. 163–190). New York, NY: Springer.

Profetto-McGrath, J., Smith, K. B., Day, R. A., & Yonge, O. (2004). The questioning skills of tutors and students in a context based baccalaureate nursing program. *Nurse Education Today, 24,* 363–372.

Reid, T. P., Hinderer, K. A., Jarosinski, J. M., Mister, B. J., & Seldomridge, L. A. (2013). Expert clinician to clinical teacher: Developing a faculty academy and mentoring initiative. *Nurse Education In Practice, 13,* 288–293. doi:10.1016/j.nepr.2013.03.022

Rhodes, M. T., Meyers, C. C., & Underhill, M. L. (2012). Evaluation outcomes of a dedicated education unit in a baccalaureate nursing program. *Journal of Professional Nursing, 28,* 223–230. doi:10.1016/j.prof.2011.11.019

Rowles, C. J., & Russo, B. L. (2009). Strategies to promote critical thinking and active learning. In D. M. Billings & J. A. Halstead (Eds.), *Teaching in nursing: A guide for faculty* (pp. 238–261). St. Louis, MO: Saunders.

Shirey, M. (2006). Faculty issues. Stress and burnout in nursing faculty. *Nurse Educator, 31,* 95–97.

Smedley, A., & Penney, D. (2009). A partnership approach to the preparation of preceptors. *Nursing Education Perspectives, 30,* 31–36.

Stolder, M. E., Rosemeyer, A. K., & Zorn, C. R. (2008). In the shelter of each other: Respite care for students as a partnership model. *Nursing Education Perspectives, 29,* 295–299.

Suresh, P., Matthews, A., & Coyne, I. (2013). Stress and stressors in the clinical environment: A comparative study of fourth-year student nurses and newly qualified general nurses in Ireland. *Journal of Clinical Nursing, 22,* 770–779. doi:10.1111/j.1365-2702.2012.04145.x

Tang, F., Chou, S., & Chiang, H. (2005). Students' perceptions of effective and ineffective clinical instructors. *Journal of Nursing Education, 44,* 187–192.

Tullmann, D. F., Shilling, A. M., Goeke, L. H., Wright, E. B., & Littlewood, K. E. (2013). Recreating simulation scenarios for interprofessional education: An example of educational interprofessional practice. *Journal of Interprofessional Care, 27,* 426–428. doi:10.3109/13561820.2013.790880

Weidman, N. A. (2013). The lived experience of the transition of the clinical nurse expert to the novice nurse educator. *Teaching & Learning In Nursing, 8*(3), 102–109. doi:10.1016/j.teln.2013.04.006

Wetherbee, E., Nordrum, J., & Giles, S. (2008). Effective teaching behaviors of APTA-credentialed versus noncredentialed clinical instructors. *Journal of Physical Therapy Education, 22,* 65–74.

Whalen, K. S. (2009). Work-related stressors experienced by part-time clinical affiliate nursing faculty in baccalaureate education. *International Journal of Nursing Education Scholarship, 6,* Article30. doi:10.2202/1548-923X.1813

Wolf, Z. R., Bender, P. J., Beitz, J. M., Wieland, D. M., & Vito, K. O. (2004). Strengths and weaknesses of faculty teaching performance reported by undergraduate and graduate nursing students: A descriptive study. *Journal of Professional Nursing, 20,* 118–128.

Wyte-Lake, T., Tran, K., Bowman, C. C., Needleman, J., & Dobalian, A. (2013). A systematic review of strategies to address the clinical nursing faculty shortage. *Journal of Nursing Education, 52,* 245–252. doi:10.3928/01484834-20130213-02

CHAPTER 6

Ethical and Legal Issues in Clinical Teaching

Clinical teaching and learning take place in a social context. Teachers, students, staff members, and patients have roles, rights, and responsibilities that are sometimes in conflict. These conflicts create legal and ethical dilemmas for clinical teachers. This chapter discusses some ethical and legal issues related to clinical teaching and offers suggestions for preventing, minimizing, and managing these difficult situations.

ETHICAL ISSUES

Ethics are standards of conduct based on beliefs about what is good and bad, obligations related to good and bad acts, and principles underlying decisions to conform to these standards. Ethical standards make it possible for nurses, patients, teachers, and students to understand and respect each other. Contemporary bioethical standards are related to respect for human dignity, autonomy, and freedom; beneficence; justice; veracity; privacy; and fidelity (Husted & Husted, 2008; Oermann & Gaberson, 2014). These standards are important considerations for all parties involved in clinical teaching and learning.

Learners in a Service Setting

If the word *clinical* means "involving direct observation of the patient," clinical activities must take place where patients are. Traditionally, learners encounter patients in health care service settings, such as acute care, extended care, and rehabilitation facilities. With the increasing focus on controlling health care costs and primary prevention, however, patients increasingly receive health care in the home, community, and school environments. Whatever the setting, patients are there to receive health care, staff members have the responsibility to provide care, and students are present to learn. Are these purposes always compatible?

Although it has been more than three decades since Corcoran (1977) raised ethical questions about the use of service settings for learning activities, those concerns still are valid. In the clinical setting, nursing students or new staff members are learners who are somewhat less skilled than experienced practitioners. Although their activities are observed and guided by clinical teachers, learners are not expected to provide cost-effective, efficient patient care services. On the other hand, patients expect quality service when they seek health care; providing learning opportunities for students is not usually their priority. The ethical standard of *beneficence* refers to the duty to help, to produce beneficial outcomes, or at least to do no harm (Husted & Husted, 2008). Is this standard violated when the learners' chief purpose for being in the clinical environment is to learn, not to give care?

Patients who encounter learners in clinical settings may feel exploited or fear invasion of their privacy; they may receive care that takes more time and creates more discomfort than if provided by expert practitioners. The presence of learners in a clinical setting also requires more time and energy of staff members, who are usually expected to give and receive reports from students, answer their questions, and demonstrate or help with patient care. These activities may divert staff members' attention from their primary responsibility for patient care, interfere with their efficient performance, and affect their satisfaction with their work.

Because achieving the desired outcomes of clinical teaching requires learning activities in real service settings, teachers must consider the rights and needs of learners, patients, and staff members when planning clinical learning activities. The clinical teacher is responsible for making the learning objectives clear to all involved persons and for ensuring that learning activities do not prevent achievement of service goals. Patients should receive adequate information about the presence of learners in the settings where they are receiving care before giving their informed consent to participate in clinical learning activities. The teacher should ensure the learners' preparation and readiness for clinical learning as well as his or her own presence and competence as an instructor, as discussed in Chapter 4.

Student–Faculty Relationships

Respect for Persons

As discussed in Chapter 1, an effective and beneficial relationship between clinical teacher and student is built on a base of mutual trust and respect. Although both parties are responsible for maintaining this relationship, the clinical teacher must initiate it by demonstrating trust and respect for students. A trusting, respectful relationship with students demonstrates the teacher's commitment to ethical values of respect for human dignity and autonomy. Because civil behavior is learned, teachers must model discretion, attentiveness, respectful communication, and professional behavior in all encounters with students, colleagues, patients, and staff members in the clinical setting (Altmiller, 2012).

Fairness and Justice

The ethical standard of justice refers to fair treatment—judging each person's behavior by the same standards. Clinical teachers must evaluate each student's performance by the same standard. Students may perceive a clinical teacher's behavior as unfair when the teacher appears to favor some students by praising, supporting, and offering better learning opportunities to them more than others. In a study of student perceptions of incivility, Altmiller (2012) found that students identified the power gradient between students and teachers as a source of potential and actual unequal treatment. They cited experiences of gender, ethnic, and racial bias and discrimination, and feared that the teacher's authority and power would discourage teachers from restraining those biases. Developing social relationships with some students could be perceived as favoritism by other students (Gardner & Suplee, 2010, p. 190). Teachers often find it difficult to set appropriate role boundaries for teacher–student relationships. While their primary role is that of teacher, they also want to model caring behavior to students, be supportive to students who are struggling, and be approachable and student-friendly (Poorman, Mastorovich, & Webb, 2011). However, in their desire to "make visible [their] concern for students" (Poorman et al., p. 373), teachers may cross the line into inequitable treatment based on personal feelings. The teacher's relationships with students can be friendly and warm but should be collegial without being personal and social.

For these reasons, nurse educators should be prudent about their use of social networking sites such as Facebook and Twitter. Faculty members have used Twitter to communicate with students, build relationships with them, and enhance their learning. For example, clinical teachers may use Twitter for instant messaging to inform students about a change in plans (such as cancellation of clinical learning activities or a change of location) and to communicate with preceptors who may not have easy access to their e-mail during work hours (Skiba, 2008). However, these uses of social networking sites should be separate from the teacher's personal use of these technologies. Befriending students on their Facebook page and following them on Twitter implies an egalitarian relationship that does not acknowledge the power advantage that faculty members hold (Oermann & Gaberson, 2014). Inviting students to sign up as friends or followers to a Facebook or Twitter account that the teacher uses for social interaction with peers invites their discovery of information that the teacher might prefer to be private.

Keeping these disadvantages in mind, teachers can use these networking sites to facilitate clinical learning. A clinical teacher might establish a Twitter account and lock it, then invite students to follow. Using this account as a filter for information, the faculty member can teach followers mini-lessons and update them on relevant topics. For example, the teacher may maximize teachable moments that occur outside of the clinical learning environment (Kryder, 2009; Skiba, 2008), such as sharing a new idea from a conference, alerting students to the publication of a relevant article in a current issue of a professional nursing journal, or suggesting that students view a particular television show that relates to content they are studying. The clinical teacher might send a weekly tweet to students with a question or brainteaser related to the competencies they are attempting to master. Because some students may have to pay for individual text messages, based on their wireless account type, it is best to inform students well in advance that you will be using this technology and invite those who have concerns to talk to you privately (Skiba, 2008).

Additionally, clinical teachers should discuss guidelines for nurses' appropriate use of social media with students. The teacher's appropriate use of social media can serve as an example of professional behavior for students when discussing the importance of enforcing professional boundaries in relationships with patients. Misuse of social media becomes a source of regulatory concern when role boundary violations occur (Spector & Kappel, 2012). The American Nurses Association's *Principles for Social Networking and the Nurse* (2011) and the National Council of State Boards of Nursing's (NCSBN) *A Nurse's Guide to the Use of Social Media* (2011) provide guidelines to nurses on using social media appropriately.

Students' Privacy Rights

When students have a succession of clinical instructors, it is common for the instructors to communicate information about student performance. Learning about the students' levels of performance in their previous clinical assignment helps the next instructor to anticipate their needs and to plan appropriate learning activities for them. Although students usually benefit when teachers share such information about their learning needs, personal information that students reveal in confidence should not be shared with other teachers. The U.S. Family Educational Rights and Privacy Act of 1974, as amended, restricts disclosure of students' academic information to individuals who have a legitimate need to know; written permission from students is necessary to discuss their performance with anyone else. Evaluative statements about student performance should not be shared with other faculty members, but information about a student's need for a particular learning activity or more practice with a specific skill is necessary for a teacher to provide the appropriate guidance (Gardner & Suplee, 2010, p. 191).

Additionally, when sharing information about students, teachers should focus on factual statements about performance without adding personal judgments. Characterizing or labeling students is rarely helpful to the next instructor, and such behavior violates ethical standards of privacy as well as respect for persons.

Because clinical teachers in nursing education programs are professional nurses, they sometimes experience conflict regarding their knowledge of students' health problems. As nurses, they might tend to respond in a therapeutic way if a student revealed personal information about a health concern, but as teachers, their primary obligation is to a teacher–student relationship. Absent any existing institutional policy or compelling evidence that the personal information should be disclosed to protect the safety of the student or other person, educators should follow the principle of what action would best promote student learning.

Clinical teachers who are aware of a student's health problem should also avoid making special exceptions for this student that would not be available to other students. Students who need special accommodations because of a health problem should request them from the institution's office of disability services. If accommodations are granted, the clinical teacher should discuss with the student how they will be made available (Gardner & Suplee, 2010, p. 192). See the discussion on students with disabilities later in this chapter.

Competent Teaching

Applying the ethical standard of beneficence to teaching, students have a right to expect that their clinical teachers are competent, responsible, and knowledgeable. As discussed in Chapter 5, clinical competence, including expert knowledge and clinical skill, is an essential characteristic of effective clinical teachers. In addition, clinical teachers must be competent in facilitating students' learning activities, including planning appropriate assignments and giving specific, timely feedback on individual student performance. Examples of unethical behavior related to clinical teacher competence include not being available for guidance in the clinical setting and not planning sufficiently for a clinical learning activity that maximizes student learning.

Academic Dishonesty

Although cheating and other forms of dishonest behavior are believed to be common in the classroom environment, academic dishonesty can occur in clinical settings as well. Academic dishonesty is defined as intentional participation in deceptive practices regarding the academic work of self or others. Dishonest acts include lying, cheating, plagiarizing, altering or forging records, falsely representing oneself, and knowingly assisting another person to commit a dishonest act (Tippett et al., 2009). While we discuss academic dishonesty as an ethical violation, it can also be classified as a legal issue when it serves as the basis of a disciplinary action.

Examples of academic dishonesty in the clinical setting include:

- *Cheating:* A student copies portions of a classmate's case study analysis and presents the assignment as her own work. Similarly, a student who asks for a staff member's assistance to calculate a medication dose but tells the instructor that he did the work alone is also cheating.
- *Lying:* A student tells the instructor that she attempted a home visit to a patient but the patient was not at home. In fact, the student overslept and missed the scheduled time of the visit.
- *Plagiarism:* While preparing materials for a patient teaching project, a student paraphrases portions of a published teaching pamphlet without citing the source.
- *Altering a document:* A staff nurse orientee appends information to the documentation of nursing care for a patient on the previous day without noting it as a late addition.

■ *False representation:* As a family nurse practitioner student begins a physical examination, the patient addresses the student as "doctor." The student continues with the examination and does not tell the patient that he is a nurse.
■ *Assisting another in a dishonest act:* Student A asks Student B to cover for her while she leaves the clinical agency to run a personal errand. The teacher asks Student B if he has seen Student A; Student B says that he thinks she has accompanied a patient to the physical therapy department.

Although some of the previous examples may appear to be harmless or minor infractions, dishonest acts should be taken seriously because they can have harmful effects on patients, learners, faculty–student relationships, and the educational program. Clinical dishonesty can jeopardize patient safety if learners fail to report errors or do not receive adequate guidance because their competence is assumed (Bavier, 2009). Mutual trust and respect form the basis for effective teacher–learner relationships, and academic dishonesty can damage a teacher's trust in students. Dishonest acts that are ignored by teachers contribute to an environment that supports academic dishonesty, conveying the impression to students that this behavior is acceptable or at least excusable (Tippett et al., 2009). Additionally, honest students resent teachers who fail to deal effectively with cheating.

Students who are dishonest in school are more likely to conceal or deny errors in the workplace or violate professional conduct standards (Smith, 2012). For this reason, most nurse faculty members are conscientious about holding students accountable to standards of integrity and imposing severe consequences as permitted by policy. However, student appeals of these decisions are often overturned or modified by grade appeal panels comprising faculty members from nonclinical disciplines who may not understand the serious implications for patient safety (Bavier, 2009).

Clinical academic dishonesty usually results from one or more of the following factors:

■ *Competition, desire for good grades, and heavy workload.* Competition for good grades in clinical nursing courses may result from student misunderstanding of the evaluation framework. If students believe that a limited number of good grades are available, they may compete fiercely with their classmates, sometimes leading to deceptive acts in an attempt to earn the highest grades. Additionally, many nursing students have additional pressures related to employment and family responsibilities; they may feel overloaded and unable to meet all of the demands of a rigorous nursing education program without resorting to cheating. "Higher education is increasingly a high stakes environment where a student's retention in or progression through a program, [retention of a] scholarship or loan, parental approval, or other significant factor is dependent on academic success" (Tippitt et al., 2009, p. 239).

■ *Emphasis on perfection.* As discussed in Chapter 2, clinical teachers often communicate the expectation that good nurses do not make mistakes. Although nurse educators attempt to prepare practitioners who will perform carefully and skillfully, a standard of perfection is unrealistic. Students naturally make mistakes in the process of learning new knowledge and skills, and punishment for mistakes, in the form of low grades or a negative performance evaluation, will not prevent these errors. In fact, it is the fear of punishment that often motivates students to conceal errors, and errors that are not reported are often harmful to patient safety (Kohn, Corrigan, & Donaldson, 2000).

■ *Poor role modeling.* The influence of role models on behavior is strong. Nursing students and novice staff nurses who observe dishonest behavior of teachers and experienced staff members may emulate these examples, especially when the dishonest acts have gone unnoticed, unreported, or unpunished (Tippitt et al., 2009).

Clinical teachers can use a variety of approaches to discourage academic dishonesty. They should be exemplary role models of honest behavior for learners to emulate (Tippitt et al., 2009). They should acknowledge that mistakes occur in the learning process and create a learning climate that allows students to make mistakes in a safe environment with guidance and feedback for problem solving.

In a study of how nurse educators determine passing or failing nursing student clinical behaviors, Tanicala, Scheffer, and Roberts (2011) concluded that

> With the growing focus in health care on creating a culture of safety, versus the current approach of blame and punishment in both practice and education, . . . nursing clinical education must engage in a culture shift . . . from individual student error to analyzing errors from an educational perspective. (p. 160)

However, students need reassurance that, if humanly possible, teachers will not allow them to make errors that would harm patients. Finally, each nursing education program should develop a policy that defines academic dishonesty and specifies appropriate penalties for violations. This policy should be communicated to all students, reviewed with them at regular intervals, and applied consistently and fairly to every violation (Tippitt et al., 2009).

When enforcing the academic integrity policy, it is important to apply ethical standards to protect the dignity and privacy of students. A public accusation of dishonesty that is found later to be ungrounded can damage a student's reputation. The teacher should speak with the student privately and calmly, describe the student's behavior and the teacher's interpretation of it, and provide the student with an opportunity to respond to the charge. It is essential to keep an open mind until all available evidence is evaluated, because the student may be able to supply a reasonable explanation for the behavior that the teacher interpreted as cheating.

LEGAL ISSUES

It is beyond the scope of this book to discuss and interpret all federal, state, and local laws that have implications for clinical teaching and evaluation, and the authors are not qualified to give legal advice to clinical teachers regarding their practice. We recommend that clinical teachers refer questions about the legal implications of policies and procedures to the legal counsel for the institution in which they are employed; concerns about a teacher's legal rights in a specific situation are best referred to the individual's attorney. However, this section discusses common legal issues that often arise in the practice of clinical teaching.

Students With Disabilities

Two federal laws have implications for the education of learners with disabilities. The Rehabilitation Act of 1973, Section 504, prohibits public postsecondary institutions that receive federal funding from denying access or participation to individuals with disabilities. The Americans with Disabilities Act (ADA) of 1990 and the ADA Amendment Act of 2008 guarantee persons with disabilities equal access to educational opportunities if they are otherwise qualified for admission. A qualified individual with a disability is one who has a physical or mental impairment that substantially limits one or more of that individual's major life activities, and that the individual has a record of or is regarded as having such impairment. In nursing education programs, qualified individuals with disabilities are those who meet the essential eligibility requirements for participation, with or without modifications (Southern Regional Education Board [SREB], n.d.).

A common goal of nursing education programs is to produce graduates who can function safely and competently in the roles for which they were prepared. For this reason, it is appropriate for those who make admission decisions to determine whether applicants could be reasonably expected to develop the necessary competence. The first step in this decision process is to define the core performance standards necessary for participation in the program. Because nursing is a practice discipline, core performance standards include cognitive, sensory, affective, and psychomotor competencies. The SREB recommended that such lists of core performance standards be shared with all applicants to nursing education programs to allow them to make initial judgments about their qualifications (SREB, n.d.).

Persons with disabilities who are admitted to nursing education programs are responsible for informing the institution of the disability and requesting reasonable accommodations. Each nursing education program must determine on an individual basis whether the necessary modifications can be reasonably made. Reasonable accommodations for participating in clinical learning activities might include:

- Allowing additional time for a student with a qualified learning disability to complete an assignment
- Allowing additional time to complete the program
- Scheduling clinical learning activities in facilities that are readily accessible to and usable by individuals who use wheelchairs or crutches
- Providing the use of an amplified stethoscope for a student with a hearing impairment

Reasonable accommodations do not include lowering academic standards or eliminating essential technical performance requirements (Smith, 2012). However, nurse educators need to distinguish essential from traditional functions by discussing such philosophical issues as whether individuals who will never practice bedside nursing in the conventional manner should be admitted to nursing education programs.

Disabilities may be visible (e.g., limited mobility, visual or hearing deficit, physical or functional loss of a limb) or invisible (e.g., learning disability, behavioral health problem, chronic illness). As previously discussed, clinical teachers should not attempt to determine whether accommodation is indicated, nor should they decide on the specific type of accommodation necessary. The disabilities services officer of the educational institution determines whether the student is a qualified individual with a disability and, if so, whether the disability requires accommodations. This officer then issues a formal, written description of the required clinical accommodations, usually to the student, who decides whom to share it with. Accommodation statements should not be shared with others without the student's written permission (Gardner & Suplee, 2010, pp. 48–49). The purpose of accommodation is to provide the student with a disability the means to compensate for it so that full participation in the clinical learning activity is possible. Many nursing faculty members voice concerns about the capacity of students with physical disabilities to perform physical tasks associated with nursing practice. A clinical teacher of a student with a physical disability should carefully analyze a planned learning activity to identify the essential elements necessary to produce desired outcomes, keeping in mind that much of the professional nurse's work is intellectual. Is it more important for a nursing student to demonstrate the ability to reposition a patient or to demonstrate the ability to assess the patient's skin integrity and pulmonary and circulatory function, recognize the need for repositioning, delegate the task to a licensed or unlicensed staff member and supervise that person as necessary, and evaluate the patient outcomes? Students with disabilities are the best sources of information about their disabilities and the limitations that they present, adaptations they have learned to compensate for them, and what accommodations have worked in the past. After appropriate accommodations are provided, however, students with disabilities must be evaluated according to the same criteria as other students.

Due Process

Another legal issue related to clinical teaching is that of student rights to due process. The 14th Amendment of the United States Constitution specifies that the state cannot deprive a person of life, liberty, or property without due process of law. With regard to the rights of students to due process, however, this constitutional protection extends only to those enrolled in public institutions. Students at private institutions may base a claim against the school on discrimination or contract law (Smith, 2012). For example, if a private school publishes a code of student rights and procedures for student grievances in its student handbook, those documents may be regarded as part of a contract between the school and the student. In paying and accepting tuition, the student and the school jointly agree to abide by this code of rights and set of procedures. A student may sue on the basis of breach of contract if the school does not follow the stated due process procedures.

Courts hold different standards for due process based on whether it applies to academic or disciplinary decisions. Academic decisions pertain to issues related to performance and academic standing, such as assigning a failing grade in a course, delaying progress, and dismissal from a program because of failure to maintain acceptable academic standing. Academic due process concerns both the *process* used to inform students of their academic standing and the *basis* for a decision regarding academic standing. Thus, *procedural due process* relates to the fairness of the process used to make academic decisions, and *substantive due process* relates to the basis for those decisions. A student appeal of an academic decision may allege a violation of either type of due process rights, but courts do not usually intervene in faculty members' evaluation of student academic or clinical performance. "Applying the principle of judicial deference, courts examining cases pertaining to faculty's evaluation of students usually uphold the faculty's decision, if there was an adherence to standard academic norms and the procedures used were fair and reasonable" (Smith, 2012, p. 5). The following legal principles apply to substantive due process (Smith, 2012):

- Students must be informed in advance about the academic standards that will be used to judge their performance.
- Student performance should be evaluated using the stated standards or criteria and grades assigned according to the stated policy. A teacher's academic decision should be based on a genuine substantive evaluation of the student's performance. All students should be evaluated according to the same standards; academic decisions should not be arbitrary or capricious.

If a student believes that a grade or other academic decision is unfair, the stated appeal or grievance process should be followed. Usually, the first level of appeal is to the teacher or group of teachers who assigned the grade. If the conflict is not resolved at that level, the student usually has the right of appeal to the administrator to whom the teacher reports. The next level of appeal is usually to a student standing committee or appeal panel of nursing faculty members. Finally, the student should have the right to appeal the decision to the highest level administrator in the nursing education program and then to the appropriate academic administrators at the parent institution.

Procedural due process concerns the fairness of the process by which academic decisions are made. Students should be notified about their academic deficiencies and the related consequences well before grading decisions are made. Ideally, notification occurs orally and in writing. To further protect students' procedural due process rights, the teacher should provide constructive feedback about their performance, suggest specific improvements, and provide a timeframe within which those improvements must be made. Evaluation of clinical performance is as much an academic decision as is assessment of classroom work, and the same procedural due process protections should be followed.

Of course, if students exhaust every level of appeal and are still not satisfied with the outcome, they have the right to seek relief in the court system. It is important to note that the courts will allow such a lawsuit to go forward only if there is evidence that the student has first exhausted all internal school remedies. However, if the educational program faculty and administrators have followed substantive due process procedures as described above, it is unlikely that the academic decision will be reversed. In particular, the courts will likely exercise judicial deference to the educational program if the student's complaint concerns a requirement of passing an exit examination to graduate because of the potential consequence to the program of a low NCLEX® pass rate (Smith, 2012). In due process appeals to a court of law, the burden of proof that academic due process was denied rests with the student. With regard to due process for academic decisions, the key to resolving conflict and minimizing faculty liability is in maintaining communication with students whose performance is not meeting standards.

Disciplinary decisions such as dismissal on the basis of misconduct or dishonesty require a higher level of due process than is required for academic actions. Unlike academic decisions that require professional judgments and are therefore beyond the scope of judicial review, disciplinary actions can be reviewed by the courts' traditional fact-finding procedures (Smith, 2012).

Disciplinary decisions are made when a student violates the law or regulation by engaging in prohibited activity. All colleges and universities have rules, standards, conduct codes, and policies that students are expected to meet, usually published in the institutional catalog and student handbook. Nursing education programs often have specific expectations regarding adherence to professional codes of conduct that are consistent with but go above and beyond the rules and standards of the parent institution. These publications must also explicate the procedures that will be followed if these rules are violated (Smith, 2012).

Disciplinary due process includes the following components:

- The student is provided with adequate written notice, including specific details concerning the misconduct. For example, a notice may inform the student that she failed to attend a required clinical activity; that neither the faculty member nor nursing unit secretary was informed of the anticipated absence, in violation of school policy on professional conduct; and that, because this incident represented the third violation of professional conduct standards, the student would be dismissed from the program according to the sanctions provided in the policy.

guidance when they are uncertain what to do. Therefore, it is not true that students practice under the faculty member's license.

Teachers are not liable for negligent acts performed by their students as long as the teacher has (1) selected appropriate learning activities based on objectives; (2) determined that students have prerequisite knowledge, skills, and attitudes necessary to complete their assignments; and (3) provide competent guidance. However, teachers are liable for their negligent actions if they make assignments that require more knowledge and skill than the learner has developed or if they fail to guide student activities appropriately. The NCSBN Model Rules (2012b) include statements about the grounds for disciplining an RN. These include failure to competently guide student clinical learning activities as a clinical teacher. Even if the clinical teacher was not negligent in making assignments or guiding student learning, he or she is likely to be named as a defendant in any lawsuit arising from a nursing student's alleged negligence or malpractice. For this reason, clinical teachers should carry sufficient individual professional liability insurance to cover the costs of defending themselves, even if their employers provide insurance coverage for faculty members.

If a student demonstrates clinical performance that is potentially unsafe, the student and the teacher who made the assignment may be liable for any subsequent injury to the patient. However, because time for learning must precede time for evaluation, is it fair for the teacher to assign a failing grade in clinical practice before the end of the course, when to do so would prevent the student's access to learning opportunities for which he or she has paid tuition? In this case, denying access to clinical learning activities because of unsafe practice or inadequate clinical reasoning should not be considered an academic grading decision. Instead, it is an appropriate response to protecting the rights of patients to safe, competent care—a disciplinary decision (Gardner & Suplee, 2010, p. 197).

The teacher's failure to take such protective action potentially places the teacher and the educational program at risk for liability. Instead of denying the student access to all learning opportunities, removal from the clinical setting should be followed by a substitute assignment that would help the student to remove the deficiency in knowledge, skill, or attitude. For example, the student might be given a library assignment to acquire the information necessary to guide safe patient care, or an extra skills laboratory session could be arranged to allow more practice of psychomotor skills. A set of standards on safe clinical practice and a school policy that enforces the standards are helpful guides to faculty decision making and action while protecting student and faculty rights. Exhibit 6.1 is an example of safe clinical practice standards, and Exhibit 6.2 is an example of a policy that enforces these standards.

Exhibit 6.1

STANDARDS OF SAFE CLINICAL PRACTICE

XXXXXX UNIVERSITY
SCHOOL OF NURSING
BSN PROGRAM
STANDARDS OF SAFE CLINICAL PRACTICE

In clinical practice, students are expected to demonstrate responsibility and accountability as professional nurses with the goal of health promotion and prevention of harm to self and others. The School of Nursing faculty believes that this goal will be attained if each student's clinical practice adheres to the Standards of Safe Clinical Practice. Safe clinical performance always includes, but is not limited to, the following behaviors:

1. Practice within boundaries of the nursing student role and the scope of practice of the registered nurse.
2. Comply with instructional policies and procedures for implementing nursing care.
3. Prepare for clinical learning assignments according to course requirements and as determined for the specific clinical setting.
4. Demonstrate the application of previously learned skills and principles in providing nursing care.
5. Promptly report significant client information in a clear, accurate, and complete oral or written manner to the appropriate person or persons.

ACKNOWLEDGMENT

I have read the XXXXXX University School of Nursing Standards of Safe Clinical Practice and I agree to adhere to them. I understand that these standards are expectations for my clinical practice and will be incorporated into the evaluation of my clinical performance in all clinical courses. Failure to meet these standards may result in my removal from the clinical area, which may result in clinical failure.

_____

Signature and Date

Exhibit 6.2

POLICY ON SAFE CLINICAL PRACTICE

XXXXXX UNIVERSITY
SCHOOL OF NURSING
BSN PROGRAM
SAFE CLINICAL PRACTICE POLICY

POLICY

During enrollment in the XXXXXX University School of Nursing BSN Program, all students, in all clinical activities, are expected to adhere to the Standards of Safe Clinical Practice. Failure to abide by these standards will result in disciplinary action, which may include dismissal from the nursing program.

PROCEDURES

1. Students will receive a copy of the Standards of Safe Clinical Practice, and they will be reviewed during the Annual Nursing Assembly at the beginning of each academic year. At that time, students will be required to sign an agreement to adhere to the standards. Each student will retain one copy of the agreement, and one copy will be filed in the student's file.
2. Violation of these standards will result in the following disciplinary action:
   a. First Violation
      1. Student will be given an immediate oral warning by the faculty member. The incident will be documented by the faculty member on the *Violation of Standards of Safe Clinical Practice* form. One copy of this form will be given to the student, and one copy will be kept in the student's record.
      2. At the discretion of the faculty member, the student may be required to leave the clinical unit for the remainder of that day. The student may be given an alternative assignment.
      3. If this violation is of a serious nature, it may be referred to the associate dean and the dean of nursing for further disciplinary action as in b and c below.
   b. Second Violation
      1. The faculty member will document the incident on the *Violation of Safe Clinical Practice* form. Following discussion of the incident with the student, the faculty member will forward a copy of the form to the associate dean for review and recommendation regarding further action.
      2. The recommendation of the associate dean will be forwarded to the dean of nursing for review and decision regarding reprimand or dismissal. This disciplinary action process will be documented and placed in the student's record.
   c. If the student has not been dismissed and remains in the program following the above disciplinary action, any additional violation will be documented and referred as above to the associate dean and the dean of nursing for disciplinary action, which may include dismissal from the program.
   d. The rights of students will be safeguarded as set forth in the XXXXXX University *Code of Student Rights, Responsibilities, and Conduct* published in the current *XXXXXX University Student Handbook*.

Documentation and Record Keeping

Teachers should keep records of their evaluations of student clinical performance. These records may include anecdotal notes, summaries of faculty–student conferences, progress reports, and summative clinical evaluations. These records are helpful in documenting that students received feedback about their performance, areas of teacher concern, and information about student progress toward correcting deficiencies (Di Leornardi & Oermann, 2010).

An anecdotal note is a narrative description of the observed behavior of the student in relation to a specific learning objective. The note may also include the teacher's interpretation of the behavior, recorded separately from the description. Limiting the description and optional interpretation to a specified clinical objective avoids recording extraneous information, which is an ineffective use of the teacher's time. Anecdotal notes should record both positive and negative behaviors so as not to give the impression that the teacher is biased against the student. Students should review these notes and have an opportunity to comment on them; used in this way, anecdotal notes are an effective means of communicating formative evaluation information to students (Di Leonardi & Oermann, 2010; Oermann & Gaberson, 2014). Some sources recommend that both teacher and student sign the notes.

Writing anecdotal notes for every student, every day, is unnecessarily time consuming. An effective, efficient approach might be to specify a minimum number of notes to be written for each student in relation to specified objectives. A student whose performance is either meritorious or cause for concern might prompt the instructor to write more notes.

Records of student–teacher conferences are likewise summaries of discussions that focused on areas of concern, plans to address deficiencies, and progress toward correcting weaknesses. These conferences should take place in private and should address the teacher's responsibility to protect patient safety, concern about the student's clinical deficiencies, and a sincere desire to assist the student to improve. During the conference, the student has opportunities to clarify and respond to the teacher's feedback. At times, an objective third party such as a department chairperson or program director may be asked to participate in the conference to witness and clarify the comments of both teacher and student. The conference note should record the date, time, and place of the conference; the names and roles of participants; and a summary of the discussion, recommendations, and plans. The note may be signed only by the teacher or by all participants, according to institutional policy or guidelines.

Because they contain essentially formative evaluation information, anecdotal notes and conference notes should not be kept in the student's permanent record. Teachers should keep these documents in their private files, taking appropriate precautions to ensure their security, until there is no reasonable expectation that they will be needed. In most cases, when the learner successfully completes the program or withdraws in good academic standing, these records can be discarded (again, taking appropriate security precautions). It is unlikely that successful learners will appeal favorable academic decisions. However, it is recommended that anecdotal records and conference notes be kept for longer periods when there is a chance that the learner may appeal the grade or other decision. The statute of limitations for such an appeal is a useful guide to deciding how long to keep those materials. It is recommended that teachers consult with legal counsel if there is a question about institutional policy on retention of records.

HIPAA Requirements

The U.S. Health Insurance Portability and Accountability Act (HIPAA) of 1996 created new challenges for clinical nurse educators. Because of privacy concerns regarding disclosure of individually identifiable health information covered by this legislation, many health care facilities have adopted policies and procedures that may pose barriers to clinical teaching and learning.

Because individually identifiable health information is increasingly recorded, stored, and accessed in electronic form, concerns about the potential transfer of this information to a personal digital assistant (PDA) and then to other devices may be a barrier to student use of PDAs in clinical settings (Zurmehly, 2010). However, if PDA use by nursing students in clinical settings is primarily to access electronic reference books, this is not a HIPAA violation (Thompson, 2005). Additionally, if patient information must be entered into a student's PDA, a software program that encrypts data may be used to de-identify data (Kuiper, 2008).

Most health care organizations require nursing education programs to provide documentation that their students have been oriented to the requirements of HIPAA. If numerous clinical sites are used by a program, this requirement can be onerous if each agency requires students to attend or complete its own HIPAA orientation. Nursing education administrators may be able to negotiate with all clinical agencies to agree on the basic content of the required orientation, recognizing that the requirement could be met in various ways. Students are typically asked to sign a verification that they have been oriented to HIPAA requirements and that they agree to abide by those requirements. This orientation and verification should be repeated at regular intervals (e.g., yearly or each semester).

Because health care agencies also usually require nursing education programs to provide verification that nursing students have met specified health requirements, this verification process may create HIPAA concerns. If the nursing education program collects, receives, or transmits students' individually identifiable health information, it could be deemed responsible for maintaining reasonable and appropriate administrative, technical, and physical safeguards to ensure the integrity and confidentiality of the information and to protect against any reasonably anticipated threats to the security of the information and unauthorized uses or disclosures of it. Some clinical agencies request specific health data as evidence that students have met clinical health requirements, such as a rubella titer result. However, if the nursing education program complies with this request and the agency misuses the information in any way, both the education program and the clinical agency risk claims of unauthorized release or use of protected information about individual students.

Many nursing education programs avoid these potential complications by requiring a licensed health care provider to verify that a student has met all specified clinical health requirements. This verification, including dates for immunizations and a signed statement that the student's general health is adequate to allow full participation in the nursing program, is kept in the nursing education program files, but the raw data remain the property of the student and his health care provider. Another approach to resolving these concerns is to have all nursing students examined and tested by the student health service of the parent institution, with the raw data stored in that office and notification to the nursing education program that the clinical health requirements have or have not been met. It is wise to seek the advice of the school, college, or university counsel about how requirements for verification of students' health status by clinical agencies should be handled so that an appropriate policy can be developed and implemented.

SUMMARY

Because clinical teaching and learning take place in a social context, the rights of teachers, students, staff members, and patients are sometimes in conflict. These conflicts create legal and ethical dilemmas for clinical teachers. This chapter discussed selected ethical and legal issues related to clinical teaching.

Ethical standards such as respect for human dignity, autonomy, and freedom; beneficence; justice; veracity; privacy; and fidelity are important considerations for all parties involved in clinical teaching and learning. Students must learn to apply these standards to nursing practice, and teachers must apply them in their relationships with students as well as their teaching and evaluation responsibilities.

Specific ethical issues related to clinical teaching and learning include the presence of learners in a service setting, the need for faculty–student relationships to be based on justice and respect for persons, students' privacy rights, teaching competence, and academic dishonesty. Legal issues that have implications for clinical teaching and learning include educating students with disabilities, student rights to due process for academic and disciplinary decisions, standards of safe clinical practice, student and teacher negligence and liability, documentation and record keeping regarding students' clinical performance, and potential violations of HIPAA requirements with regard to student health information.

Suggestions were offered for preventing, minimizing, and managing these difficult ethical and legal situations. Laws and institutional policies often provide guidelines for action in specific cases. However, these suggestions should not be construed as legal advice, and teachers are advised to seek legal counsel in regard to specific questions or problems.

Exhibit 6.3

CNE EXAMINATION TEST BLUEPRINT CORE COMPETENCIES

1. **Facilitate Learning**

   E. Practice skilled oral and written (including electronic) communication that reflects an awareness of self and relationships with learners (e.g., evaluation, mentorship, and supervision)
   K. Demonstrate personal attributes that facilitate learning (e.g., caring, confidence, patience, integrity, respect, and flexibility)
   P. Act as a role model in practice settings

2. **Facilitate Learner Development and Socialization**

   A. Identify individual learning styles and unique learning needs of learners with these characteristics
      4. at-risk (e.g., educationally disadvantaged, learning and/or physically challenged, social, and economic issues)
   B. Provide resources for diverse learners to meet their individual learning needs
   D. Create learning environments that facilitate learners' self-reflection, personal goal setting, and socialization to the role of the nurse

   (continued)

E. Foster the development of learners in these areas:
    3. affective domain

3. Use Assessment and Evaluation Strategies

    B. Enforce nursing program standards related to
        1. admission
        2. progression
        3. graduation

    K. Advise learners regarding assessment and evaluation criteria
    L. Provide timely, constructive, and thoughtful feedback to learners

5. Pursue Continuous Quality Improvement in the Academic Nurse Educator Role

    H. Practice according to legal and ethical standards relevant to higher education and nursing education

6. Engage in Scholarship, Service, and Leadership

    C. Function effectively within the organizational environment and the academic community
        3. Integrate the values of respect, collegiality, professionalism, and caring to build an organizational climate that fosters the development of learners and colleagues

---

REFERENCES

Altmiller, G. (2012). Student perceptions of incivility in nursing education: Implications for educators. *Nursing Education Perspectives, 33,* 15–20.

American Nurses Association (2011). *Social networking principles toolkit.* Retrieved from www.nursingworld.org/socialnetworkingtoolkit

Bavier, A. R. (2009). Holding students accountable when integrity is challenged. *Nursing Education Perspectives, 30,* 5.

Corcoran, S. (1977). Should a service setting be used as a learning laboratory? An ethical question. *Nursing Outlook, 25,* 771–774.

Di Leonardi, B. C. & Oermann, M. H. (2010). Teaching in a clinical setting. In L. Caputi (Ed.), *Teaching nursing: The art and science* (pp. 82–141). Glen Ellyn, IL: College of DuPage Press.

Family Educational Rights and Privacy Act, 20 U.S.C. § 1232g; 34 CFR Part 99.

Gardner, M. R., & Suplee, P. D. (2010). *Handbook of clinical teaching.* Sudbury, MA: Jones and Bartlett.

Health Insurance Portability and Accountability Act of 1996. Public Law 104–191.

Husted, G. L., & Husted, J. H. (2008). *Ethical decision making in nursing and health care: The symphonological approach* (4th ed.). New York, NY: Springer.

Kohn, L., Corrigan, J., & Donaldson, M. (2000). *To err is human: Building a safer health system.* Washington, DC: National Academy Press, Institute of Medicine.

Kryder, C. (2009). Medical communicators: Did you tweet today? *AMWA Journal, 24*, 78–79.

Kuiper, R. (2008). Use of personal digital assistants to support clinical reasoning in undergraduate baccalaureate nursing students. *CIN: Computers, Informatics, Nursing, 26*, 90–98.

National Council of State Boards of Nursing, Inc. (2011). *A nurse's guide to the use of social media*. [Brochure]. Retrieved from https://www.ncsbn.org/NCSBN_SocialMedia.pdf

National Council of State Boards of Nursing, Inc. (2012a). *Model nurse practice act*. Retrieved from https://www.ncsbn.org/12_Model_Act_090512.pdf

National Council of State Boards of Nursing, Inc. (2012b). *Model rules*. Retrieved from https://www.ncsbn.org/12_Model_Rules_090512.pdf

Oermann, M. H., & Gaberson, K. B. (2014). *Evaluation and testing in nursing education* (4th ed.). New York, NY: Springer.

Poorman, S. G., Mastorovich, M. L., & Webb, C. A. (2011). Helping students who struggle academically: Finding the right level of involvement and living with our judgments. *Nursing Education Perspectives, 32*, 369–374.

Skiba, D. J. (2008). Nursing education 2.0: Twitter & tweets. *Nursing Education Perspectives, 29*, 110–112.

Smith, M. (2012). *The legal, professional, and ethical dimensions of higher education in nursing* (2nd ed.). New York, NY: Springer.

Southern Regional Education Board. (n.d.). *The Americans with Disabilities Act: Implications for nursing education.* Retrieved from http://www.sreb.org/page/1390/the_americans_with_disabilities_act.html

Spector, N., & Kappel, D. (2012). Guidelines for using electronic and social media: The regulatory perspective. *Online Journal of Issues in Nursing, 17*(3), Manuscript 1. Retrieved from http://www.medscape.com/viewarticle/780050_print

Tanicala, M. L., Scheffer, B. K., & Roberts, M. S. (2011). Pass/fail nursing student behaviors Phase I: Moving toward a culture of safety. *Nursing Education Perspectives, 32*, 155–161.

Thompson, B. W. (2005). Infobytes: HIPAA guidelines for using PDAs. *Nursing 2005, 35*(11), 24.

Tippitt, M. P., Ard, N., Kline, J. R., Tilghman, J., Chamberlain, B., & Meagher, P. G. (2009). Creating environments that foster academic integrity. *Nursing Education Perspectives, 30*, 239–244.

Zurmehly, J. (2010). Personal digital assistants (PDAs): Review and evaluation. *Nursing Education Perspectives, 31*, 179–182.

Strategies for Effective Clinical Teaching

CHAPTER 7

Crafting Clinical Learning Assignments

One of the most important responsibilities of a clinical teacher is crafting clinical assignments that are related to desired outcomes, appropriate to students' levels of knowledge and skill, and challenging enough to motivate learning. Although directing a learner to provide comprehensive nursing care to one or more patients is a typical clinical assignment, it is only one of many possible assignments, and not always the most appropriate choice. This chapter presents a framework for selecting clinical learning assignments and discusses several alternatives to the traditional total patient care assignment.

PATIENT CARE VERSUS LEARNING ACTIVITY

When planning assignments, clinical teachers typically speak of selecting patients for whom students will provide care. However, as discussed in Chapter 1, the primary role of the nursing student in the clinical area is that of learner, not nurse. Although it is true that nursing students need contact with patients in order to apply classroom learning to clinical practice, caring for patients is not synonymous with learning. In a classic study of the use of the clinical laboratory in nursing education, Infante (1985) took the position that nursing students are *learning to care* for patients; they are not nurses with *responsibility for patient care.* Providing patient care does not guarantee transfer of knowledge from the classroom to clinical practice; instead, it often reflects work requirements of the clinical agency.

Many faculty members assume that caring for patients always constitutes a clinical assignment for students on every level of the nursing education program. Even in their earliest clinical courses, nursing students typically have responsibility for patient care while learning basic psycho-motor and communication skills. However, given the high patient acuity level in most acute care settings, beginning-level nursing students are not ready to provide total care for the typical patient in such environments, and this early responsibility for patient care often creates anxiety that interferes with learning.

As discussed in Chapter 2, changes in health care, technology, society, and education influence the competencies needed for professional nursing practice. Learning outcomes necessary for safe, competent nursing practice today include cognitive skills of problem solving, decision making, critical thinking, and clinical reasoning, in addition to technical proficiency. If nurse educators are to produce creative, independent, assertive, and decisive practitioners, they cannot assume that students will acquire these competencies through patient care assignments. To produce these outcomes, clinical teachers should choose clinical assignments from a variety of learning activities, including participation in patient care.

FACTORS AFFECTING SELECTION OF CLINICAL ASSIGNMENTS

The selection of learning activities within the context of the clinical teaching process was discussed earlier. Clinical activities help learners to apply knowledge to practice, develop skills, cultivate professional values, and become socialized to the role of professional nurse. Clinical assignments should be selected according to criteria such as the learning objectives of the clinical activity; needs of patients; availability and variety of learning opportunities in the clinical environment; and the needs, interests, and abilities of learners (Di Leonardi & Oermann, 2010).

Learning Outcomes

The most important criterion for selection of clinical assignments is usually the desired learning outcome. The teacher should structure each clinical activity carefully in terms of the learning objectives, and each clinical activity should be an integral part of the course or educational program. In some nursing education programs, one set of course objectives applies to both the classroom and clinical learning outcomes; in others, separate but related sets of objectives are created to reflect the different emphases of "knowing that" (classroom learning outcome) and "knowing how" (clinical learning outcome).

Whatever method of specifying desired outcomes is used, it is essential that the clinical teacher, students, and staff members understand the purpose and goals of each clinical activity. Depending on the level of the learner, students may have difficulty envisioning how broad program or course outcomes can be achieved in the context of a specific clinical environment. It is the clinical teacher's role to translate these outcomes into specific clinical objectives and to select and structure learning activities so that they relate logically and sequentially to the goals (Di Leonardi & Oermann, 2010). The clinical teacher should share with each student the rationale for his or her specific clinical assignment to help students to focus on the learning opportunities presented by each unique assignment.

Learner Characteristics

As previously discussed, the learner's educational level or previous experience; aptitude for learning; learning style; and specific needs, interests, and abilities should also influence the selection of clinical assignments. The teacher must consider these individual differences; all learners do not have the same needs, so it is unreasonable to expect them to have the same learning assignments on any given day (Di Leonardi & Oermann, 2010; Gardner & Suplee, 2010).

For example, Student A learns skills at a slower pace than other students at the same level. The instructor should plan assignments so that this student has many opportunities for repetition of skills with feedback. If the objective is to learn the skills of medication administration, most students might be able to learn those skills in a reasonable amount of time in the context of providing care to one or more patients. Student A might learn more effectively with an assignment to administer all medications to a larger group of patients over the period of a day or more, without other patient care responsibilities. When the student has acquired the necessary level of skill, the next clinical assignment might be to administer medications while learning other aspects of care for one or more patients.

Students who are able to achieve the objectives of the essential curriculum (see Chapter 1) rather quickly might receive assignments from the enrichment curriculum that allow them to focus on their individual needs. For example, a student who is interested in exploring perioperative nursing might be assigned to follow a patient through a surgical procedure, providing preoperative care, observing or participating in the surgery, assisting in immediate postoperative care in the postanesthesia care unit, and presenting a plan for home care in a postclinical conference. Taking learners' interests and professional development goals into account when planning enrichment activities will motivate students and individualize their learning experiences.

Needs of Patients

Patient needs and care requirements should also be considered when planning clinical assignments for students. In relation to the learning objective, will the nursing care activities present enough of a challenge to the learner? Are they too complex for the learner to manage?

Even if patients signed consents for admission to the health care facility that included an agreement to the participation of learners in their care, their wishes regarding student assignment and those of their family members should be respected (Di Leonardi & Oermann, 2010). At times of crisis, patients and family members may not wish to initiate a new nurse–patient relationship with a nursing student or new employee orientee. Nursing staff members who have provided care to these patients can often help the clinical teacher determine whether student learning needs and specific patient and family needs can both be met through a particular clinical assignment.

As mentioned previously, the patient acuity level in a given clinical setting affects the selection of learning opportunities for nursing students. When the acuity level is high, it may not be possible for a clinical teacher to assign every student to learn to care for patients with many complex needs. In this case, some students may be assigned to apply their knowledge to the care of two or more relatively stable patients to develop their prioritization and time management skills, or two or more students may be assigned to plan, organize, deliver, evaluate, and document care for one patient with complex needs (Gardner & Suplee, 2010). Variations in student–patient ratio assignment options are described in more detail later in this chapter.

Timing of Activities and Availability of Learning Opportunities

Because the purpose of clinical learning is to foster application of theory to practice, clinical learning activities should be related to what is being taught in the classroom. Ideally, clinical activities are scheduled concurrently with relevant classroom content so that learners can make immediate transfer and application of knowledge to nursing practice. However, there is little evidence of a relationship between clinical learning outcomes and the structure, timing, and organization of clinical learning activities.

The availability of learning opportunities to allow students to meet objectives often affects clinical assignments. The usual schedule of activities in the clinical facility may determine the optimum timing of learning activities. For example, if the learning objective for a new nursing student is "Identify sources of information about patient needs from the health record," it would be difficult for students to gain access to patient records at the beginning or end of a shift. Thus, scheduling learners to arrive at the clinical site at midmorning may allow better access to the resources necessary for learning.

Some clinical settings, such as outpatient clinics and operating rooms, are available to both patients and students only on a daytime, Monday through Friday, schedule. In other settings, however, scheduling clinical learning activities during evening or nighttime hours or on weekend days may offer students better opportunities to meet certain objectives. If the learning objective is "Implement health teaching for the parents of a premature or ill neonate," the best time for students to encounter parents may be during evening visiting hours or on weekends. Using these time periods for clinical activities may also prevent two or more groups of learners from different educational programs being in the same clinical area simultaneously, affecting the availability of learning opportunities.

Of course, learning activities at such times may conflict with family, work, and other academic schedules and commitments for both teachers and students. In some cases (for example, with the use of preceptors), it is not necessary for the teacher to be present in the clinical setting with learners, thereby allowing more flexible scheduling of clinical activities. However, flexibility is necessary to take advantage of learning opportunities when they are available.

The clinical teacher should broadly interpret the objectives for a clinical course to take full advantage of the learning opportunities in each clinical setting. If the instructor knows what concepts the students are learning in the classroom, he or she can find various clinical learning opportunities in different settings. For example, if the focus is wound healing, students could have learning activities involving patients with postoperative wounds, pressure ulcers, traumatic wounds, or arterial or venous chronic leg ulcers. It is not necessary for every student to have a similar learning opportunity if all learning activities enable students to apply the same concept in practice (Gardner & Suplee, 2010). In postclinical conference, students can be guided to discuss the various ways in which they applied a particular concept or principle; this debriefing activity will broaden their clinical knowledge and help them to identify similarities and differences among the various patient responses to a common alteration in health status.

OPTIONS FOR LEARNING ASSIGNMENTS

The creative teacher may craft clinical assignments from a wide variety of learning activities. Several options for making assignments are discussed.

Teacher-Selected or Learner-Selected Assignments

Although it is the teacher's responsibility to specify the learning objective, learners should have choices of learning activities that will help them achieve the objective. Having a choice of assignment or at least a choice between options selected by the teacher motivates students to be responsible for their own learning and fully engage in the learning activity. Allowing learners to participate in selecting their own assignments may also reduce student anxiety.

Of course, the teacher should offer guidance in selecting appropriate learning activities through questions or comments that require students to evaluate their own needs, interests, and abilities. Sometimes teachers need to be more directive; a student may choose an assignment that clearly requires more knowledge or skill than the student has developed. In this case, the teacher must intervene to protect patient safety as well as to help the student make realistic plans to acquire the necessary knowledge and skill. Other students may choose assignments that do not challenge their abilities; the teacher's role is to support and encourage such students to take advantage of opportunities to achieve higher levels of knowledge and skill (Gardner & Suplee, 2010, p. 65).

Skill Focus Versus Total Care Focus

As previously discussed, the traditional clinical assignment for nursing students is to give total care to one or more patients. However, not all learning objectives require students to practice total patient care (National League for Nursing [NLN], 2008). For example, if the objective is, "Assess patient and family preparation for postoperative recovery at home," the student does not have to provide total care to the postoperative patient in order to meet the objective. The student could meet the objective by interviewing the patient and family, observing a case manager's assessment of the patient and family's readiness for discharge or a physical therapist's assessment of the patient's ability to perform physical activities, and reviewing the patient's records. Additionally, total patient care is an integrative activity that can be accomplished effectively only when students are competent in performing the component skills (NLN, 2008).

As previously discussed, all students do not need to be engaged in the same learning activities at the same time. Depending on their individual learning needs, some students might be engaged in activities that focus on developing a particular skill, while others could be practicing more integrative activities such as providing total patient care.

For example, if students are learning physical assessment skills, some students could be assigned to practice auscultation by listening to breath, heart, and abdominal sounds of a variety of patients without having the responsibility of performing other patient care activities. In postclinical conference, these students should share their insights about the commonalities and differences among their assessment findings and relate them to the patient's history and pathophysiology. A different group of students could perform assessment rounds during the next clinical practice day.

One advantage to assigning some students to learning activities that do not involve total patient care is that the clinical teacher is more available for closer guidance of students when they are learning to care for patients with complex needs. Staggering assignments in this way helps the clinical teacher better meet the learning needs of all students (Gardner & Suplee, 2010, pp. 60–61).

Student–Patient Ratio Options

Although the traditional clinical assignment takes the form of one student to one patient, there are other assignment options (Di Leonardi & Oermann, 2010). These options are:

- *One student/one patient or multiple patients.* One student is responsible for certain aspects of care or for comprehensive care for one or more patients. The student works alone to plan, implement, and evaluate nursing care. This type of assignment is advantageous when the objective is to integrate many aspects of care after the student has learned the individual activities.
- *Multiple students/one patient.* Two or more students are assigned to plan, implement, and evaluate care for one patient. Each learner has a defined role, and all collaborate to meet the learning objective. Various models of dual or multiple assignment exist. For example, three students would read the patient record, review the relevant pathophysiology, and collaborate on an assessment and plan of care. Student A reviews information concerning the patient's medications, administers and documents all scheduled and p.r.n. (when-needed) medications, and manages the intravenous infusions. Student B focuses on providing and documenting all other aspects of patient care. Student C evaluates the effectiveness of the plan of care, assists with physical care when needed, interacts with the patient's family, and provides reports to appropriate staff members. Members of the learning team can switch roles on subsequent days. This assignment strategy is particularly useful when patients have complex needs that are beyond the capability of one student, although it can be used in any setting with a large number of students and a low patient census.

Other advantages include reducing student anxiety and teaching teamwork and collaborative learning.

■ *Multiple students–patient aggregate.* A group of students is assigned to complete activities related to a community or population subgroup at risk for certain health problems. For example, a small group of students might be assigned to conduct a community assessment to identify an actual or potential health problem in the aggregate served by the clinical agency. Clinical activities would include interviewing community residents and agency staff members, identifying environmental and occupational health hazards, documenting the availability of social and health services, and performing selected physical assessments on a sample of the aggregate. The student group would then analyze the data and present a report to the agency staff and community members. Advantages of this assignment strategy include promoting a focus on the community as client, teaching collaboration with other health care providers and community members, and reinforcement of group process.

Management Activities

Some clinical assignments are chosen to enable learners to meet outcomes related to nursing leadership, management and improvement of patient care, and health care organizational goals. Undergraduate nursing students are usually introduced to concepts and skills of leadership and management in preparation for their future roles in complex health care systems. These students often benefit from clinical assignments that allow them to develop skill in planning and managing care for a group of patients. For example, a senior baccalaureate student may enact the role of team leader for other nursing students who are assigned to provide total care for individual patients. The student team leader may receive reports about the group of patients from agency staff, plan assignments for the other students, give reports to those students, supervise and coordinate work, and communicate patient information to staff members.

Master's and doctoral students may be preparing for management and administrative roles in health care organizations; their clinical activities might focus on enacting the roles of first-level or middle manager, patient care services administrator, clinical nurse leader, or case manager. New staff nurse employees usually need to be oriented to the role of charge nurse; assignments to help them learn the necessary knowledge, skills, and attitudes should include practice in this role. Often, such clinical assignments involve the participation of a preceptor (Chapter 13, "Using Preceptors as Clinical Teachers and Coaches").

Guided Observation

Observation is an important skill in nursing practice, and teachers should provide opportunities for learners to develop this skill systematically. Observing patients in order to collect data is a prerequisite to problem solving, clinical reasoning, and clinical decision making. To make accurate and useful observations, the student must have knowledge of the phenomenon and the intellectual skill to observe it: the what and how of observation. As a clinical learning assignment, observation should not be combined with an assignment to provide care. If students do not have concurrent care responsibilities, they are free to choose the times and sometimes the locations of their observations. The focus should be on observing purposefully in order to meet a learning objective.

Observation also provides opportunities for students to learn through modeling. By observing another person performing a skill, the learner forms an image of how the task or behavior is to be performed, which serves as a guide to learning. For this reason, it is helpful to schedule learners to observe in a clinical setting before they are assigned to practice activities. However, scheduling an observation before the learner has acquired the prerequisite knowledge is unproductive; the student may not be able to make meaning out of what is observed.

Written observation guidelines can be used effectively to prepare learners for the activity and to guide their attention to important data during the observation. Exhibit 7.1 is an example of an observation guide to prepare students for a group observation activity in an operating room. Note the explicit expectations that, before the observation, students will read, think critically, and anticipate what they will see. The presence of a clinical teacher or other resource person to answer questions and direct students' attention to pertinent items or activities is also helpful. Students may be asked to evaluate the observation activity by identifying learning outcomes, what they did and did not like about the activity, and the extent to which their preparation and the participation of the instructor was helpful. Exhibit 7.2 is a sample evaluation tool for an observation activity.

Service Learning

Another option for clinical learning assignments is service learning. Service learning differs from volunteer work, community service, fieldwork, and internships. Volunteer and community service focus primarily on the service that is provided to the recipients, and fieldwork and internships primarily focus on benefits to student learning. Service learning intentionally combines the benefits to the community with student learning in ways that are mutually satisfying (Bassi, 2011). Service learning is an academic credit-earning learning activity in which students:

- participate in an organized service activity that meets identified community needs and
- reflect on the service activity to gain a deeper understanding of course content, a broader appreciation of the discipline, and an enhanced sense of responsibility as a citizen (Bassi, 2011).

Exhibit 7.1

EXAMPLE OF AN OBSERVATION GUIDE

Operating Room Observation Guide

Purposes of the Observation Activity

1. To gain an overview of perioperative nursing care in the intraoperative phase.
2. To observe application of principles of surgical asepsis in the operating room.
3. To distinguish among roles of various members of the surgical team.

General Information

You are expected to prepare for this observation and to complete an observation guide while you are observing the surgical procedure. Please read your medical –surgical nursing textbook, pp. 195 to 200, for a general understanding of nursing roles in the intraoperative phase.

Bring this observation guide and a pen or pencil on the day of your observation. The guide will be collected and reviewed by the instructor at the end of the observation activity.

Most likely, you will observe either a coronary artery bypass graft or an aortic valve replacement. Please review the anatomy of the heart, specifically the coronary vessels and valves. In addition, read the following pages in your medical–surgical nursing textbook: coronary artery disease, pp. 1058 to 1059 and 1069 to 1085; valvular heart disease (aortic stenosis), pp. 1131 to 1132 and 1135 to 1139.

After you have completed your reading assignment, attempt to answer the questions in the first section of the observation guide (Preparation of the Patient) related to preparations that take place before the patient comes to the operating room. Don't be afraid to make some educated guesses about the answers; we will discuss them and supply any missing information on the day of your observation.

Complete the remaining sections of the observation guide during your observation. The instructor will be available to guide the observation and to answer questions.

(continued)

Preparation of the Patient

1. Who is responsible for obtaining the consent for the surgical procedure? Why?
2. Who identifies the patient when he or she is brought into the operating room? Why?
3. What other patient data should be reviewed by a nurse when the patient is brought to the operating room? Why?
4. Who transfers the patient from transport bed to the operating room bed? What safety precautions are taken during this procedure?
5. What is the nurse's role during anesthesia induction?
6. What team members participate in the Universal Protocol? Identify elements of the protocol that protect the safety of this patient.
7. When is the patient positioned for the surgical procedure? Who does this? What safety precautions are taken? What special equipment may be used?
8. What is the purpose of the preoperative skin preparation of the operative site? When is it done? What safety precautions are taken?
9. What is the purpose of draping the patient and equipment? What factors determine the type of drape material used? What safety precautions are taken? Who does the draping? Why?
10. What nursing diagnoses are commonly identified for patients in the immediate preoperative and early intraoperative phases?

Preparation of Personnel

1. Apparel: Who is wearing what? What factors determine the selection of apparel? How and when do personnel don and remove apparel items? What personal protective equipment is used and why?
2. Hand antisepsis: Which personnel use hand antisepsis techniques to prepare for the procedure? When? Which method is used?
3. Gowning and gloving: What roles do the scrub person and the circulator play?

Roles of Surgical Team Members

1. Surgeons and assistants (surgical residents, interns, medical students)
2. Nurses and surgical technologists
3. Anesthesia personnel
4. Others (perfusion technologist, radiologic technologist, pathologist, etc.)

Maintenance of Aseptic Technique

1. Movement of personnel
2. Sterile areas and items
3. Nonsterile areas and items
4. Handling of sterile items

Equipment

1. Lighting: Who positions it? How? When?
2. Monitoring: What monitors are used? Who is responsible for setting up and watching this equipment?

(continued)

3. Blood/other fluid infusion: Who is responsible for setting up and monitoring this equipment?
4. Electrosurgical unit: What is this equipment used for? Who is responsible for it? What safety precautions are taken?
5. Suction: What is this equipment used for? Who is responsible for setting up and monitoring it?
6. Smoke evacuator: What is this equipment used for? Who is responsible for setting up and using it?
7. Patient heating/cooling equipment: What is this equipment used for? Who is responsible for setting up and monitoring it?
8. Other equipment

Intraoperative Nursing Diagnoses

1. What nursing diagnoses are likely to be identified for this patient in the intraoperative period?

Conclusion of Procedure

1. What elements of the Universal Protocol are implemented at this time?
2. How is the patient hand-over communication conducted? What personnel are involved? Were the essential elements included?
3. What nursing diagnoses are likely to be identified for this patient in the early postoperative period?

Benefits of service learning to students include developing skills in communication, critical thinking, and collaboration; developing a community perspective and commitment to health promotion in the community; awareness of diversity and cultural dynamics; and increased student engagement, fostering civic engagement and social justice, developing leadership abilities, and professional development and self-discovery (Groh, Stallwood, & Daniels, 2011). Benefits to the community include having control of the service provided and recipients of service becoming better able to serve themselves and be served by their own actions.

The Pew Health Professions Commission (1993) report, *Health Professions Education for the Future,* recommended that service learning be incorporated into university nursing education to meet the increasing demand of community-based health care needs. As nursing education programs include more community-based learning activities, opportunities to incorporate service learning increase. Meaningful community-based service learning opportunities are based on relationships between the academic unit and the community to be served. For such partnerships to work effectively, there must be a good fit between the academic unit's mission and goals and the needs of the community.

Exhibit 7.2

EXAMPLE OF STUDENT EVALUATION OF A GUIDED OBSERVATION ACTIVITY

Student Evaluation of Operating Room Observation

1. To what extent did you prepare for this learning activity?
   ___ I completed all assigned readings and attempted answers to all questions on the first section of the observation guide.
   ___ I completed all assigned readings and attempted to answer some of the observation guide questions.
   ___ I completed some of the assigned readings and attempted to answer some of the observation guide questions.
   ___ I didn't do any reading, but I tried to answer some of the observation guide questions before I came to the operating room.
   ___ I didn't do any reading, and I didn't answer any observation guide questions before I came to the operating room.

2. How would you rate the overall value of this learning activity?
   ___ It was excellent; I learned a great deal.
   ___ It was very good; I learned more than I expected to.
   ___ It was good; I learned about as much as I expected to.
   ___ It was fair; I didn't learn as much as I expected to.
   ___ It was poor; I didn't learn anything of value.

3. How would you rate the value of the observation guide in helping you to prepare for and participate in the observation?
   ___ Extremely helpful in focusing my attention on significant aspects of perioperative nursing care.
   ___ Very helpful in guiding me to observe activities in the operating room.
   ___ Helpful in guiding my observations but at times distracted my attention from what I wanted to watch.
   ___ Only a little helpful; it seemed like a lot of work for little benefit.
   ___ Not at all helpful; it distracted me more than it helped me to observe what was going on in the operating room.

4. How would you rate the helpfulness of the instructor who guided your operating room observation?
   ___ Excellent; helped me to analyze, synthesize, and evaluate the activities I observed.
   ___ Very good; answered my questions and focused my attention on important activities.
   ___ Good; was able to answer some questions, attempted to make the activity meaningful to me.
   ___ Fair; I probably could have learned as much without an instructor present.
   ___ Poor; distracted me or interfered with my learning; I could have learned more without an instructor present.

(continued)

5. What was the most meaningful part of this learning activity for you? What was the most important or surprising thing you learned?
6. What was the least meaningful part of this observation activity? If there is something that you would change, suggest a specific change to make it better.

As is true for any other clinical learning activity, planning for a service-learning activity begins with the teacher's decision that such learning activities would help students to achieve one or more course outcomes. The teacher should determine how much time to allot to this activity, keeping in mind that the time spent in service learning would replace and not add to the total time available for other clinical activities for that course.

Before students participate in a service-learning activity, they may prepare a learning contract that includes:

- The name of the community agency or group
- The clients or recipients of that agency's or group's services
- The services to be provided by the student
- A service objective related to a need that has been identified by the community or the community recipient of the proposed service
- A learning objective that is related to a course outcome, goal, or competency that the activity would help the student to achieve

Students may seek community groups and agencies where they believe they could meet their learning needs, or the instructor may develop a list of such agencies and groups appropriate for a specific course, from which students may choose a site. Examples of community settings and agencies that would be appropriate for service learning include daycare centers, extended care or assisted living centers, senior centers, Meals on Wheels, the American Red Cross, Head Start, and a camp for children with disabilities, among many others.

As another option, a group of students enrolled in the same course could be placed in a community setting to participate in a designated population-based project relevant to the course objectives. For example, Bassi (2011) described a service-learning activity in which a group of nursing students participated in a tobacco-prevention project at an elementary school in their community. The students' service was counted as their final course project for their public health nursing course. Benefits of this service-learning activity included:

- Creation of a partnership between the nursing education program and the elementary school community

- Student attainment of desired course outcomes of understanding and addressing community health needs
- Increased student confidence in their patient teaching abilities
- Students' sense of accomplishment and satisfaction with the opportunity to give back to the community. (Bassi, 2011)

Because service learning is more than expecting students to use some of their clinical practice hours for service projects, clinical teachers should plan to spend as much time planning these activities as they do traditional clinical learning activities. Even though the teacher will not be present with the students during the learning activity, the teacher must allow time to read and give feedback to students' reflective journal entries about their experiences or to participate in face-to-face individual or group reflective sessions. Teachers may require students to do presentations about their service-learning projects, which the teachers would observe and evaluate—another time requirement to consider. Faculty members must also continue to interact with members of the community to evaluate the outcomes of service learning from the perspective of the recipients of service and to continually nurture the partnerships that were established.

SUMMARY

This chapter presented a framework for selecting clinical learning assignments. Clinical teachers should select clinical assignments that are related to desired learning outcomes, appropriate to students' levels of knowledge and skill, and challenging enough to motivate learning. Providing comprehensive nursing care to one or more patients is a typical clinical assignment, but it is not always the most appropriate choice.

Clinical teachers typically speak of selecting patients for clinical assignments. However, the primary role of the nursing student in the clinical area is that of learner, not nurse. Caring for patients is not synonymous with learning. Nursing students are *learning to care* for patients; they are not nurses with *responsibility for patient care*. In fact, early responsibility for patient care often creates anxiety that interferes with learning.

Factors affecting the selection of clinical assignments include the learning objectives of the clinical activity; needs of patients; availability and variety of learning opportunities in the clinical environment; and the needs, interests, and abilities of learners. The most important criterion for selection of clinical assignments is usually the desired learning outcome. Each clinical activity should be an integral part of the course or educational program, and it is essential that the clinical teacher, students, and staff members understand the goals of each clinical activity. Learning activities are selected and structured so that they relate logically and sequentially to the desired outcome.

Individual learner characteristics such as education level; previous experience; aptitude for learning; learning style; and specific needs, interests, and abilities should also influence the selection of clinical assignments. All learners do not have the same needs, so it is unreasonable to expect them to have the same learning assignments on any given day. Students who are able to achieve the objectives of the essential curriculum might quickly receive assignments from the enrichment curriculum that allow them to focus on their individual needs and interests.

Patient needs and care requirements should also be considered when planning clinical assignments. The nursing care activities required by a patient may not present enough of a challenge to one learner and may be too complex for another. Patient wishes regarding student assignment should be respected. Nursing staff members who have provided care to these patients can often help the clinical teacher determine whether student learning needs and specific patient and family needs can both be met through a particular clinical assignment.

Another factor affecting the selection of clinical assignments is the timing and availability of learning opportunities. Ideally, clinical learning activities are scheduled concurrently with relevant classroom content so that learners can apply knowledge to nursing practice immediately. The usual schedule of activities in the clinical facility may determine the optimum timing of learning activities. Some clinical settings are available to both patients and students only at certain times. In other settings, however, scheduling clinical activities during evening or nighttime hours or on weekends provides better learning opportunities.

Alternatives for making clinical assignments include selection by teacher or learner, focus on particular skills or integrative patient care, various student–patient ratio options, management activities, guided observation, and service learning. Advantages and drawbacks of each alternative were discussed.

Exhibit 7.3

CNE EXAMINATION TEST BLUEPRINT CORE COMPETENCIES

1. **Facilitate Learning**

    A. Implement a variety of teaching strategies appropriate to
        1. content
        2. setting
        3. learner needs
        4. learning style
        5. desired learner outcomes

(continued)

E. Practice skilled oral and written (including electronic) communication that reflects an awareness of self and relationships with learners (e.g., evaluation, mentorship, and supervision)

H. Create opportunities for learners to develop their own critical thinking skills

K. Demonstrate personal attributes that facilitate learning (e.g., caring, confidence, patience, integrity, respect, and flexibility)

P. Act as a role model in practice settings

2. **Facilitate Learner Development and Socialization**

B. Provide resources for diverse learners to meet their individual learning needs

D. Create learning environments that facilitate learners' self-reflection, personal goal setting, and socialization to the role of the nurse

E. Foster the development of learners in these areas:
   1. cognitive domain
   2. psychomotor domain
   3. affective domain

3. **Use Assessment and Evaluation Strategies**

L. Provide timely, constructive, and thoughtful feedback to learners

4. **Participate in Curriculum Design and Evaluation of Program Outcomes**

H. Collaborate with community and clinical partners to support educational goals

REFERENCES

Bassi, S. (2011). Undergraduate nursing students' perceptions of service-learning through a school-based community project. *Nursing Education Perspectives, 32,* 162–167.

Di Leonardi, B. C., & Oermann, M. H. (2010). Teaching in a clinical setting. In L. Caputi (Ed.), *Teaching nursing: The art and science* (pp. 82–141). Glen Ellyn, IL: College of DuPage Press.

Gardner, M. R., & Suplee, P. D. (2010). *Handbook of clinical teaching in nursing and health sciences.* Sudbury, MA: Jones and Bartlett.

Groh, C. J., Stallwood, L. G., & Daniels, J. J. (2011). Service-learning in nursing education: Its impact on leadership and social justice. *Nursing Education Perspectives, 32,* 400–405.

Infante, M. S. (1985). *The clinical laboratory in nursing education* (2nd ed.). New York, NY: Wiley.

National League for Nursing. (2008). *NLN think tank on transforming clinical nursing education.* New York, NY: Author.

Pew Health Professions Commission. (1993). *Health professions education for the future: Schools in service to the community.* San Francisco, CA: UCSF Center for the Health Professions.

CHAPTER 8

Self-Directed Learning Activities

Some outcomes of clinical courses may be met by students through self-directed learning activities. These activities may involve instructional media such as videos on DVDs and CDs, computer-assisted instruction (CAI), virtual reality, web-based methods, learning objects, independent study, and others. Faculty members have a wealth of instructional technologies to integrate in their clinical courses for students to acquire the prerequisite knowledge and skills, for review, and for learning new concepts and skills, among other uses.

Many individual differences among nursing students influence how they learn. Some students enter a clinical course with extensive knowledge and skills, while others may lack the prerequisite behaviors for engaging in the learning activities. Differences in learning styles, preferences for teaching methods, cultural and ethnic backgrounds, and pace of learning all suggest a need for self-directed activities that reflect these individual variations among learners. With these activities, the responsibility for learning rests with the student.

There are varied types of self-directed activities for use in clinical teaching. Many of these activities are based on multimedia and instructional technology; others, such as a literature review and critique, may not incorporate media. Self-directed activities may be required for completion by all students to meet the outcomes of the clinical course or for use by individual students for reinforcement of learning, continued practice of skills, and remedial instruction. This chapter reviews self-directed learning activities appropriate for clinical teaching. The reader should recognize, however, that the activities involving multimedia are changing rapidly, and new technologies are continually being introduced for teaching and learning in clinical practice.

USING SELF-DIRECTED LEARNING ACTIVITIES

Self-directed learning activities are what the term suggests—activities directed by the students themselves. Although they may be planned by the teacher as part of the clinical activities or recommended to meet specific learning needs, self-directed activities are intended for completion by the students on their own. These activities are typically self-contained units of instruction that students complete independently, often in a setting of their choice, and according to their own time frame. CAI, for instance, may be completed in a computer or learning laboratory, at home, or in virtually any location in which students can use a mobile computing device at a time convenient for the student. The learner may move through the instruction at a fast or slow pace depending on the learning needs, and may repeat content and activities until the competency is achieved. Many self-directed activities also include pre- and posttests for students to assess their progress and learning at the end of the instruction.

Self-directed activities may be planned for completion by all students to meet certain clinical outcomes or by students on an individual basis to reflect their particular learning needs. For some clinical courses and rotations, all students may be required to complete self-directed activities as a means of acquiring essential knowledge for practice and developing course competencies. These activities, then, would be integrated in the clinical course during its development.

When students lack prerequisite knowledge and skills or when remedial instruction is warranted for some students but not others, self-directed activities provide a means of meeting these learning needs without requiring all students to complete the same learning activities. In these instances, the self-directed activities assist individual students in gaining the knowledge and skills they need for practice. Self-directed activities, therefore, are an important adjunct to clinical teaching.

Along with allowing students to learn in a setting of their choice and at a time convenient for them, self-directed activities encourage them to assume responsibility for their own learning, an important outcome of nursing programs. As students progress through a nursing program, they may encounter outcomes that they are unable to meet because they lack the prerequisites for learning or need to review or practice their skills further. By identifying personal learning needs and seeking opportunities to meet them, students begin to develop skills they can use in the future, when confronted with questions about nursing practice they are unable to answer and competencies they need to develop. Nursing education programs provide the knowledge and competencies for entry into practice, but nurses need to be self-directed so they can keep current in their practice.

Although beneficial for students, self-directed learning requires their commitment and motivation. The teacher may plan strategies, such as regular reflective journal submissions, to monitor student progress in completing the learning activities, provide feedback, and assist students in developing self-discipline. In some courses, faculty members may establish time frames for completion of certain activities to better monitor progress and assure completion by the end of the clinical course.

Using Self-Directed Activities for Cognitive Skill Development

Self-directed activities that depict clinical situations and patient care scenarios are particularly effective for promoting problem-solving and higher level thinking skills. After viewing the clinical situation presented in media, multimedia, or through other technologies, students may be asked to:

- Identify the problems and issues to be solved and provide a supporting rationale.
- Identify alternative problems that might be possible in the clinical situation.
- Differentiate relevant and irrelevant information.
- Develop careful and pointed questions to further clarify the problems and issues.
- Identify additional data needed for decision making.
- Identify multiple approaches for solving the clinical problems and issues, possible alternative approaches, and advantages and disadvantages of each.
- Compare the various decisions possible in a clinical situation and their outcomes.
- Decide on the approach they would use or decision they would make and provide a rationale underlying their thinking.
- Examine how key concepts and theories apply to the clinical situation depicted in the media or multimedia.
- Analyze the clinical scenario using concepts and theories described in class, in readings, and through other learning activities as a way of transferring learning to clinical practice.
- Identify assumptions made and how these influenced thinking.
- Articulate different points of view. (Oermann & Gaberson, 2014)

Using Self-Directed Activities for Values Development

Media and multimedia are effective for teaching students professional nursing values and for students to examine their beliefs and values that might influence their patient care. By viewing clinical situations depicted in video clips, at websites, and in other types of media, students can gain awareness of other people's circumstances and their own values and beliefs. Students enter nursing programs with personal values and preset ideas that may influence their care and decisions they make in clinical practice. Analysis of scenarios shown in media provides a safe way for students to become more aware of their own value systems and beliefs. Through open-ended questions and a safe environment in which to discuss beliefs and feelings, students can begin to explore their values and how they might affect decisions in clinical practice.

PLANNING SELF-DIRECTED ACTIVITIES

Although self-directed activities are completed by students independently, the teacher is responsible for planning those activities as part of the clinical course or recommending them for students to meet individual learning needs. Self-directed learning activities, similar to other types of clinical activities, should be consistent with the outcomes of the clinical course or competencies that students develop in that course. The main reason for their use in a course is their potential to assist students in achieving certain outcomes.

In planning self-directed activities, the teacher should consider the resources needed for their implementation. These resources include costs for developing materials, purchasing commercially available materials, and supporting software and hardware; equipment needed; space, such as computer and other laboratories, considering the numbers of students in the program; other requirements associated with using a particular technology; and resources needed by students. Many of these activities are now done on the web and are easily integrated into course management systems; however, students' computer resources need to be taken into account. The time required for completion is another consideration in planning these activities for a course. The teacher should monitor the time students take for each activity so this information is available for planning at a later time.

One way of ensuring effective planning and use of self-directed activities in a clinical course is to follow the acronym PLAN:

Plan activities that assist students in meeting the outcomes of the clinical course, individual learning needs, or both.

Link these activities with the resources of the nursing program and those needed by students.

Assess prerequisite knowledge and skills for initiating the self-directed activities, students' progress as they complete them, and learning outcomes.

Never assume that students will learn at the same rate and in the same way; allow for individualization in types of learning activities, rates of learning, and outcomes.

When incorporating self-directed activities in clinical courses, students should have directions regarding specific activities to complete and due dates if required in the clinical course. It is also helpful to students to indicate how these particular activities promote achievement of the outcomes of the course and how they will be assessed, if at all.

TYPES OF SELF-DIRECTED LEARNING ACTIVITIES

It is beyond the scope of this chapter to describe in detail all of the self-directed activities available for clinical teaching, particularly when considering the rapid growth of computer, web-based, and other instructional technologies. Although a number of self-directed methods are reviewed in this chapter, they are only a sampling of these methods and discussion of how they might be used in clinical teaching. In this chapter, self-directed activities are categorized as instructional media, multimedia, learning objects, and independent study. There are different ways of grouping these methods for presentation; this categorization represents only one way. The reader should also recognize that many of these methods use more than one technology; for instance, a computer simulation may include video, audio, and other media.

Instructional Media

Many types of instructional media are available for clinical teaching. Media include static models or visual representations such as photographs, charts, posters, and handouts; moving visuals such as DVDs; and audio media such as CDs, real audio, and podcasts. Exhibit 8.1 provides a list of different instructional media that can be used in clinical teaching.

Instructional media promotes learning through different senses, facilitating comprehension of difficult concepts and complex skills. Media that depict patient scenarios help students understand how concepts and theories are used in clinical practice and give them an idea of what a clinical situation is like. This vicarious experience prepares learners for the reality of clinical practice. It also allows students to think critically about a situation and possible decisions that could be made.

Exhibit 8.1

TYPES OF INSTRUCTIONAL MEDIA

Models

Nonprojected still visuals
  Brochure and pamphlet
  Diagram
  Handout and other types of written materials
  Photograph
  Poster

Projected still visuals
  Document camera
  Digital camera
  Overhead transparency
  Slide
  Whiteboard

Audio technologies
  Audiotape
  CD
  Podcast
  Real audio

Video technologies
  CD
  DVD
  Film
  Video on the web

Multimedia
  CD-ROM
  CAI and other computer technology
  DVD
  Podcast
  Virtual reality
  The web

Another important use of instructional media in clinical teaching is the ability to present clinical situations involving ethical dilemmas and value conflicts for students to analyze. When media are used in this way, students gain experience in analyzing and responding to an ethical dilemma before encountering it in actual practice. Instructional media for this purpose also provides a means for students to examine their values and beliefs that may influence care of patients and their interactions with staff and others in the practice setting.

Instructional media effectively shows clinical situations that would be inaccessible to students. With technological skills, instructional media provides a way of demonstrating the use of equipment and how to carry out a procedure in the clinical setting, emphasizing critical elements of performance.

Multimedia

Multimedia, another type of instructional media, includes CAI; CD-ROMs, DVDs, and similar technologies; virtual reality; websites; and many others. Multimedia are the combination of video, audio, text, and/or graphics. Multimedia, similar to media, may be used by all students to meet clinical learning outcomes or by individual students. Many multimedia programs are interactive, providing feedback to students on their responses and engaging students actively in the learning process. The most important characteristic of multimedia is its ability to deliver effective and flexible instruction that attracts learners' interest, keeps their attention, and accommodates different learning styles.

Prior to using any multimedia for clinical teaching, the teacher should evaluate their content, including accuracy, organization, clarity in presenting the content, and comprehensiveness; relevance to the clinical course and clinical learning outcomes; usefulness for meeting individual student needs; currency in terms of clinical practice; extent of interaction between student and multimedia; cost; and resources needed for effective implementation (Exhibit 8.2). One other aspect of this evaluation relates to the appropriateness of the content for the clinical setting; with some multimedia, students may need to adapt interventions and procedures to their own clinical settings.

Exhibit 8.2

EVALUATION OF MEDIA AND MULTIMEDIA FOR CLINICAL TEACHING

Is the instructional media:

- Relevant to the clinical course? Relevant to clinical learning outcomes? Relevant to clinical settings where students have practice?
- Useful for meeting individual student needs?
- Able to be modified or adapted to better meet the objectives and learner needs?
- Of high technical quality (e.g., graphics, sounds, etc.)?

(continued)

- The student is provided the opportunity for a fair, impartial hearing on the charges. Students have the right to speak on their own behalf, to present witnesses and evidence, and to question the other participants in the case (usually teachers and administrators). Using the example above, the student might present evidence that she did attempt to call the faculty member to report her absence; this evidence could include the date and time of the call, the name of the person with whom she spoke, and a copy of a telephone bill verifying the date, time, and number called. Although the student and the faculty member are entitled to the advice of legal counsel, neither attorney may question or cross examine witnesses.
- The student has the right to appeal an unfavorable decision by the hearing panel to an appeals panel or a designated administrator. Usually, this administrator or, ultimately, the university or college president has the authority to make the final decision (Smith, 2012).

If the final decision is to uphold the dismissal, students have the right to seek remedy from the court system if they believe that due process was not followed. However, in disciplinary cases, the burden of proof that due process was denied rests with the student.

Negligence, Liability, and Unsafe Clinical Practice

When determining whether a given action meets the criteria for professional negligence, the overall standard of care is what an ordinary, reasonable, and prudent person would have done in the same context. The standard of care for a nursing student is not what another nursing student would have done; students are held to the same standards of care as registered nurses (RNs). The NCSBN Model Nurse Practice Act (2012a), Article V, Section 10 includes the statement that the nurse practice act does not prohibit the practice of nursing by a student in an approved nursing education program as long as the student "is under the auspices of the program [and] . . . acts under the supervision of an RN serving for the program as a faculty member or teaching assistant" (p. 7). Another section of the Model Act (Article VII, Section 2) states that each nurse is required to know and adhere to the requirements of the nurse practice act, that nurses are accountable for their decisions based on their education and experience, and that nurses must practice with reasonable skill and safety. The concept of personal liability also applies to cases of professional negligence. Each person is responsible for his or her own behavior, including negligent acts. Students are liable for their own actions as long as they are performing according to the usual standard of care for their education and experience, and they seek

Is the content:

- Accurate?
- Organized logically?
- Presented clearly?
- Comprehensive?
- In sufficient depth for clinical course and learners?
- Up to date and consistent with current practice guidelines and recommendations?

Does the instruction:

- Provide for interaction with the student?
- Give immediate feedback and reinforcement?
- Maintain student interest?
- Allow for entering and exiting the program as needed?
- Adapt for individual student needs?

Is the cost (to the student or nursing education program or both) worth the investment?

Are there sufficient resources for implementation?

CAI

There are many types of CAI programs for use in nursing education. CAI may be used to present new content important for clinical practice, to promote application of concepts and theories to simulated clinical situations, as a review prior to clinical practice, and to provide remedial instruction for individual students. With some CAI, students can practice problem solving and decision making in simulated scenarios. One main use of CAI is to guide students in applying concepts that they are learning in face-to-face and online courses to clinical situations and gaining experience in thinking through those situations before encountering them in clinical practice.

There are many CAI programs, and teachers need to be aware of what is available in their nursing education programs, clinical settings, or on the web when they plan their courses. With this information, clinical teachers can integrate CAI within clinical courses and recommend specific programs to students when they need additional instruction or review. Often CAI programs incorporate questions for feedback to students, indicating which answers and decisions are correct or incorrect and why. The questions and answers also provide reinforcement for learning as students progress through the instruction. When not included with the CAI, faculty members can develop ways to provide feedback for student self-assessment. Another advantage of CAI is that students can pace themselves through the instruction.

Two types of CAI include tutorials and simulations.

- *Tutorials* instruct students on new concepts and generally include questions to review the content. Students then get feedback based on their responses. Tutorials using branching techniques allow students to move forward to learn new content or backward if remedial instruction is needed. For clinical teaching, tutorials may be used to present new content for practice or for remedial instruction.
- *Simulations* present a real-life situation for analysis and decision making. With a simulation, students make a series of clinical decisions similar to those needed in actual practice and receive immediate feedback on them. With some simulations, the learners' decisions influence subsequent information presented. Simulations are particularly appropriate for gaining practice in identifying data to collect, analyzing data in a simulated clinical situation, identifying problems and interventions, evaluating outcomes, and developing critical thinking and technological skills.

Human patient simulators (HPSs) are being used increasingly in nursing education programs. These provide opportunities for students to develop knowledge and competencies for clinical practice, make clinical decisions in real time, develop technological skills not possible in many clinical settings, practice in a safe environment, develop collaboration skills, and achieve many other clinical outcomes (Campbell & Daley, 2009; Dillon, Noble, & Kaplan, 2009; Jeffries, McNelis, & Wheeler, 2008; Kardong-Edgren, Starkweather, & Ward, 2008). Students may schedule individual or small group practice sessions in simulation labs with appropriate HPSs after being oriented to the use of the equipment. Because feedback is important in skill development, a lab supervisor or teaching assistant may be present, especially if the simulation lab policies prohibit student use of equipment without guidance. Another way of providing feedback is for the student to videorecord the practice session and review it later either privately, with peers, or with a clinical teacher. However, this activity is self-directed because the student is responsible for scheduling and completing the activity, and may be responsible for identifying the need for this additional practice. Simulations are discussed more extensively in Chapter 9.

CD-ROMs, DVDs, and Related Technologies

Many CD-ROMs, DVDs, and related technologies are available for use in clinical teaching across all levels of nursing education. Some of these resources teach skills such as measuring vital signs, administering medications, and inserting and discontinuing IVs. For example, the multimedia program *IV Therapy* (FITNE Inc., 2009), which is available online or as a CD-ROM, teaches students about various delivery systems for IVs; uses videos to show how to start, maintain, and discontinue IVs; and explains complications of IV therapy and the nurse's role in preventing them.

As discussed in Chapter 10, many textbook publishers provide supplemental student learning resources on CD or via the web. These resources are designed to be used independently by students to explore their individual interests or facilitate additional practice of skills. Standardized testing and remediation packages also provide opportunities for self-directed learning, especially in response to knowledge gaps identified by the assessment procedures.

With these types of multimedia programs, faculty members can expose students to care of patients and clinical situations that they may not have an opportunity to experience in the clinical setting. For example, not all students in a course may have a chance to care for a child with a critical illness or an adult patient on dialysis. By viewing a CD-ROM or DVD on care of these patients, students can acquire essential knowledge, learn about typical interventions and why they are used in the patient's care, review related medication and treatments, and analyze related clinical scenarios. They can be completed by students independently, not taking in-class or online instruction time.

Virtual Reality

In virtual reality, scenes that represent a real situation are displayed on a computer screen, and learners have an opportunity to actively participate in them. Visualization on the computer screen simulates what the patient or procedure would look like in an actual clinical situation. Often the virtual reality system includes software packages with different scenarios to enhance students' learning and practice of skills. As students practice procedures, they receive audible feedback about their technique and decisions.

Schmidt and Stewart (2009) described how they introduced a virtual environment called Second Life in their accelerated nursing program, using it in their online courses as part of their class sessions, for discussions and meetings with students, and for other purposes. Eventually, the faculty intends to develop various clinical scenarios for analysis by students. In Chapter 10, virtual reality is described in more detail with examples of how it can be used in clinical education.

The Web

The web is a multimedia platform for accessing information that is organized in relationship to other information, enabling students to retrieve it quickly and easily through different paths. The web gives learners access to evidence and literature related to patient care, enables them to find answers to questions about patient problems and clinical situations, and allows students to find information appropriate for their own learning needs and interests. The web provides a wealth of instructional resources that can be used in clinical teaching, such as illustrations, photos, digital imaging, and video clips. When learning about a clinical concept, students can be directed to a website to view that concept.

Many courses in nursing are now web-based, allowing teachers to make their web courses multisensory and multidimensional, incorporating audio, video, photos, animation, and other multimedia in them. The web has opened many opportunities for self-directed activities to support clinical learning. Students may communicate with each other in the clinical group and with the teacher through e-mail, Twitter, instant messaging, discussion boards, and computer conferences. They may also analyze cases and clinical issues in online discussions in small groups set up by the teacher.

Students may be directed to websites related to the clinical objectives or to explore specific clinical issues faced in their practice. In the beginning of a clinical course, for example, students may explore sites relevant to the area of clinical practice, such as oncology nursing, and evaluate each site for its usefulness in caring for these patients, in patient education, and for their own learning. If resources are available, self-directed activities on the web are limited only by the teacher's and students' creativity and willingness to explore new technologies.

Mobile Computing Devices and Personal Digital Assistants

The use of handheld technology continues to increase rapidly in society in general, health care, and higher education. Therefore it should be no surprise that current nursing students own and use at least one of these devices. The presence of personal digital assistants (PDAs), smartphones, and tablet devices in the classroom and in clinical areas is a source of concern and even alarm among some nurse educators (Skiba, 2011). However, because most nursing students today are digital natives and are more familiar with the technology than their teachers are, they may have been using it for self-directed learning in both classroom and clinical settings for some time. The literature supports the use of PDAs as effective teaching-learning tools (Zurmehly, 2010), and mobile learning technology allows students to participate in "situated, contextual, just-in-time, participatory, and personalized learning" (Skiba, 2011, p. 195). Clinical teachers should harness the power of this technology and use it to engage students in self-directed clinical learning.

Mobile learning on handheld devices is useful as a self-directed learning tool because:

- In clinical and simulation lab settings, students can access what they need to learn when they need to learn it within a particular context
- It promotes active, collaborative learning, self-efficacy, and student engagement
- It supports the achievement of the intended program outcome of being a lifelong learner
- It is appropriate for all learning styles—verbal, visual, auditory, and kinesthetic
- It helps to build communities of practice beyond the classrooms and clinical settings provided to students
- Most students already know how to use the devices. (Skiba, 2011; Wyatt et al., 2010; Zurmehly, 2010)

However, some disadvantages of using these devices in clinical learning must be acknowledged (Skiba, 2011; Zurmehly, 2010). These include:

- Cost of the devices and the data plans required to use them.
- Teachers often are not as familiar with the devices as their students are, and thus fail to see the potential in their use for self-directed learning. The need for faculty development in this area is evident.
- Policies in clinical agencies may prohibit or block use of mobile technology, limiting the learning spaces in which they can be used.
- The potential for distraction by interrupting a self-directed learning activity with personal matters (e.g., phone calls, e-mails, messages).

- Wi-fi access might not be available in every potential learning space, including many community and patient home settings. Although portable wi-fi "hot spots" are available for mobile devices, these add to the cost of the technology.

Suggestions for using mobile technology in self-directed clinical learning activities include:

- Facilitating student orientation to clinical learning sites (Zurmehly, 2010). Students can be directed to a clinical facility's website to obtain driving directions, public transportation information, parking options, building maps or floorplans, and similar information.
- Promoting the use of these devices to obtain up-to-date clinical information, including recommended practices, guidelines, consensus statements, and position statements, at the point of care to allow students to provide care consistent with high-quality, reliable scientific evidence (De Natale & Malloy, 2012; Doran et al., 2010).
- Use of mobile devices to access information from databases and reference books, especially in regard to up-to-the-minute, accurate information about drugs and public health concerns, which may prevent health care errors, reduce health care–acquired infections, and enhance public health surveillance (Zurmehly, 2010).

GUIDELINES FOR USING MULTIMEDIA

With the wealth of multimedia available for clinical teaching, the teacher should first evaluate the quality and appropriateness of the multimedia for the intended learning outcomes. Not all multimedia are of high quality, nor are they all appropriate for the objectives or meeting learner needs. Other guidelines for using multimedia for clinical teaching are:

- Evaluate the currency of the multimedia content and its congruence with recommended clinical practices and guidelines.
- Prepare objectives to be achieved through completion of the multimedia.
- Consider assigning or recommending selected parts of a multimedia program that are most appropriate for the learning outcomes rather than the entire program.

- When parts of a multimedia program are used and when students complete multiple learning activities, provide written guidelines for them to follow that include the sequence for completing the activities. These guidelines direct students through varied activities and segments of a program, similar to a map.
- Plan for some of the activities involving multimedia to be completed in pairs or small groups. Small group discussions about the content and possible answers to questions posed in the multimedia and the exchange of ideas about problems, approaches, and multiple ways of viewing clinical situations encourage problem solving, decision making, critical thinking, and collaborative learning and practice. These discussions can be conducted online.
- Consider carefully the resources needed for effective implementation of the multimedia. For programs completed in a computer or learning laboratory, students can work in pairs and small groups to ease the burden for adequate hardware and software.
- Develop questions for students to answer as they progress through the multimedia and at the end of the instruction if feedback questions and a posttest are not already included. If the teacher intends for the multimedia to be used independently by students, then answers with a rationale should be included with the questions. The teacher should first review the multimedia program, because many will have questions integrated throughout for student response. Questions may also be written to link the multimedia to the specific clinical objectives and help students relate the content to the clinical setting and types of clients for whom they are learning to care.
- Provide an opportunity for students to evaluate the multimedia from a learner's perspective in terms of quality and usefulness in developing knowledge and skills for clinical practice.

FACULTY DEVELOPMENT

In many nursing education programs and clinical settings, nurse educators are not prepared to use new technologies in their teaching. There is a need in this area for faculty development, and educators should be alert to initiatives designed to introduce technologies in nursing education and prepare faculty for their use. There are web-based resources that faculty members can use to get ideas about multimedia and other technologies for teaching and to keep current. For example, EDUCAUSE is a nonprofit organization that promotes the use of technologies in higher education (www.educause.edu).

LEARNING OBJECTS

Learning objects are small units of learning that are reusable—that is, one learning object may be used in different situations and courses and enhanced for more complex learning. With learning objects, the outcomes and content to be learned can be divided into small units of instruction that can be reused in different learning situations. Although learning objects are self-contained and can thus be completed independently, they can also be grouped together into broader and more extensive collections of content.

Learning objects are developed to teach a single learning concept or objective (Lymn, Bath-Hextall, & Wharrad, 2008). Many types of learning objects can be designed for use in clinical courses such as digital photographs of patients, conditions, procedures, and clinical situations; video clips to teach clinical concepts; case studies for analysis with critical thinking questions; hyperlinks to web pages and Internet resources; simulations; interactive games; and units of content taught with multimedia.

Learning objects are valuable resources for use in distance education clinical courses and other web-based courses. They can be stored in repositories or libraries of learning objects. Because they can be reused, faculty members can access these repositories as they are planning their clinical courses and can direct students to them to meet individual learning goals. MERLOT (Multimedia Educational Resource for Learning and Online Teaching; healthsciences.merlot.org/index.html) is a free resource for faculty members and students that contains links to online learning objects in nursing with peer reviews and assignments.

INDEPENDENT STUDY

Independent study allows students freedom in deciding their own learning goals, strategies for learning, and how the learning outcomes will be assessed as part of the clinical course. The teacher and student typically collaborate on the objectives to be met through independent study so that they relate to the clinical goals and are reasonable within the time frame. A contract may be established between the teacher and student outlining the goals to be met through the independent study project, types of learning activities to be completed, assessment methods and products of learning to be submitted as part of the clinical course, and dates for completion of these. Independent study is particularly useful when students want to explore a new area of clinical practice or a patient problem and interventions in depth.

SUMMARY

Many clinical objectives and competencies may be met by students through self-directed learning activities. Whether planned by the teacher as part of the clinical activities or recommended to meet specific learning needs, self-directed activities are intended for completion by the students on their own. These activities are typically self-contained units that students complete independently, often in a setting of their choice and according to their own time frame. Self-directed activities encourage them to assume responsibility for their own learning, an important outcome of nursing programs.

Self-directed activities may be completed by all students to meet certain clinical competencies or by students on an individual basis to reflect their particular learning needs. Similar to other types of learning activities, they should be consistent with the outcomes of the clinical course.

In planning self-directed activities, the teacher should consider the resources needed for their implementation. These resources include costs for developing materials, purchasing commercially available materials, and supporting software and hardware; equipment needed; space such as computer laboratory space; other requirements associated with a particular technology; and resources needed by students. The time required for completion is another consideration in planning these activities for a course.

Self-directed activities are categorized as instructional media such as models, still visuals, audio, video, or multimedia, including CAI, CD-ROM, DVDs, virtual reality, and the web; learning objects; and independent study. Instructional media promotes learning through different senses, making it easier to comprehend difficult concepts. Instructional media that depicts patient care scenarios helps students understand how concepts and theories are used in practice and gives them an idea of what a clinical situation is like. This vicarious experience prepares learners for the reality of clinical practice. Many new instructional technologies can be used for clinical teaching. It is up to the teacher to be creative and willing to integrate these into clinical courses.

Other types of self-directed activities are learning objects and independent study. Learning objects are small units of learning that are reusable—that is, one learning object may be used in different situations and courses. Independent study allows students freedom in deciding on their own learning goals, strategies for learning, and how the outcomes will be assessed as part of the clinical course.

| Exhibit 8.3 |

CNE EXAMINATION TEST BLUEPRINT CORE COMPETENCIES

1. **Facilitate Learning**

   A. Implement a variety of teaching strategies appropriate to
      1. content
      2. setting
      3. learner needs
      4. learning style
      5. desired learner outcomes

   B. Use teaching strategies based on
      1. educational theory
      2. evidence-based practices related to education

   C. Modify teaching strategies and learning experiences based on consideration of learners'
      2. past clinical experiences
      3. past educational and life experiences
      4. generational groups (i.e., age)

   D. Use information technologies to support the teaching-learning process

   N. Use knowledge of evidence-based practice to instruct learners

2. **Facilitate Learner Development and Socialization**

   B. Provide resources for diverse learners to meet their individual learning needs

   D. Create learning environments that facilitate learners' self-reflection, personal goal-setting, and socialization to the role of the nurse

   E. Foster the development of learners in these areas
      1. cognitive domain
      2. psychomotor domain
      3. affective domain

6. **Engage in Scholarship, Service, and Leadership**

   A. Function as a change agent and leader
      5. Implement strategies for change within the nursing program
      7. Adapt to changes created by external factors

REFERENCES

Campbell, S. H., & Daley, K. M. (2009). *Simulation scenarios for nurse educator: Making it real*. New York, NY: Springer Publishing.
De Natale, M. L., & Malloy, S. E. (2012). The use of position statements in teaching best practices in nursing. *Nursing Education Perspectives, 33*, 378–380.

Dillon, P. M., Noble, K. A., & Kaplan, L. (2009). Simulation as a means to foster collabora-tive interdisciplinary education. *Nursing Education Perspectives, 30,* 87–90.

Doran, D., Haynes, B., Kushniruk, A., Straus, S., Grimshaw, J., McGillis, L . . . Jedras, D. (2010). Supporting evidence-based practice for nurses through information technologies. *Worldviews on Evidence-Based Nursing, 7,* 4–15. doi:10.1111/j.1741-6787.2009.00181.x

FITNE Inc. (2009). *IV therapy.* Retrieved from http://www.fitne.net/vlrc4/iv_therapy.jsp

Jeffries, P. R., McNelis, A. M., & Wheeler, C. A. (2008). Simulation as a vehicle for enhanc-ing collaborative practice models. *Critical Care Nursing Clinics of North America, 20,* 471–480.

Kardong-Edgren, S., Starkweather, A., & Ward, L. (2008). The integration of simu-lation into a clinical foundations of nursing course: Student and faculty perspec-tives. *International Journal of Nursing Education Scholarship, 5*(1), article 26. doi:10.2202/1548-923X.1603

Lymn, J., Bath-Hextall, F., & Wharrad, H. (2008). Pharmacology education for nurse prescribing students: A lesson in reusable learning objects. *BMC Nursing, 7*(2). doi:10.1186/1472-6955-7-2

Oermann, M. H., & Gaberson, K. B. (2014). *Evaluation and testing in nursing education* (4th ed.). New York, NY: Springer Publishing.

Schmidt, B., & Stewart, S. (2009). Implementing the virtual reality learning environment: Second Life. *Nurse Educator, 34,* 152–155.

Skiba, D. (2011). Mobile devices: Are they a distraction of another learning tool? *Nursing Education Perspectives, 32,* 195–197.

Wyatt, T. H., Krauskopf, P. B., Gaylord, M. N., Ward, A., Huffstutler-Hawkins, S., & Goodwin, L. (2010). Cooperative m-learning with nurse practitioner students. *Nursing Education Perspectives, 31,* 109–113.

Zurmehly, J. (2010). Personal Digital Assistant (PDAs): Review and evaluation. *Nursing Education Perspectives, 31,* 179–182.

CHAPTER 9

Clinical Simulation

Teresa Shellenbarger and Debra Hagler

Clinical simulation and mannequin-based human patient simulation have become widely accepted and integrated as a part of clinical nursing education (Chronister & Brown, 2012; Neill & Wotton, 2011). Simulation activities that mimic reality allow students to develop technical skill proficiency in a safe, nonthreatening environment while contributing to student learning, enhancement of critical thinking, and problem-solving skills (Garrett, MacPhee, & Jackson, 2010; Sittner, Hertzog, & Fleck, 2013).

This use of clinical simulation comes at a time when nurse educators face numerous challenges that impact clinical teaching. An increased interest in nursing as a career has led to more applications to nursing education programs, but the number of nursing faculty members remains inadequate to meet the demand (American Association of Colleges of Nursing, 2012), creating capacity limits in classrooms and clinical settings. In addition, the health care environment has grown in complexity due to the increasing presence of technology in hospitals and, subsequently, patients with higher acuity levels who are older, frailer, and have greater comorbidity. Patients are also spending less time in the hospital, so students have less exposure to patients in the acute care hospital environment and fewer opportunities to maintain and improve their skills. Finally, a shortage of clinical space, particularly in specialty clinical areas such as obstetrics, pediatrics, and intensive care units, often limits nursing student activities to observation rather than hands-on patient care and may also restrict the number of students placed on those units for clinical learning experiences (Jeffries, Settles, Milgrom, & Woolf, 2010; Kardong-Edgren, Wilhaus, Bennett, & Hayden, 2012). Nurse educators are thus challenged to prepare students for a complex environment where they must think critically, act quickly, and communicate effectively with multidisciplinary team members. This chapter discusses how simulation can be used to enhance clinical teaching to ensure a better prepared nursing workforce. It also discusses the importance of debriefing as a critical component of clinical simulation.

BACKGROUND

Simulation using a clinical scenario "involves a student or group of students providing care for a patient who is represented by a mannequin, an actor, or an SP" (standardized patient; Jeffries, 2012, p. 3) in a realistic clinical environment. Students can demonstrate psychomotor skills, clinical reasoning, clinical judgment, problem solving, and critical thinking through techniques such as role-playing and the use of devices such as interactive videos or mannequins. Simulation allows teachers to take specific information—such as a patient's personal characteristics; health information; family components; and physical, mental, and emotional state—and weave it into a real-life scenario that enhances a student's comprehension of the material because it is meaningful (Jeffries, 2012). In the case of clinical nursing scenarios, simulation provides an opportunity to suspend belief of what is real to produce a low-risk, hands-on opportunity to practice a clinical situation involving patient monitoring, management, communication, and multidisciplinary collaboration.

In the past, simulation activities have been documented in a variety of disciplines, such as medicine, aviation, psychology, and education (Lusk & Fater, 2013). In nursing, simulation has been used for teaching in all clinical areas. Traditionally, medical–surgical and emergency resuscitations were the most commonly used scenarios in nursing programs as identified in the National Council of State Boards of Nursing (NCSBN) National Simulation Survey (Kardong-Edgren et al., 2012). Other specialty areas in nursing education, such as pediatrics, geriatrics, obstetrics, and hospice or palliative care, are now using simulation as part of the clinical experience (Johnson et al., 2012; Parker et al., 2011; Pullen et al., 2012; Simonelli & Paskausky, 2012). Simulation may never replace direct student contact with human patients, but it has the potential to make student and teacher time in clinical settings more valuable and cost effective.

The use of human patient simulators (HPSs) has become common practice in many nursing education programs. Using simulation-based pedagogy allows students to integrate psychomotor skill performance, critical thinking, clinical judgment, and communication skills while gaining self-confidence prior to entering the clinical setting. In addition, simulation offers an opportunity for evaluation and assessment of student skills with options for remediation and continued learning (Durham & Alden, 2010). The active learning component of simulation also appeals to many of today's millennial generation students, helping them to maintain engagement in the learning process and retain the material learned.

Various organizations have recognized simulation's value as a teaching technique. The Commission on Collegiate Nursing Education (CCNE) accreditation standards encourages the use of innovative teaching methods and the introduction of technology and informatics to improve student learning (CCNE, 2009). The National League for Nursing (NLN) has also provided long-standing leadership and support for simulation in nursing education, conducting a national multisite multimethod study investigating the innovative use of simulation to teach nursing care of ill adults and children (Jeffries & Rizzolo, 2006). NLN's leadership continued with the development of the Simulation Innovation Resource Center (SIRC). SIRC provides education and training about simulation while also allowing participants an opportunity to engage in dialogue with colleagues about simulation and providing resources for the development and integration of simulation into the curriculum (NLN, 2013). Lastly, the NLN Leadership Development Program for Simulation Educators offers an opportunity for experienced simulation nurse educators to examine issues related to research in simulation, curricular integration, and the role of simulation in interprofessional education (NLN, 2011). Another organization, the International Association for Clinical Simulation and Learning (INACSL), has developed simulation standards and publishes a monthly journal focusing on clinical simulation in nursing.

Additionally, the NCSBN recognizes the increased emphasis on simulation in nursing education. The NCSBN conducted a national survey to assess simulation use in the United States. Phase II of the study will investigate the role and outcomes of simulation (NCSBN, 2013). Nursing experts acknowledge the value of simulation as a teaching–learning approach that mimics reality but these experts also emphasize the need for nursing student clinical experiences with real patients, thus encouraging clinical teachers to use all available learning opportunities.

TYPES OF SIMULATORS

There are different levels of sophistication as well as a variety of types of simulators that teachers must consider when planning simulation use in nursing education. The level of simulators, categorized according to the fidelity or how closely it represents a realistic situation, can be described as low, moderate or high. Low-fidelity simulators use static tools, are less precise reproductions, and lack the realism of a clinical situation, but offer opportunities for procedural skill practice. These low-fidelity simulators are sometimes referred to as "task-trainers" (Nehring, 2010). Examples of low-fidelity simulation may involve the use of a disembodied pelvis for catheter insertion simulation or a gel pad for intramuscular injection practice. Moderate-fidelity simulators offer a more realistic reproduction of a clinical situation and provide some feedback to the student. A mannequin that produces heart and lung sounds, but does not offer the realism of chest movement, is an example of a moderate-fidelity simulator. Moderate-fidelity simulators allow students to complete an assessment but without interactive features. High-fidelity simulators produce the most lifelike scenarios. These full-size mannequins react to student manipulations in real time and in realistic ways, such as speaking, coughing, and demonstrating chest movements and pulses.

SPs represent another type of simulation used in nursing education. This form of simulation uses live actors with scripts that portray patients and require nursing students to engage in nursing care activities with the SP in an environment that simulates patient care areas (Durham & Alden, 2010). Nursing education programs affiliated with academic health centers may have SPs available to them since SPs are commonly used in medical education. Practice with SPs can provide invaluable learning opportunities for students, especially advanced practice nurses, as they refine their history-taking and clinical investigation skills (Durham & Alden, 2010). However, for students who do not have this option available, other well-planned simulation experiences can help to meet their needs. Visual and performing arts students, improvisation group members, nursing alumni, or retired professionals (e.g., actors, physicians, nurses, teachers), may be able to role-play as patients, family members, or interdisciplinary health care professionals to enhance simulation realism.

USING SIMULATION AS A TEACHING–LEARNING STRATEGY

Most nursing programs are integrating some form of simulation into their curriculum. This integration may be a result of external pressure (visiting prospective students who ask to see the HPSs), administrators who recognize the need, or nurse educators who desire to keep up with the technology-driven millennial generation of students. Still, well-designed research is necessary to demonstrate how the use of simulation creates the desired outcomes in student learning and how simulation can best translate into clinical practice.

Jeffries et al. (2010) suggested four key elements for nurse educators teaching with simulation: student-centered learning, simulation objectives and focus, simulation fidelity, and guided reflection. Additionally, teachers need adequate training for the development of appropriate clinical scenarios, implementation of the simulation, and evaluation of the pedagogy. Faculty development related to simulation must be a critical factor to consider when implementing clinical simulation for teaching–learning purposes.

EDUCATIONAL PRACTICES

Today's millennial generation of nursing students require a teaching pedagogy that is based on collaboration and group work, incorporates technology, and provides a realistic immersion in the experience (Pardue & Morgan, 2008); simulation meets these needs. By engaging learners directly in the simulation, active learning can occur. Providing constructive feedback during the debriefing session, allowing students to view a recording of their performance, or getting suggestions and critiques from classmates who may be viewing them in a nearby classroom all provide feedback for enhanced student performance (Durham & Alden, 2010).

Acknowledging that students learn through many different styles, simulation allows the incorporation of different teaching strategies to appeal to these diverse needs. But is simulation simply a teaching method? Does it have the potential to affect learning and student outcomes? Several educational theories support simulation education, including constructivism learning theory, adult learning theory, brain-based learning theory, social cognitive learning theory, experiential learning theory, and novice-to-expert theory (Rodgers, 2007, pp. 71–109; Rothgeb, 2008, p. 490). Parker and Myrick (2009) urged nurse educators to reconsider the use of high-fidelity HPSs within the broad context of nursing pedagogy (process, critical thinking, clinical judgment), rather than approaching it as simply a teaching method. Kaakinen and Arwood (2009) argued that simulation is more than just a series of goals, objectives, methods, and student outcomes that evaluate simple skill acquisition taught by doing. In a review of the literature, Kaakinen and Arwood (2009) examined 120 simulation manuscripts to determine whether nursing faculty members were using simulation as a teaching method or as a way to design learning opportunities. Of those articles, 94 described simulation as a teaching method or strategy; of the 16 that used learning as a purpose to design the simulation, only two considered learning to be a cognitive task (p. 11). Kaakinen and Arwood's main assumption for the review was that simulation would focus on learning, but they found that "the majority of the simulation studies in this review did not consider student learning as cognitive and social processes that occur through a planned experience" (p. 12), and "none of the studies used research about how the brain acquires or learns concepts" (p. 17).

PREPARING FOR SIMULATION

In order to realize the full benefit of clinical simulation, teachers need to ensure that students participating in simulation experiences in clinical nursing laboratories see this as a realistic environment and consider various factors when preparing the clinical scenario for simulation. Specific policies and procedures related to clinical simulation recording and the confidentiality of the recording need to be developed. Students need to be orientated to the mannequin and the simulated environment. Additionally, ground rules for professional behavior and attire (e.g., uniform, scrubs, lab coats) will enhance the realness of the experience (Jeffries et al., 2010).

Teachers need to consider many factors when preparing the clinical scenario used for simulation. Exhibit 9.1 provides a listing of recommendations for inclusion in the clinical scenario design. Program outcomes and course objectives should provide some direction for the type of simulation needed. For example, if a clinical or course objective focuses on

---

Exhibit 9.1

CLINICAL SCENARIO DESIGN CONSIDERATIONS

- Participant preparation
- Prebriefing
- Patient information
- Participant objectives
- Environmental conditions
- Support items to enhance realism
- Participant roles and expectations
- Progression outline
- Debriefing
- Evaluation

Source: Adapted from Meakim et al. (2013).

client assessment, teachers might decide to create a simulation that has a patient experiencing shortness of breath, decreased oxygen saturation, and abnormal breath sounds. During the simulation, students could use their critical thinking and problem-solving skills to explore the respiratory status of the patient and complete a respiratory assessment. The Standards of Best Practice developed by INACSL suggest some best practices for participant objectives and include: addressing the learning domains, corresponding to participant's knowledge and experience, congruency with program outcomes, incorporating evidence, viewing the client holistically, and being achievable within an appropriate timeframe (Lioce et al., 2013).

CHOOSING FIDELITY

Another planning consideration involves the most appropriate level of fidelity. Teachers should not automatically select a high-fidelity simulator. Basic skills practice can be easily achieved by lower levels of simulation fidelity. Beginning students may be overwhelmed by the high-fidelity mannequin. It may be better to introduce novice students to lower level–fidelity mannequins, allowing them to practice skills before moving on to more complex situations and higher fidelity simulators, while advanced students may require simulations involving complex care or emergent situations that would be best suited for a high-fidelity simulator mannequin. The level of technology used in clinical simulation also depends on several other factors: teacher familiarity with the technology, the technology available, and support for use of technology. Clinical teachers should use the resources and expertise available to provide an optimal simulation experience. Nursing education programs that have access to simulation specialists or information technology (IT) support (ideally, designated IT staff members) may have an easier time incorporating simulation into clinical education. In addition, college or university services that support academic excellence with resources and specialists can assist with faculty development, and other departments can help incorporate components that will make the simulation feel more real. Faculty members in a university department of communication may be able to assist nursing clinical teachers with the dialogue component of scenarios. Performing arts faculty members and students can add to the contextual experience by role-playing anxious family members; nursing education colleagues might apply some of their rich clinical experience by portraying a spouse, parent, or child of the HPS.

PLANNING CONSIDERATIONS

Past simulation and educational experiences, level of student (e.g., first year prelicense students versus advanced practice nurses), and number of clinical students should also be part of the simulation planning considerations. Will all students actively participate in the simulation activities or will a select group of students play an active role serving as the nurse or other health care provider in the simulation scenario while others observe? Have the students participated in simulation activities before or are they new to this experience and need a full orientation to the mannequins and simulation environment? Does the simulation build on prior knowledge or is it intended to teach new content? Is the simulation an adjunct for clinical learning, an alternate activity in case of an absence from clinical learning activities, or a replacement for activities at a clinical facility? These factors will impact the amount of time and preparation that may be required for the simulation experience.

Another planning consideration is the focus and purpose of the simulation. Is the simulation planned to provide students with practice opportunities or is the simulation intended to evaluate student performance? Simulated patient experiences are often used for advanced practice nursing students to demonstrate skills needed for practice and are thus used for competency evaluation. Teachers need to consider the high-stakes testing component of simulation as they plan for simulation use. Lastly, consider the time for simulation, including lab availability, teacher time, and student time, making sure to include time for introduction, student preparation, simulation implementation, and debriefing. Once these areas have been considered, then further scenario development or selection can occur.

SCENARIO SELECTION

Once some of these preliminary decisions about the simulation have been determined, then teachers can create the scenario. Scenario development incorporates evidence and professional standards, but is at heart a creative process. The use of a simple storyboard template can provide structure without being overwhelming for teachers who are developing their first scenarios. An example of a storyboard for a simple simulation for beginning-level clinical nursing students (see Exhibit 9.2) includes the specific objectives for the simulation activity, the types of cues that the patient and other team members may provide to the students, expected actions, and suggested debriefing and reflection topics. The use of a storyboard template by teachers as they develop scenarios will increase consistency among

Exhibit 9.2

EXAMPLE STORYBOARD FOR "HARRY HAS A LOW BLOOD-GLUCOSE LEVEL: A SCENARIO FOR BEGINNING-LEVEL STUDENTS"

Simulation-Specific Objectives
Critical Thinker

1. Interpret subjective and objective symptoms of hypoglycemia.
2. Identify abnormal blood glucose levels.

Evidence-Based Practitioner

3. Demonstrate proper use of a glucometer by obtaining blood sample and recording results.
4. Explain blood glucose results to the patient.

Innovative Professional

5. Demonstrate respect for the patient and family.

Simulator Settings/ Other Actions	Verbal Cues	Expected Student Actions	Notes for Reflection
Vital Statistics: T 97.5° F., P 88, R 18, BP 167/88 Report blood glucose below 65.	*Harry* ■ Oriented to own identity and birth date but is disoriented to time and place. ■ Complains of feeling sweaty and a little strange. ■ Gives permission to have blood sugar checked. *Daughter* ■ Asks for information about the nurse's actions. ■ Verifies Harry's identity if asked.	When student enters room: ■ Wash hands, wear gloves appropriately. ■ Introduce self. ■ Identify patient using two identifiers. ■ Inform client of purpose of interaction. ■ Perform brief head-to-toe assessment. ■ Use therapeutic communication during assessment. When student exits the room: ■ Wash hands.	■ How did you know you were caring for the correct patient? ■ What questions did the patient or family have about diabetes? How did it feel when you tried to answer them? ■ Did you check the patient orders? What should you do about the low blood glucose? ■ What do you think you might say to a provider if you call to report a blood glucose level?

(continued)

■ Expresses concern about father's state if students do not begin to identify patient's condition.	■ Assure that call light is in place. ■ State when a care provider will check on patient next. During care: ■ Check and document blood glucose.

Adapted from the Arizona State University Educational Simulation Program.

teachers across a curriculum as well as encourage them to start with basic information (e.g., identifying three to five simulation objectives and learning outcomes). It is important to identify essential learning outcomes, taking into consideration social and demographic trends specific to the geographic area, and incorporating cultural sensitivity, spirituality, and ethical considerations. The level of the students, specific course objectives, and teacher clinical expertise all need to be considered when specifying an appropriate learning outcome. Other suggestions for creating scenarios include reviewing course evaluations, licensure and certification exam results by subject area, communication with clinical facilities, and other program evaluation data to identify essential learning needs of students (Chambers, 2006). Drawing on common situations seen at clinical sites or relying on past clinical cases will help provide ideas for scenario creation. If you are drawing ideas or information from actual patients, make sure case details are generic and that patient privacy is not compromised by revealing too much personal or identifiable information. Sometimes scenarios are a compilation of many patients seen in clinical practice. Incorporate unique aspects of care that can be vividly portrayed in simulations. For example, simulations that use a cluttered, dusty, and insect-infested home during a home health simulation; stressed, arguing parents as part of a pediatric simulation; or a homeless patient with poor literacy skills, comorbidities, and limited support systems can effectively portray challenging situations that nurses face in practice. Regardless of the method used to create scenarios, ensure that they are student-centered, interactive, and related to outcomes.

Many nursing education programs access or purchase existing scenarios from publishers, simulation manufacturers, other nursing education programs, and national nursing organizations. These already-developed materials aid teachers by providing well-constructed scenarios with the completed template of essential information and support data needed to implement the simulation. When using prepackaged scenarios, it is important to check alignment with course and program outcomes and needs. Sometimes tailoring these scenarios to align with individual program needs may be necessary. Regardless of the origin of the scenario, check to ensure that the scenario uses life-like situations that are appropriate for the level of students and clinical course.

OTHER CONSIDERATIONS

Once the scenario is written, teachers must schedule time with lab staff members (equipment managers and IT experts for programming the equipment) for a rehearsal of the simulation on paper and then in real time. Reviewing scenarios for accuracy, current evidence-based practice guidelines, and unnecessary distracters will ensure the quality of the simulation experience for all and help to identify needed resources (e.g., teacher and staff support, props, space, and time). It is necessary to practice the scenario, and it is ideal if students or teachers are present for a practice session prior to implementing the live scenario with the students. Lastly, prepare the mannequin or simulated patient with props and include appropriate moulage or a reproduction of special effects so that students can see, feel, smell, and hear in a life-like clinical environment.

Because electronic health record (EHR) use and its relationship to patient safety and staff efficiency and vigilance has been documented (Valentine, 2005; Weir, Hoffman, Nebeker, & Hurdle, 2005), teachers should consider use of this technology as part of simulation. Some nursing programs are experimenting with the use of EHRs as a tool to enhance clinical simulation. Students can use the academic EHR to access simulated patient records and document care provided during a simulation, thus giving students an opportunity to develop these essential informatics skills needed for new graduates (Gardner & Jones, 2012). Creating a database of mock patient records as part of the EHR that can be accessed and used during simulation will enhance realism while allowing students to access longitudinal patient data and help ensure that students develop the knowledge and skills needed to function in a technology-rich clinical environment. This hands-on approach of using an EHR during simulation will provide additional practice opportunities and help students make the transition to EHR use in the clinical setting.

IMPLEMENTING SIMULATION

In addition to appropriate scenario planning, adequate student preparation for the simulation can contribute to the success and learning in the simulation. Students may have an assignment prior to the simulation, such as reading relevant background information on pathophysiology or medications that will be used during the simulation, completing preparation worksheets, reviewing Internet resources, or viewing a video or online presentation. Providing students with a brief history of the patient and the diagnosis will then allow students to answer some key questions in preparation for the simulation experience. Exhibit 9.3 provides some sample questions that can be used to prepare for the simulation. Clinical teachers can conduct this presimulation preparation in a variety of ways; students can complete individual written assignments or they can participate in oral discussions with the clinical group. A formal presimulation preparatory group meeting with the students is also an opportunity to review expectations about student performance, remind students about confidentiality of the experience, and obtain signatures for videorecording consents.

The simulation should begin with a briefing about the simulation. This is an opportunity for the teacher to assess student preparation for

---

Exhibit 9.3

SAMPLE PREPARATORY QUESTIONS FOR SIMULATIONS

1. What physical assessments should be completed as a priority for this patient?
2. What questions will you ask the patient so you can fully explore and understand the health problem?
3. What data or information do you still need in order to understand and provide appropriate care for this patient?
4. What lab or diagnostic tests will you review and what might you expect to find?
5. What are the patient's medications (drug classification, dosage, route, administration, nursing implications)?
6. What teaching will be necessary?
7. What might be important to discuss with the family or significant others?
8. What other social, emotional, religious, psychological, or environmental issues need to be considered when planning your care?
9. What will be your priority nursing actions?
10. What other health care providers should be contacted?
11. What nursing interventions will be necessary?

the experience, check on essential student knowledge, review background information about the patient (HPS), provide instructions, and assign roles for the simulation. Many times the simulation begins with a report or review of background information about the patient in the form of a handoff or change of shift report. It may also include a brief review of the relevant patient health history. Students begin the scenario and enact the assigned roles, which may include primary nurse, charge nurse, medication nurse, or other supportive staff. Sometimes students or others serve in ancillary or supportive roles that help to enhance the realism of the simulation. This is also an opportunity to collaborate with other disciplines such as students from medicine, speech therapy, respiratory therapy, or dieticians who can serve in their respective roles during the simulation. The teacher, controlling the simulation from a separate room, if feasible, uses the preplanned scenario to respond to student actions during the simulation. Teachers may use either preprogrammed patient vocal responses or spontaneously respond to student questions and actions on behalf of the simulated patient. Teachers should allow students to make mistakes, problem solve throughout the scenario, and find their own way. Many nursing education programs use videorecording capabilities that allow for a recording of all events of the scenarios. These recordings can be used for debriefing after the simulation.

Depending upon clinical group size, learning goals, and time available, teachers may choose to have some students observe the scenario and provide suggestions and insight during debriefing. Students may experience anxiety when the simulation is videorecorded or when they are performing before others during a simulation (Nielsen & Harder, 2013). The literature suggests strategies that may assist in decreasing anxiety during simulation, including: providing a supportive learning environment that allows students to make mistakes, mentoring, group planning for care, cueing, assuring confidentiality, providing teacher support, and proper simulation orientation (Elfrink, Nininger, Rohig, & Lee, 2009; Ganley & Linnard-Palmer, 2012; Gore, Hunt, Parker, & Raines, 2011; Nielsen & Harder, 2013). Use of these strategies may help reduce the anxiety during simulation.

DEBRIEFING AND GUIDED REFLECTION

The last, but perhaps most important, area of clinical simulation involves debriefing and providing an opportunity for guided reflection on the simulation. Debriefing has been identified as crucial for students' learning and satisfaction with their simulation experience; however, it requires adequate time and some preplanning to be effective. Jeffries (2005, p. 101) proposed that debriefing "reinforces the positive aspects of the experience and encourages reflective learning, which allows the participant to link theory to practice and research, think critically, and discuss how to intervene professionally in very complex situations." Debriefing allows the students to make meaning of the experience, critique performance while reinforcing learning, and figure out how to apply information to practice (Chronister & Brown, 2012; Overstreet, 2010).

Because debriefing can be critical for student learning, teachers need to carefully plan and consider the methods, format, and approach used while also ensuring that they can effectively facilitate this activity. Exhibit 9.4 provides suggestions for best practices for effective debriefing.

Teachers may choose between a structured or unstructured approach to debriefing. Structured debriefing involves development of prepared questions that can be used to guide the debriefing session. These questions typically arise from simulation objectives and serve as a prompt to focus the debriefing discussion. Caution must be exercised to allow the unfolding of the discussion and to avoid restricting the interactive and reflective activities so crucial in debriefing. Teachers must allow enough flexibility so that they can respond to unexpected developments during simulation and incorporate them into the debriefing activities. On the other hand, unstructured debriefing is a more spontaneous approach that allows the discussion about the clinical simulation to unfold and go where the participants take it. This free-flowing approach may deviate from the learning objectives, so teachers need to be able to refocus students as needed (Dreifuerst, 2009).

Oral or written format, or a combination of both, may be used to accomplish debriefing. Oral debriefing or discussions about simulation can be public or private. Public debriefing allows observers, typically other clinical students who observed the simulation, to participate in the debriefing process. Student observers can provide valuable insight and

Exhibit 9.4

EFFECTIVE DEBRIEFING PRACTICES

1. Facilitated by a person competent in the process of debriefing.
2. Conducted in an environment that is conducive to learning and supports confidentiality, trust, open communication, self-analysis, and reflection.
3. Facilitated by a person who observes the simulated experience.
4. Based on a structured framework for debriefing.
5. Congruent with the participants' objectives and outcomes of the simulation-based learning experience.

Source: Adapted from Decker et al. (2013).

suggestions after watching the simulation. They may notice actions that the students in the nurse's role may not be aware of and can offer insight from their unique perspective of observer. Sometimes the debriefing process can be sensitive and anxiety-provoking, particularly if the student performance is deficient or problems were encountered, or when video playback of the simulation is reviewed. Teachers may choose to complete private debriefing with only those students playing an active role in the simulation.

Regardless of the approach used for oral debriefing, teachers should anticipate and plan for the amount of time needed to debrief. Time used for debriefing varies and the published literature does not reveal sufficient research to make definitive evidence-based recommendations on this topic. Gore, Van Gele, Ravert, and Mabire (2012) conducted a survey of the INACSL members to identify current simulation practices and found that in the United States, respondents spend equal time on simulation and debriefing; however, international respondents reported debriefings that were twice as long as the simulations. Further research in this area is needed, but as a general guideline for planning purposes, teachers should consider spending at least the same amount of time on debriefing as they do with the simulation.

Oral debriefing typically follows immediately at the conclusion of the scenario. This timing for debriefing is helpful in that students are able to recall recent events and discuss them while they are still current. However, some students may benefit from some additional time to process the simulation events and think about the experience, or they may prefer to privately reflect about the experience in writing rather than orally in a public forum. Journaling activities can be assigned to encourage students to personally reflect on the experience. Electronic activities such as blogging (in a private rather than public format) or threaded electronic discussions can also be used to engage students who are digital natives and promote reflection after simulation. Either structured or unstructured approaches can be used. For example, students can be asked to compose a reflective journal entry that uses a broad prompt, such as "Write about what you learned from the simulation." Or, they can write more specifically about what went well and what could be improved. Structured prompts could direct students to write about specific examples of actions during the simulation. For example, "What were you thinking when the patient complained of shortness of breath during the simulation? What actions did you take and what else could you have done to address this situation?"

Teachers must also consider the use of technology for the debriefing, such as whether and how to incorporate video playback of the simulation. Chronister and Brown (2012) reported that oral discussion led by the teacher is a traditional approach to debriefing. They conducted a research study using a comparative crossover design to evaluate the effectiveness of different debriefing approaches on student skill and knowledge retention. Although they used only a small convenience sample, they found that quality of skill improvement was higher for students in the video-assisted oral debriefing group than the oral-only debriefing group. Reed, Andrews, and Ravert (2013) compared debriefing with and without video with nursing students following an intensive care simulation. Although the sample size was small, they found no evidence to indicate superiority of any specific debriefing method.

Conflicting opinions exist regarding debriefing and video use. Gore et al. (2012) reported significant differences between United States and international INACSL respondents regarding the incorporation of videorecording use as part of debriefing. In the United States, participants reported that students were not required to view the simulation videorecordings. If teachers and students cannot quickly access pertinent video clips to use for immediate debriefing training and support are needed. In the meantime, teachers could consider methods to allow students to view the video at another time. Caution should be exercised to prevent inappropriate distribution of the video and potential violation of student confidentiality. Video review can be required as part of the written journaling activities previously discussed. Limited research is available to provide clear guidance about best uses of video replay; however, use of select video snippets of the simulation would help to remind students of what happened during the simulation and could lead to rich debriefing discussions. Further studies exploring the use and effectiveness of videorecording and understanding how to best use this resource to aid student learning are needed.

Once decisions about the method, format, and approach to debriefing are complete, the teacher needs to implement activities that will ensure an appropriate climate for debriefing. The instructor's role during debriefing is that of facilitator, coach, or guide—not lecturer and monopolizer of debriefing conversations. At the beginning of a debriefing session the teacher should review the objectives of the simulation, discuss confidentiality as well as teacher expectations for students' participation in evaluating themselves and their peers, and share the general format of the debriefing session (Anderson, n.d.). Teachers must work to establish a trusting environment because students may feel vulnerable and anxious, particularly if video playback is used (Nielsen & Harder, 2013). Sensitive issues need to be openly discussed in a constructive and supportive manner. Once the ground rules of the debriefing session are complete, then discussion about the events and experiences can begin. As students share their impressions and reflections, teachers should listen, redirect discussion as appropriate, and encourage participation. The use of probing open-ended questions will help to engage students in reflective conversations. Exhibit 9.5 provides some sample questions that can be incorporated into simulation debriefing. Use what, how, and why questions to promote student discussion and higher level thinking. Sometimes teachers may need to clarify inaccuracies or correct misinterpretations in a manner that provides positive feedback about performance but also gives students suggestions for areas to strengthen or change.

Conclude the debriefing session with some closing statements about what students identified as effective and efficient, areas they need to work on, and take-away learning messages to summarize the experience. Thanking students for their participation and stating the teacher's appreciation for their attention, efforts in enacting the scenario, and shared reflections provides positive reinforcement and shows respect for their efforts. Asking students to identify content that helped them succeed in the scenario and where they received it (classroom, presentations, scenario preparation) will guide the teacher to further course and curricular improvements.

EVALUATING SIMULATIONS

The final aspect of clinical simulation, evaluating simulations, involves multiple components. As the simulation unfolds, teachers can easily identify

---

Exhibit 9.5

SAMPLE DEBRIEFING QUESTIONS

- Was there anything you missed on report or was there other information that you needed so you could act more effectively?
- What knowledge do you still need to manage the situation more effectively?
- What areas require further practice?
- What went well?
- What would you do differently the next time? Why?
- Why do you think the patient responded in the manner that he or she did?
- What were you thinking about during the simulation?
- Why did you complete the nursing actions in the order that you did?
- How could you have acted differently to meet the patient's needs more effectively and efficiently?
- What problems did you identify?
- How did you prioritize your care?

areas that are working and areas that are problematic. The dynamic process of the simulation allows for some modification during use, but careful note-taking during the scenario, as well as after the debriefing session with students, will document changes necessary to enhance the effectiveness of the simulation for the future. Another method commonly used for simulation evaluation involves asking for student feedback or reactions to the experience. This evaluation can occur in a group debriefing session or individually by each student in a written format. This data, while not directly linked to performance, will provide valuable information about the simulation experience, allowing teachers to consider further revisions and improvements. Reviewing student feedback with teachers and simulation specialists who assisted with the technology component of simulation soon after the scenario is completed provides the best opportunities for change and revision.

There are a variety of ways to assess student performance and determine whether the simulation enabled attainment of the learning objectives. To evaluate student performance, computer-generated logs can be created by the automated setting of a high-fidelity HPS, with an option for the teacher to type comments while students are performing the scenario. In addition, videorecording of the scenarios will provide concrete information about students' actions, knowledge, and skill. These evaluation methods reflect students' performance and whether they met the objectives and demonstrated the skills and knowledge identified as important outcomes for that scenario. This type of learning can also be assessed with skills checklists, rating scales, or other performance indices. Student behaviors can be assessed for items such as level of independence, prompting, accuracy, timeliness, and appropriate sequence of activities. Debriefing is enriched with this information because students are provided with concrete, constructive, and immediate feedback in an objective manner.

Sometimes simulation is used during class time to reinforce content and engage the students, in which case it probably involves more than one student with classmates observing (either live or a recording). In this situation, peer observers can be given an assignment that instructs them to observe for specific actions or activities. Because a simulation can often be complex, assigning students specific areas to observe can allow students to focus more effectively. For example, one student can watch the simulation and note safety measures and another student may watch for communication skills; students can then share their impressions and evaluation about these areas during debriefing. Teachers may find it helpful to agree on and detail the behaviors in a particular scenario that best demonstrate achievement of the defined objectives. Exhibit 9.6 provides an example of how specific actions in a multipatient scenario are related to the overall objectives for a simulation activity.

Exhibit 9.6

EXAMPLE OF A MULTIPATIENT SIMULATION SPECIFIC BEHAVIORS FEEDBACK FORM

SIMULATION: Adult health multipatient scenario—A day in the life of three patients on a cardiac telemetry unit.

Student Outcomes:

Critical Thinker

The student will:

1. Use clinical judgment to provide high-quality, evidence-based patient care.
2. Discuss the rationale for prioritization of activities based on report, patient chart, and assessment.

Evidence-Based Practitioner

The student will:

3. Manage care of multiple patients.
4. Demonstrate assessment, including focused assessments as indicated by patient history (for instance, identify and interpret lab value changes).
5. Prioritize care of multiple patients and families based on competing critical, urgent, and routine needs.
6. Demonstrate safe, effective patient care including treatments, medications, and comfort care.
7. Communicate effectively with interprofessional team, patient, and family.
8. Initiate and perform interventions appropriate for patients as deviations from the norm arise.
9. Evaluate interventions and act accordingly.
10. Request assistance using appropriate and thorough communication skills.
11. Complete appropriate documentation.

Innovative Professional

The student will:

12. Demonstrate reflection on own performance and learning.
13. Provide useful and constructive feedback to fellow participants.

Simulation Patients:

Patient 1: Coder Johnson: 77-year-old man who was found in his room by the staff of a long-term care facility complaining of chest pain, shortness of breath, and nausea. He was admitted to the ICU 2 weeks ago. He survived a cardiac arrest after admission and he has been on the ventilator for 10 days, but he was extubated yesterday. He is alert and oriented.

Diagnosis: S/P acute myocardial infarction

(continued)

Medical History: Normally alert and active, oriented to time and place. Hypertension, increased cholesterol (currently untreated by medication)

Social History: A nephew visits every morning before going to work.

Patient 2: Rosalee Sweetwater: 54-year-old woman admitted from the ED with chest pain

Diagnosis: R/O MI

Medical History: Insulin-dependent diabetes mellitus, peripheral vascular disease, and hypertension.

Social History: Patient is a Native American who lives on a reservation, with her daughter and husband. She has two grown children and five grandchildren. Family history of diabetes, coronary artery disease, and hypertension.

Allergies: Penicillin and Lopressor

Patient 3: Harry Chester: 89-year-old man

Diagnosis: Community-acquired pneumonia

Past Medical History: COPD, non-insulin dependent diabetes, atrial fibrillation, early Alzheimer's disease.

Social History: Married, lives with wife who provides his home care with the support of their three children. He is a World War II veteran. Hobbies include, carpentry and jigsaw puzzles

Allergies: Latex

FEEDBACK FORM (Adult Health Multipatient Simulation)

Purpose: To give students meaningful feedback related to the adult health immersion simulation experience. The core elements are based on the clinical performance rubric and objectives of this simulation. The specific behavioral markers listed are based on the data for the patients in these simulations.

Directions for use: During the simulation, note the presence and quality of the specific behavioral markers listed below. The student may do some things well and some things not so well within each core element. Think holistically about each core element as you consider the cumulative impact of the behaviors. Discuss the core elements and the pertinent behaviors during guided reflection.

Core elements with behavioral markers for the adult health immersion simulation. Note comments regarding specific observations for use in the post-scenario guided reflection.

Prioritize care of multiple patients and families (Objectives 2, 5) as indicated by:
- Manage pain appropriately
- Respond to alarms (ventricular tachycardia, IV)

(continued)

- Assess Coder Johnson's swallowing before breakfast arrives
- Delegate or perform blood glucose assessment before insulin administration
- Determine breakfast intake by 9:30
- Delegate morning comfort care with any special instructions
- Delegate assisting Harry Chester to eat

Use clinical judgment to provide evidence-based patient care (Objectives 1, 4, 9, 12) as indicated by statements of rationale related to:
- Coder Johnson:
  - Identify need for a swallow study
  - Notice low K+ value and need for potassium before administering furosemide
- Rosalee Sweetwater:
  - Identify impending renal failure, explain new orders and required care
- Harry Chester:
  - Identify safety concerns related to confusion
  - Notice use of MS Contin in the long-term care facility, associate medication use with potential side effects and withdrawal given the current medication orders. (Exemplary level)

Manage a multipatient assignment (Objective 3) as indicated by:
- Initial assessment of all patients by 8:30
- Provision of insulin to Rosalee Sweetwater and Harry Chester before breakfast but after obtaining current blood glucose values
- Provision of all necessary medications within required time frames

Demonstrate safe, effective patient care, including treatments, medication, and comfort care (Objectives 6, 8) as indicated by:
- Hand washing and patient identification with each patient contact
- Follow hub-scrub policy prior to IV medication administration
- Use gloves appropriately (e.g., when assessing dressing, providing Foley catheter emptying, and changing incontinence briefs)
- Manage equipment (IV controller, bed, monitor, etc.)
- Coder Johnson:
  - Replace nasal cannula if off
  - Carry out swallow study following the protocol in the chart
  - Secure central line dressing if needed

(continued)

- Administer potassium in a safe concentration for a central or peripheral IV line
- Assess urine output after furosemide
■ Rosalee Sweetwater:
- Do *not* give Ampicillin
- Give insulin SQ
- Administer new antibiotic ordered
- Discontinue IV fluids
- Administer 0900 meds, note duplicate order
■ Harry Chester:
- Assure side rails are used correctly
- Change or delegate change of incontinence brief
- Teach use of incentive spirometer
- Assess breakfast intake

Communicate effectively with patient, family, and interprofessional team
(Objectives 7, 10, 11, 13) as indicated by:
■ Identify self, state purpose for each encounter
■ Coder Johnson:
- Assure family member concerning rationale for nurse presence for care
- Explain need for swallow test before eating due to recent extubation
- Provide report to physician based on situation, background, assessment, and recommendation (SBAR), including lack of antihypertension medication and current blood pressure
- Read back and verify new orders, document on chart
- Report ventricular tachycardia occurrence using SBAR
■ Rosalee Sweetwater:
- Provide SBAR-based report to physicians including lab values, weight gain, urine appearance and output, allergy to penicillin
- Read back and verify new orders
- Explain to family about renal disease and dialysis if asked
- Document in electronic health record (medications, assessment as assigned)
■ Harry Chester:
- Reorient as necessary
- Provide SBAR report and referral to case manager concerning Harry's wife

(continued)

- Provide clear and organized report at 10:00 (to be video recorded for student self-evaluation)
- Document assigned system assessments and medication administration, and verify orders received

Adapted from Arizona State University Educational Simulation Program.

Various tools have been used as part of simulation evaluation and research. In a recent review of published simulation evaluation instruments, Adamson, Kardong-Edgren, and Willhaus (2013) reported the repeated use of four tools to evaluate simulation performance and learning: the Sweeny-Clark Simulation Performance Evaluation Tool, the Clinical Simulation Evaluation Tool, the Lasater Clinical Judgment Rubric, and the Creighton Simulation Evaluation Instrument. Widespread use of these tools contributes valuable reliability and validity evidence about their appropriateness for evaluating student performance. Further research is needed to effectively determine how simulation impacts learning, behavior and, ultimately, patient care.

FUTURE IMPLICATIONS

Many aspects of simulation pedagogy have been covered in this chapter. Some areas for future research and innovation are addressed briefly below.

- Consider creating partnerships with local agencies, collaborating with other nursing education programs or health care facilities, or negotiating with regional simulation centers for simulation activities (Metcalfe, Hall, & Carpenter, 2007).
- Work with other related professions to conduct interprofessional simulation activities. Evaluate the effectiveness of these interprofessional educational experiences.
- Conduct research demonstrating the efficacy of simulation in nursing education and attainment of learning outcomes. How can simulation be used as an educational tool to meet the desired student learning outcomes and clinical competencies, and how will we measure its efficacy in those areas? Further research is needed to provide sound evidence-based support for simulation activities such as the most effective methods for debriefing.
- Teacher support, resources, and curricular integration require administrative support and affordable simulation software and

evaluation systems that streamline faculty efforts. As simulation continues to advance, ongoing faculty training on the latest developments is essential to keep teachers up-to-date on simulation advances.

- More research and support is necessary for the use of EHRs and scenario implementation.
- Move from small-scale, single-site descriptive studies about simulation to robust multisite experimental designs using strong methodology, adequate sample sizes, and measurement tools that produce reliable results on which to base valid academic decisions.

SUMMARY

Clinical simulation has become widely integrated into clinical nursing education. Simulation activities allow students to develop psychomotor skills, clinical reasoning, clinical judgment, problem solving, and critical thinking through techniques such as role-playing and the use of devices such as interactive videos or mannequins. In addition, simulation offers an opportunity for evaluation and assessment of student skills with options for remediation and continued practice and refinement. Nursing experts acknowledge the value of simulation as a teaching–learning method that mimics reality but also emphasize the need for nursing student clinical experiences with real patients.

Simulators can be categorized as low-, moderate-, or high-fidelity in relation to how closely they represent a realistic situation. Low-fidelity simulators, sometimes referred to as "task-trainers," lack the realism of a clinical situation but offer opportunities for procedural skill practice. Moderate-fidelity simulators allow students to practice multiple psychomotor skills but without interactive features. High-fidelity simulators produce the most lifelike scenarios. These full-size mannequins react to student manipulations in real time and in realistic ways, such as speaking, coughing, and demonstrating chest movements and pulses. Simulations with SPs use live actors with scripts who portray patients, and require nursing students to engage in nursing care activities with the SPs in an environment that simulates patient care areas.

Key elements for nurse educators teaching with simulation include student-centered learning, simulation objectives and focus, simulation fidelity, and guided reflection. Teachers need adequate training for the development of appropriate clinical scenarios, implementation of the simulation, and evaluation of the pedagogy.

Teachers should ensure that students participating in simulation experiences view them as realistic environments by establishing ground rules for professional behavior and attire. Specific policies and procedures related to clinical simulation recording and the confidentiality of the recordings should be developed.

Factors to consider when choosing or preparing clinical scenarios used for simulation include program outcomes and course objectives, the purpose of the activity, the most appropriate level of fidelity, the number and educational level of the students, time available, teacher familiarity with the technology, the technology available, and support for use of the technology. Scenario development should incorporate creativity and available scientific evidence for practice, and should be student-centered, interactive, and related to desired outcomes. The use of a simple storyboard template can provide structure for scenario development; an example was given in the chapter. Scenarios may also be accessed or purchased from publishers, simulation manufacturers, other nursing education programs, and national nursing organizations. Already-developed scenarios aid inexperienced teachers by providing the completed template of essential information and support data needed to implement the simulation, but it is important to check alignment of the materials with course and program outcomes and needs.

The use of EHRs can be incorporated into scenarios to enhance clinical simulation. Students can use the academic EHR to access simulated patient records and document care provided during a simulation. Creating a database of mock patient records as part of the EHR that can be accessed and used during simulation will enhance realism.

Preparation for using simulation also includes practice sessions prior to implementing the live scenario with the students, and preparing the mannequin or SP with props and special effects so that students perceive a life-like clinical environment. Student preparation may include reading relevant background information and a brief patient history and diagnosis, completing preparation worksheets, reviewing Internet resources, viewing a video or online presentation, and answering some key questions in preparation for the simulation activity. This presimulation preparation can be an individual written assignment or oral group discussion.

After a short briefing, students enact their assigned roles and the teacher uses the preplanned scenario to respond to student actions on behalf of the simulated patient. Videorecording allows observation by others during the simulation and provides a recording that can be used for debriefing after the simulation. Debriefing after the simulation activity provides an important opportunity for guided reflection on the positive aspects of the experience to reinforce learning, and encourages critical thinking, making meaning of the experience, and critique of student performance. Suggestions were offered for reducing student anxiety about being observed and video-recorded during simulations. Various options for conducting debriefings were presented, including individual or group, immediate or delayed, structured or unstructured, private or public, and oral or written. The instructor's role during debriefing is that of facilitator, coach, or guide.

The evaluation of clinical simulations involves multiple data sources, including teachers' notes during the simulation and debriefing and group or individual student feedback and reactions to the activity. Computer-generated logs generated by high-fidelity HPSs and videorecordings of scenarios can also be assessed with skills checklists, rating scales, or other performance indices. Further research substantiating educational practices with simulation is needed to guide best practices.

Exhibit 9.7

CNE EXAMINATION TEST BLUEPRINT CORE COMPETENCIES

1. **Facilitate Learning**

   A. Implement a variety of teaching strategies appropriate to
      1. content
      3. learner needs
      5. desired learner outcomes
      6. method of delivery

   B. Use teaching strategies based on
      1. educational theory
      2. evidence-based practices related to education

   C. Modify teaching strategies and learning experiences based on considera-tion of learners
      2. past clinical experiences
      3. past educational and life experiences

   D. Use information technologies to support the teaching-learning process
   G. Model reflective thinking practices, including critical thinking
   H. Create opportunities for learners to develop their own critical thinking skills
   I. Create a positive learning environment that fosters a free exchange of ideas
   N. Use knowledge of evidence-based practice to instruct learners
   O. Demonstrate ability to teach clinical skills
   Q. Foster a safe learning environment

   (continued)

2. **Facilitate Learner Development and Socialization**
    D. Create learning environments that facilitate learners' self-reflection, personal goal setting, and socialization to the role of the nurse
    E. Foster the development of learners in these areas:
        1. cognitive domain
        2. psychomotor domain
        3. affective domain
    F. Assist learners to engage in thoughtful and constructive self and peer evaluation

3. **Use Assessment and Evaluation Strategies**
    C. Use a variety of strategies to assess and evaluate learning in these domains:
        1. cognitive
        2. psychomotor
        3. affective

    D. Incorporate current research in assessment and evaluation practices
    E. Analyze available resources for learning assessment and evaluation
    H. Implement evaluation strategies that are appropriate to the learner and learning outcomes
    I. Analyze assessment and evaluation data
    J. Use assessment and evaluation data to enhance the teaching-learning process
    K. Advise learners regarding assessment and evaluation criteria
    L. Provide timely, constructive, and thoughtful feedback to learners

6. **Engage in Scholarship, Service, and Leadership**
    A. Function as a change agent and leader
        4. Participate in interdisciplinary efforts to address health care and education needs
            a. within the institution
            b. locally
            c. regionally

    B. Engage in scholarship of teaching
        1. Exhibit a spirit of inquiry about teaching and learning, student development, and evaluation methods
        2. Use evidence-based resources to improve and support teaching
        3. Participate in research activities related to nursing education

REFERENCES

Adamson, K. A., Kardong-Edgren, S., & Willhaus, J. (2013). An updated review of published simulation evaluation instruments. *Clinical Simulation in Nursing, 9*, e393–e405. doi:10.1016.j.ecns.2012.09.004

American Association of Colleges of Nursing. (2012). *Nursing shortage fact sheet*. Retrieved from http://www.aacn.nche.edu/media-relations/fact-sheets/nursing-shortage

Anderson, M. (n.d.). *Debriefing and guided reflection*. Retrieved from National League for Nursing website: http://sirc.nln.org/mod/resource/view.php?id=97

Chambers, K. (2006, June). *Simulation in nursing education: The basics*. Paper presented at the 4th Annual Laerdal® Northeast Simulation User's Group Meeting, Mashantucket, CT.

Chronister, C., & Brown, D. (2012). Comparison of simulation debriefing methods. *Clinical Simulation in Nursing, 8*, 281–288. doi:10.106.j.ecns.2010.12.005

Commission on Collegiate Nursing Education. (2009). *Standards for accreditation of baccalaureate and graduate degree nursing programs*. Washington, DC: Author.

Decker, S., Fey, M., Sideras, S., Caballero, S., Rockstraw, L., Boese, T., … Borum, J. C. (2013). Standards of best practice: Simulation standard VI: The debriefing process. [Supplement]. *Clinical Simulation in Nursing, 9*(6), s27–s29. doi:10.106/j.ecns.2013.04.008

Dreifuerst, K. T. (2009). The essentials of debriefing in simulation learning: A concept analysis. *Nursing Education Perspectives, 30*, 109–114. doi:10.1043/1536-5026-030.002.0109

Durham, C. F., & Alden, K. R. (2010). The nuts and bolts of using simulation. In L. Caputi (Ed.), *Teaching nursing: The art and science* (pp. 28–55). Glen Ellyn, IL: College of DuPage Press.

Elfrink, V., Nininger, J., Rohig, L., & Lee, J. (2009). The case for group planning in human patient simulation. *Nursing Education Perspectives, 30*, 83–86. doi:10.1043/1536-5026-030.002.0083

Ganley, B., & Linnard-Palmer, L. (2012). Academic safety during nursing simulation: Perceptions of nursing students and faculty. *Clinical Simulation in Nursing, 8*(2), e49–e57. doi:10.1016/j.ecns.2010.06.004

Gardner, C. L., & Jones, S. J. (2012). Utilization of academic electronic medical records in undergraduate nursing education. *Online Journal of Nursing Informatics (OJNI), 16*(2). Retrieved from http://ojni.org/issues/?p=1702

Garrett, B., MacPhee, M., & Jackson, C. (2010). High-fidelity patient simulation: Considerations for effective learning. *Nursing Education Perspectives, 31*, 309–313. doi:10.1043/1536-5026-31.5.309

Gore, T., Hunt, C., Parker, F., & Raines, K. (2011). The effects of simulated clinical experiences on anxiety: Nursing student's perspectives. *Clinical Simulation in Nursing, 7*(5), e175–e180. doi:10.106/j.ecns.2010.02.001

Gore, T., Van Gele, P., Ravert, P., & Mabire, C. (2012). A 2010 survey of the INACSL membership about simulation use. *Clinical Simulation in Nursing, 8*(4), e125–e133. doi:10.1016/j.ecns.2012.01.002

Jeffries, P. (2005). A framework for designing, implementing, and evaluating simulations used as teaching strategies in nursing. *Nursing Education Perspectives, 26*, 96–103.

Jeffries, P. R. (2012). *Simulation in nursing education: From conceptualization to evaluation* (2nd ed.). New York, NY: National League for Nursing.

Jeffries, P. R., & Rizzolo, M. A. (2006). *Designing and implementing models for the innovative use of simulation to teach nursing care of ill adults and children: A national, multisite, multi-method study*. New York, NY: National League for Nursing.

Jeffries, P. R., Settles, J., Milgrom, L., & Woolf, S. (2010). Using simulations: Guidelines and challenges. In L. Caputi (Ed.), *Teaching nursing: The art and science* (pp. 56–81). Glen Ellyn, IL: College of DuPage Press.

Johnson, E. A., Lasater, K., Hodson-Carlton, K., Siktberg, L., Sideras, S., & Dillard, N. (2012). Geriatrics in simulation: Role modeling and clinical judgment effect. *Nursing Education Perspectives, 33*, 176–180. doi:10.5480/1536-5026-33.3.176

Kaakinen, J., & Arwood, E. (2009). Systematic review of nursing simulation literature for use of learning theory. *International Journal of Nursing Education Scholarship, 6*, 1–20. doi:10.2202/1548-923X.1688

Kardong-Edgren, S., Wilhaus, J., Bennett, D., & Hayden, J. (2012). Results of the National Council of State Boards of Nursing national simulation survey: Part II. *Clinical Simulation in Nursing, 8*(4), e117–e123. doi:10.1016/j.ecns.2012.01.003

Lioce, L., Reed, C. C., Lemon, D., King, M. A., Martinez, P. A., Franklin, A. E., … Borum, J. C. (2013). Standards of best practice: Simulation standard III: Participant objectives [Supplement]. *Clinical Simulation in Nursing, 9*(6), s15–s18. doi:10.1016/j.ecns.2013.04.005

Lusk, J., & Fater, K. (2013). Postsimulation debriefing to maximize clinical judgment development. *Nurse Educator, 38,* 16–19. doi:10.1097/NNE.0b013e318276df8b

Meakim, C., Boese, T., Decker, S., Franklin, A. E., Gloe, D., Lioce, L., … Borum, J. C. (2013). Standards of best practice: Simulation standard I: Terminology [Supplement]. *Clinical Simulation in Nursing, 9*(6), s3–s11. doi:10.1016/j.ecns.2013.04.001

Metcalfe, S. E., Hall, V. P., & Carpenter, A. (2007). Promoting collaboration in nursing education: The development of a regional simulation laboratory. *Journal of Professional Nursing, 23,* 180–183. doi:10.1016/j.profnurs.2007.01.017

National Council of State Boards of Nursing. (2013). *NCSBN national simulation study.* Retrieved from www.ncsbn.org/2094.htm

National League for Nursing. (2011). *Faculty programs & resources: Leadership development program for simulation educators.* Retrieved from http://www.nln.org/facultyprograms/leadershipinstitute.htm

National League for Nursing. (2013). *Simulation innovation resource center.* Retrieved from http://sirc.nln.org/

Nehring, W. M. (2010). History of simulation in nursing. In W. M. Nehring & F. R. Lashley (Eds.), *High fidelity patient simulation in nursing education* (pp. 3–26). Boston, MA: Jones & Bartlett.

Neill, M. A., & Wotton, K. (2011). High-fidelity simulation debriefing in nursing education: A literature review. *Clinical Simulation in Nursing, 7*(5), e161–e168. doi:10.1016/j.ecns.2011.02.001

Nielsen, B., & Harder, N. (2013). Causes of student anxiety during simulation: What the literature says. *Clinical Simulation in Nursing, 9*(11), e507–e512. doi:10.1016/j.ecns.2013.03.003

Overstreet, M. (2010). Ee-chats: The seven components of nursing debriefing. *Journal of Continuing Education in Nursing, 41,* 538–539. doi:10.3928/00220124-20101122-05

Pardue, K. T., & Morgan, P. (2008). Millennials considered: A new generation, new approaches, and implications for nursing education. *Nursing Education Perspectives, 29,* 74–79.

Parker, B. C., & Myrick, F. (2009). A critical examination of high-fidelity human patient simulation within the context of nursing pedagogy. *Nurse Education Today, 29,* 322–329. doi:10.1016/j.nedt.2008.10.012

Parker, R. A., McNeill, J. A., Pelayo, L. W., Goei, K. A., Howard, J., & Gunter, D. M. (2011). Pediatric clinical simulation: A pilot project. *Journal of Nursing Education, 50,* 105–111. doi:10.3928/01484834-20101230-05

Pullen, R., McKelvy, K., Reyher, L., Thurman, J., Bencini, P., Taylor, T. D., … Robinson, L. (2012). An end-of-life care interdisciplinary team clinical simulation model. *Nurse Educator, 37,* 75–79. doi:10.109/NNE.0b013e3182461be3

Reed, S. J., Andrews, C. M., & Ravert, P. (2013). Debriefing simulations: Comparison of debriefing with video and debriefing alone. *Clinical Simulation in Nursing, 9*(12), e585–e591. doi:10.1016/j.ecns.2013.05.007

Rodgers, D. L. (2007). *High-fidelity patient simulation: A descriptive white paper report.* Retrieved from http://sim-strategies.com/downloads/Simulation%20White%20Paper2.pdf

Rothgeb, M. K. (2008). Creating a nursing simulation laboratory: A literature review. *Journal of Nursing Education, 47,* 489–494.

Simonelli, M. C., & Paskausky, A. L. (2012). Simulation stimulates learning in a childbearing clinical course. *Journal of Nursing Education, 51*, 172–175.

Sittner, B., Hertzog, M., & Fleck, M. O. (2013). Enhancing labor and delivery learning experiences through simulation. *Clinical Simulation in Nursing, 9*(11), e521–e530. doi:10.1016/j.ecns.2013.04.012

Valentine, K. (2005). Electronic medical records promote caring and enhance professional vigilance. *International Journal for Human Caring, 9*, 121.

Weir, C., Hoffman, J., Nebeker, J., & Hurdle, J. (2005). Nurse's role in tracking adverse drug events: The impact of provider order entry. *Nursing Administration Quarterly, 29*, 39–44.

CHAPTER 10

Pedagogical Technologies for Clinical Teaching

Debra Hagler

The lines between classroom and clinical teaching have become increasingly blurred, causing potential confusion for clinical teachers and curriculum developers. Intentional efforts over decades to distinguish nursing as a science have led to separation of theoretical knowledge from the practice of providing nursing care in clinical settings. Now, the previously desired distance between what students need to know and what they will actually do seems too great a rift as it threatens to impact patient safety and quality of care. The call for radical transformation in nursing education outlines the extensive efforts needed to shift the current paradigm that is separating knowledge from context (Benner, Sutphen, Leonard & Day, 2009). Frith and Clark (2013) suggested breaking down artificial boundaries in nursing education to include the boundary between theory and practice, the boundary between knowledge acquisition and knowledge use, and the boundary between classroom and clinical teaching.

Today's nurses must accept a tremendous amount of personal responsibility and liability. Fortunately, they are well positioned to take advantage of educational strategies that use technology for personal and professional development. Nursing leaders and educators must thoughtfully incorporate technology that supports learning the complex skills and competencies demanded of today's health care professionals.

TECHNOLOGY USE IN CLINICAL TEACHING

Technology has further blurred the boundaries between classroom and clinical teaching, which were previously often defined by the settings where they were located rather than what happened in the setting. It is more and more difficult to tell what differentiates a clinical course activity from a theory course activity, but maybe that is what is needed to prepare competent practicing nurses. Where once application might have been thought to be the realm of only clinical courses, increased emphasis on engaging students through active learning has led to more application-type activities in the classroom. Simulation technology provides a method for even a large classroom group in a theory course to observe and reflect on a simulated patient care scenario that may far exceed some of their clinical experiences in terms of matching course and program objectives. Students in their own homes can be in virtual worlds interacting with simulated patients and developing skills in communication and decision making that they might not be able to practice deliberately in an authentic clinical practice setting.

Clinical courses are incorporating more online and other educational technology, although the range extends from technology only as a glitzy add-on resource to extensive incorporation of the technology as the major form of instructional delivery and repeated practice. Teachers who adopt online technology learn to think differently about their teaching and reconceptualize what they do, particularly in areas such as managing the learning environment, promoting collegiality and cooperation, and supporting problem solving (Creasman, 2012). Key differences that may come with increased use of online educational technology include:

- Online activities are often asynchronous, meaning that one student's activity occurs independently from the activity of other students and independent of the clinical teacher's presence. Students may be free to interact with course materials when it is convenient for them, often around the clock.
- Online discussions are generally nonlinear, facilitated by discussion boards, blogs, and journals where students can participate in multiple conversations simultaneously.
- Online environments favor the written word, which takes longer for students to compose and may take longer for teachers to review than a face-to-face discussion. However, the written word provides a more relaxed timeline for responding thoughtfully.
- The physical separation of teacher and student may slow communication. A confusing e-mail conversation or discussion board thread can be very frustrating without the rapid clarification available during an in-person discussion.
- Students may expect that because clinical activities are available online around the clock, clinical teachers are likewise continuously

available to troubleshoot the technology or answer questions about the content. Clinical teachers may have to manage technology support needs and expectations about availability.
- The volume of information available online is seemingly endless. Teachers might be able to keep track of what information is provided in a specific textbook from edition to edition, but keeping track of what is new information available to students online every day is certainly impossible (Creasman, 2012).

Clinical skills for nursing students have traditionally been cultivated through a combination of laboratory activities and direct observation of skilled clinicians in actual clinical practice. Over time, nursing students gradually increase their role and responsibility for the care of patients under the tutelage of teachers and mentors (Gould & Bauman, 2012). Today's learners are often accustomed to multimedia environments and are comfortable using media for academic and personal activities (Danforth, 2011). In fact, students have come to expect that technology, including web- and simulation-based education, be integrated into their curricula (Campbell & Daley, 2013). The access to infinite online resources for learning supports a change in the clinical teacher's role from the direct provider of information to a facilitator and co-learner (Edwards, Perry, & Janzen, 2011).

Although simulation and virtual reality–based learning does not take place in an actual clinical environment, it does provide learners with knowledge through their lived experiences in contextually rich environments that encourage reflection. Environments that support learning activities designed to authentically replicate clinical practice settings should be seen and treated as clinical environments. In this way, these environments may support and provide a foundation for learning during future clinical experiences. When learners are integrating data and decisions in more complex situations, more elaborate technology that includes simulated patient interaction may add a level of realism that engages the student and improves the overall learning experience (Kopp & Hanson, 2012; Rystedt & Sjöblom, 2012).

Evaluation of textbooks for adoption in a particular clinical course or sharing text selections across courses has taken on a new level of complexity. Considerations for textbook adoption now include whether the book is available in print, as an e-book that students can download on their computers or mobile devices, or both. The availability of additional electronic resources for the cost of the book or for an additional student fee can increase the desirability of adopting a particular text. Supplementary electronic resources may include downloadable test banks, instructor resource manuals, slide sets with elaborate graphics, and practice exercises. Even if the teacher only uses some of the supplementary resources, time and effort can be reduced compared with developing new clinical resources. Assigning practice exercises, practice tests, or slide set reviews before face-to-face clinical activities can help learners prepare to use their clinical time well.

In some communities, nursing programs and clinical care agencies share online resources for coordinating and negotiating clinical placement scheduling. Requests are put into the system for clinical specialty rotations and student groups, then reviewed to determine how to best meet the needs of all learners using scheduling that is reasonable and feasible for the agencies. Students may be given access to online orientation modules for individual clinical sites or as a shared resource among many clinical agencies whose leaders have agreed upon shared orientation requirements. Asking students to complete some or all of the educational orientation modules online before arriving at the clinical agency is efficient for the learners, the teachers, and the agency.

SELECTING TECHNOLOGY

Clinical teachers who want to incorporate electronic or web-based resources into their courses should consider the course objectives and the characteristics of the learners. Educational technology is a tool; finding the right tool or tools for the purpose is as important in selecting educational technology as it is in performing a health assessment. Some technological tools can serve multiple learning support functions and some learning objectives can be supported by more than one tool. Wenger, White, and Smith (2009) offered general advice for teachers who are considering educational technology:

- Start with simple and inexpensive strategies
- Learn from others who have been there
- Test the tools out before you adopt them
- Watch for what is coming next

Mastering clinical practice technology that learners will continue to use through their working careers, such as electronic health records (EHRs), may be a worthwhile learning outcome in itself. However, a focus on the specific technology rather than the learning objectives can lead to a misguided instructional effort.

Most educational technology is a resource and a means to an end, a tool rather an intended program outcome. There is no requirement for using the most elaborate possible technology to support clinical learning; expensive and complicated materials and plans may not be a better fit than simple and inexpensive materials and methods for supporting a particular clinical objective. A high-level effort to use a specific nonclinical technology for completion of a single assignment is generally not worthwhile from the perspective of either the students or the teacher. Clinical teachers should take care that even while striving to support students in using new technological learning tools, the teachers do not trade their responsibility of facilitating learning based on the clinical objectives for a full-time role as the technology support specialist and mechanic.

Frith and Clark (2013) provided guidance in matching the intended type of learning to the specific choice of the technology. For example, an intention that learners will create a product such as a patient teaching pamphlet or an electronic clinical portfolio suggests the use of tools such as specific types of design software, while an intention to provide learners practice in decision making might suggest human patient simulation, virtual reality simulations, or online case study analysis (see Exhibit 10.1).

The role of individual teachers or groups of faculty members who take on the responsibility for implementing technology resources is called *technology stewardship*. Technology stewards help their community of learners choose, organize, and apply technology to meet the learners' needs. It is not unusual that students show leadership in joining the team of technology stewards, supporting their peers and teachers in beginning use of and in troubleshooting technology. Technology stewards as individuals or teams need a clear understanding of their learning community members, so that they can respond to both expressed and implied needs in context. It is helpful if stewards are technology experts, but even an awareness of possibilities and available products is sufficient to trigger the process of finding others who can help with the selection and installation of more complex programs or equipment. During adoption of a new technology, stewards serve the leadership functions of managing the direction and pace of the change. Once a new technology is implemented into practice, stewards may support upgrading practices and new applications of the technology in response to emerging needs (Wenger et al., 2009).

Clinical teachers who like to try out new ideas are often natural technology stewards, but a team approach supports successful implementation of more complex systems. Benefits to the clinical teacher of taking on the technology steward role include the satisfaction of moving an initiative forward that does not otherwise have a champion; the impact of improving learning or educational practices; the opportunity for developing leadership, teaching, and technical skills; and enhanced reputation and credibility in both the academic and the practice setting (Hagler, Kastenbaum, Brooks, Morris, & Saewert, 2013; Wenger et al., 2009).

Exhibit 10.1

LEARNING INTENTS AND SELECTION OF INSTRUCTIONAL TECHNOLOGIES

Learning Intent	What Is It?	Media Forms	Active-Learning Strategies	Support Tools
Assimilative	Students are asked to process narrative media while managing and structuring information	Content delivery in multimedia formats (readings, lectures, narrated slide presentations, etc.)	Web quests, concept mapping, mind mapping, brainstorming, participatory sense making	Learning management systems (Blackboard, Sakai, Moodle, etc.), presentation software, brainstorming tools including concept mapping software, citation/research management tools including social bookmarking software, news aggregators (e.g., Google Reader), reflective journaling software (blogs), and collaboration software (wikis that support group work, including multiauthor annotated bibliographies)
Adaptive	An environment that changes according to learner input	Clinical simulations, game-based assessment environments	Situated coaching through online learning and assessment modules	Task-centered online learning modules (including a series of questions, decision points, and requests for rationale that students must address), role-playing exercises performed in multiplayer online role-playing game environments, interactive web-based lessons and clinical cases like NovEx eLearning

Learning Intent	What Is It?	Media Forms	Active-Learning Strategies	Support Tools
Communicative	Discussing	Asynchronous or synchronous discussions, chats, text messages	Reasoning, arguing, coaching, debate, discussion, negotiation, performance, online peer critique	Electronic whiteboards, e-mail, discussion boards, chat, instant messaging, VoIP (Voice over Internet Protocol, i.e., Internet telephony applications such as Skype), video conferencing, blogs, wikis
Productive	Learners producing something	Creating, producing, writing, synthesizing, remixing, mash-ups	Patient care plan, reflective journal, literature review, portfolio, narrated slide presentation	Creative applications (Google Video, office software, InDesign, Photoshop, Sketch, and other design software), publishing environments (YouTube), computer-aided assessment tools, electronic learning environments
Experiential	Interactive activities that focus on problem solving in a variety of clinical situations	Practicing, applying, mimicking, experiencing, exploring, investigating, performing	Case studies, simulation scenarios, role-playing exercises, interprofessional team-based learning	Multimedia, interactive case study lessons (NovEx eLearning), virtual simulation labs that approximate clinical settings and conditions within a 3-D immersive environment, massively multiplayer online role-playing games

Source: Reprinted from Frith and Clark (2013). Copyright © 2013 by Springer Publishing. Reprinted with permission of the publisher.

How can a busy clinical teacher gain access to educational technology? Teachers can acquire technology through at least seven strategies:

- Use what you have—often teachers do not know what is available unless they ask
- Try free demonstration editions of software or programs
- Build on an enterprise platform—one already owned by the school
- Get a commercial platform that meets current needs
- Build your own custom platform or tool
- Use open-source software
- Patch elements together (Wenger et al., 2009)

HEALTH INFORMATION TECHNOLOGY

Students are likely to encounter EHRs in most clinical settings, but agency policy may prevent them from using some or all parts of the record. In order to assure practice with documentation, some academic programs have designed their own simulated EHRs or asked students to purchase access to a commercial EHR for educational use.

Similar to implementing EHRs in a clinical setting, educators considering EHR adoption should plan carefully for the best outcomes. Compare options diligently and take advantage of demonstrations to test usability and adaptability before selecting a system. Consider generalist and specialist needs for documentation among various levels of students who will use the system as well as technical support needs and resources available to the nursing education program. Ask for peer reviews and lessons learned from educators in other programs who have implemented the systems you are considering. Develop a generous budget for time and expenses beyond the most obvious purchase costs, because upgrades may be required for related hardware and software, and faculty development can take extended time. Identify champions to provide leadership and be patient (Krisik, 2013).

Other agency-specific types of electronic clinical communication may also be available. A bedside electronic computer communication application that provides interactive patient-specific information, such as inpatient medication lists, names and photographs of care providers, room telephone number, laboratory results, daily schedule, and a location to write notes to the care team, has potential to enhance patient-provider communication and improve the patient experience (Dykes et al., 2013). As bar-code technology has been implemented in more clinical settings (Henneman et al., 2012; Poon et al., 2010), nurse educators have adopted bar-code technology for learner practice during medication administration in clinical skills and simulation laboratories.

WEB-BASED TECHNOLOGIES

Web-based activities that support self-paced learning or content review can provide flexibility and expanded access for busy learners. Choices of web-based activities should support the intended clinical learning outcomes. Planning for facilitated reflection and integration of the learners' web experience with other clinical activities helps to underscore the value of the activities.

PUBLISHERS' SUPPLEMENTARY MATERIALS

A common source of clinical learning activities is found in the instructor resources and other supplementary materials supplied by publishers based on textbook purchase or for an additional fee. There is a wide range of the extent of these resources. Some are only websites with a list of additional recommended readings; some provide application activities and slide sets in concert with each textbook chapter. Test banks that can be uploaded into course learning management system sites are common, but extensive online workbooks with evaluation components may cost students an additional fee for use. Sets of online case simulations can be required for clinical courses similar to a textbook purchase and assigned as individual cases throughout the curriculum.

An entire online environment, The Neighborhood, with multiple characters and a range of health and health care needs is available for purchase and learner use over multiple semesters. A designed environment and community population has been used to help students integrate their classroom and clinical learning as they plan care for individuals, families, and a community (Gonzalez & Fenske, 2012).

LEARNING OBJECTS

A learning object (LO), also called a reusable learning object (RLO), is a self-contained digital educational resource that may include objectives, content, interactive learning activities, animations, narrated text, visual images, self-assessments, and feedback tools (Windle, McCormick, Dandrea, & Wharrad, 2011). LOs may be used independently in support of a smaller, more focused topic or combined with other LOs or activities to teach larger content areas. LOs are often published on the web, embedded in a learning management system, or produced as a podcast or DVD; most are less than 15 minutes long.

A number of open repositories allow educators and their learners to browse for and use LOs that fit particular learning needs and content areas. Some repositories catalog resources that meet only specific technical or pedagogical standards while others allow open posting and use. See Exhibit 10.2 for examples of learning repositories.

Exhibit 10.2

EXAMPLES OF LEARNING REPOSITORIES

Name of Repository	Website Address
Connexions—Rice University	cnx.org
EducaNext	www.educanext.org
FREE—Federal Resources for Educational Excellence	www.free.ed.gov
Harvey Project	opencourse.org/Collaboratories/harveyproject
ide@s	www.ideas.wisconsin.edu/index.cfm
iTunes U	www.apple.com/education/itunes-u
Library of Congress	www.loc.gov/library/libarch-digital.html
MERLOT	www.merlot.org
MIT OpenCourseWare	ocw.mit.edu/index.htm
MLX—Maricopa Learning Exchange	www.mcli.dist.maricopa.edu/mlx
NEAT—Nursing Education and Technology Project	webcls.utmb.edu/neat
Nursing Objects Library—Maricopa Community Colleges Nursing Program	www.mesacc.edu/dept/d31/nursing/learning_objects
Problem-Based Learning at University of Delaware	primus.nss.udel.edu/Pbl
PBS Teachers	www.pbs.org/teachers
Free e-Books by Project Gutenberg	www.gutenberg.org/wiki/Main_Page
Shareable Learning Objects from WSU College of Nursing and Health	www.wright.edu/nursing/shareableobjects
SMETE	www.smete.org/smete
SoftChalk Connect	www.softchalkconnect.com
Learning Tools	www.learningtools.arts.ubc.ca

(continued)

Name of Repository	Website Address
The Orange Grove: Florida's K20 Digital Repository	www.theorangegrove.org/index.asp
USG Share	usgshare.org/logon.do
Virginia Commonwealth University School of Nursing Learning Objects	www.nursing.vcu.edu/it/learning_objects.html
Wisc-Online	www.wisc-online.com

Source: From Frith and Clark (2013). Copyright © 2013 by Springer Publishing. Reprinted with permission of the publisher.

Some repositories, such as MERLOT (2013), provide access to simultaneous searches in the databases of multiple other repositories. Some LOs in repositories or independent websites may be covered under Creative Commons licenses (Creative Commons, 2013), which include a range of six different standardized levels of copyright permissions to the creative work.

When clinical teachers develop LOs for their own courses, it is important to keep focused on a small area of content, clearly define the scope, and incorporate strategies that facilitate ease of navigation and interactivity. Some teachers use a storyboard approach to help facilitate the development of LOs. Before beginning to create an LO that you may want to make publicly available, review the standards at several online repositories and consider the type of copyright permission you are willing to grant to others for educational or commercial uses.

MASSIVE OPEN ONLINE COURSES

Massive open online courses (MOOCs) provide an opportunity for students who are not enrolled in a particular college or university to attend an online course taught by that institution's faculty, often including nationally known expert faculty members. "Massive" describes open enrollment that can exceed 100,000 learners; some courses begin new sections only at scheduled times, while other MOOCs allow interested learners to begin at any time. The courses have assignments and exams similar to many other online courses taught in colleges and universities, and they often feature discussion boards on which tens of thousands of students can share ideas. MOOC quality varies widely and most students who enroll in MOOCs do not complete them. However, MOOCs on clinical topics can provide access to organized resources and media that supports just-in-time asynchronous learning (Kellogg, 2013) for the clinical teacher or the students.

BEST PRACTICE RESOURCES

The Internet provides access to numerous libraries and databases of evidence to support effective nursing care and promote health. Government and other public websites provide access to data that can be used to frame the significance of health problems in a given location or target population as well provide students with practice in using databases for planning population-based care. Standards of care and policy statements may provide very current access to best practice information (De Natale & Malloy, 2012). For example, students may visit the Centers for Disease Control and Prevention (CDC) website to prepare for a clinical activity in immunization or disaster preparedness, or to find out more about a particular disease or condition (CDC, 2013). Searching clinical practice guidelines at the Agency for Healthcare Research and Quality (AHRQ) site helps students locate best practices for providing care to patients with a specific disease or condition, and to compare clinical guidelines proposed by different expert groups (AHRQ, 2013).

VIRTUAL REALITY AND GAME-BASED LEARNING

Web, virtual reality, and game-based learning environments can provide important cues and learning opportunities related to the contexts and roles that students will be expected to develop and master in order to attain professional expertise and acceptance as a clinician in today's complex health care environment (Benner, Tanner, & Chesla, 2009; Gould & Bauman, 2012). The virtual world may provide students with interesting ethical questions where boundaries and discourse can be explored. Teachers can select virtual environments that reflect real-world best practices.

Nurses have long appreciated the use of stories for teaching and learning. Many virtual activities and games are based on the power of storytelling or authoring one's own story. Stories are naturally engaging and highly flexible; they can be told from multiple perspectives on a moment's notice to emphasize different key messages. Storytelling formats can range from a simple video- or audiorecording recalling an experience to a polished, highly interactive multimedia production. As Sanford and Emmott (2012) described it, narrative requires readers to produce rich and complex mental representations. It offers one of the major means through which the experiences of other people, different cultures, and distant times may be conveyed, and expands our virtual experience of the world. Typically, narratives manipulate not only our knowledge of things, but also our impressions of how people feel, judge, and react in a multitude of situations (p. xi).

This ability of a story to help us experience a novel event or a situation from a different perspective provides a way to integrate information across the cognitive, psychomotor, and affective domains. Features common to narratives and stories when used as a teaching method in any format include

- Specific rather than generic events
- Specific time and place settings
- People involved in the events
- Moment-by-moment thoughts, feelings, and sensory perceptions
- A setting, theme, plot, and resolution
- Audience members feel as if they have entered a different world (Sanford & Emmott, 2012)

Video game and virtual world scholars have come to recognize the power that narratives have in the creation of meaningful learning (Gee, 2003). Narratives help people recognize patterns and make sense of the world (Walsh, 2011). Pattern recognition is a key component marking a critical difference among novices and experts. Through their lived and situated experience, experts come to recognize patterns that often lead them to conclusions much more quickly than novices.

Narrative provides learning situations with valuable cues to direct student performance in the virtual world. Think of the narrative as the background information that would be provided to students during a case-based learning scenario. However, instead of simply providing a didactic presentation of the patient's history by reading it to students, the virtual environment unfolds based on the students' interaction with the environment as well as with others concurrently occupying the environment.

Narratives also assist game players in the negotiation and reconciliation of their identities, particularly projective identities. The projective identity emerges to represent learners' reflection on assumptions and implications associated with the reconciliation of their virtual and real-world identities. This reflection represents an essential opportunity to study aspects of cultural framing of self and other (Games & Bauman, 2011; Gee, 2003).

The virtual environment provides aspects of narrative that simply may not exist in actual clinical environments. Teachers, mentors, and preceptors do not have predictable and reliable access to disasters and crises for teaching purposes. Many clinical education settings do not provide culturally diverse environments. Virtual encounters with culture and diversity may prepare learners for actual encounters with patients and colleagues in real clinical settings. Understanding cultural framing in simulations and games is important for nursing students because they are learning how to interact in new, different, and often uncomfortable contexts where culture and diversity can play important roles (Kastenbaum, Hagler, Brooks, & Ruiz, 2011).

Narratives also provide spaces for reflection on the consequences of one's decision making. Learners can be encouraged to see the consequences of their action or inaction from multiple perspectives. The virtual world can provide different narrative endings based on learners' ongoing interaction with their environment. In this way, students are able to engage in deliberate decision making that will produce varying scenario outcomes. This type of deliberate practice is not available in the real clinical world. In actual clinical encounters, mentors and clinical teachers must often make sure that optimal care is provided to patients, so students are often relegated to the role of observer, at least on the initial patient encounter. When students care for real patients, they do not have the luxury of revisiting the same clinical encounter in order to make a better or different decision. Virtual environments allow students to take responsibility for their decisions in a situated but safe context. Teachers can monitor students' progress as they adjust their behavior and decision making to negotiate more acceptable outcomes. This allows the teacher to guide students while letting them develop competence, confidence, and expertise through reflection on past experience. In this sense, for students inhabiting the virtual world, an error simply becomes an opportunity for reflection, learning, and behavioral change.

Negotiating responsibilities related to virtual identities existing within situated narratives can involve sophisticated cognitive effort and critical thinking strategies. For example, a virtual operating room that has been engineered to provide an interactive procedural simulation could serve as an introduction and orientation to roles and expectations associated with perioperative nursing. Elements of this environment could include everything from hand antisepsis and gowning to the surgical time-out. Preprogrammed nonplayer characters in virtual environments can provide cues based on learners' actions to direct the in-world learning experience. Furthermore, learning activities in the virtual world can be engineered as situated interactions to promote designed experiences that emphasize specific curriculum objectives (Gould & Bauman, 2012).

The fluidity and malleability of virtual environments applies not only to the look and feel of virtual teaching spaces but also to learners' identities. In most virtual worlds, players interact with others and the environment by controlling avatars that represent them. The ability to try on multiple identities may be of great value for the design of learning experiences involving culture and diversity. One could imagine a lesson in which students play the role of patients belonging to a different culture from their own. In the same way, the teacher could facilitate behavioral responses from students that represent either cultural competence or cultural clichés and stereotypes (Games & Bauman, 2011; Gould & Bauman, 2012). Character design and assignment allows individuals to adopt the appearance and persona of cultural groups other than their own and experience others' situations. Reflection on this experience may help students develop understanding and skills related to culture and diversity that they can bring to future clinical practice.

Designed experiences that have the potential to evoke strong emotional responses should include guided debriefing and reflection sessions to diffuse and mitigate those responses. The debriefing not only ensures that targeted objectives have been met but also encourages further reflection by students and teachers. Video capture of in-world interactions and behavior can serve as an important tool to facilitate debriefings and further reflection.

Lessons in professional conduct related to character appearance and behavior could be further situated in a number of contexts. For example, should players in the virtual world fail to adhere to expected personal protective precautions, they may have a significant exposure, leading to illness. Clearly, the importance of activities, contexts, narratives, and characters as facets or elements of an ecology for culturally competent design are dynamic.

Virtual reality and video game–based learning opportunities solve some of the conundrums associated with fixed learning spaces like traditional nursing and mannequin-based simulation laboratories. Advancements in media technology increasingly allow educators to customize and integrate virtual reality and game-based learning into nursing and other types of clinical curricula. Within reason, students can access virtual spaces at their convenience. A number of virtual-world and gaming platforms already exist, wherein the original purpose could be changed to include clinical education. Higgins and Hannan (2013) reported on a game-based intervention to increase hand hygiene compliance in an acute health care setting. Additional options can be explored as we gain a better understanding of how clinical teachers and others can use virtual worlds and gaming most effectively in ways that promote the transfer of knowledge and desired behavioral change.

USE OF MOBILE AND HANDHELD DEVICES

Some clinical settings allow students and clinical teachers the use of cell phones and mobile devices while on site, while others do not; it is important to know the clinical policies regarding mobile devices and remind learners of the policies. Learners may be able to access in the clinical setting some or all of the technology applications by mobile phone that they can access on campus. Learning management systems often have mobile application options that provide some or all of the functions from a mobile device. Learners may download their e-textbooks on tablet PCs, phones, or e-readers to have ready access to resources for looking up current medication information or other clinical topics.

Some faculty members and clinical teachers may discourage use of mobile devices in clinical areas because they expect students to be fully prepared for clinical learning activities without consulting information resources during those activities. However, in the real world of nursing practice, nurses often receive new information that must be evaluated or verified, and learning how to access appropriate resources as needed to plan care is an important goal as students prepare to function without the guidance of instructors. For example, no nurse can be expected to know everything there is to know about every medication that may be ordered for a patient, especially when new drugs are approved, removed from the market, or have revised indications for use on an ongoing basis. If a patient's medication order is changed (e.g., new medication order, dosage, or route of administration), the nurse providing care to that patient must know how to locate and access the necessary information about the new drug order to be able to administer the medication safely or whether to question the order. Use of mobile devices in the clinical setting can facilitate this process; nursing students need to practice using this technology throughout their educational program so that they will be able to demonstrate this competency upon graduation.

Clinical teachers can help direct students to credible professional websites for clinical information and help them evaluate information found on more general websites. A recent concern related to cell phones and other technology is that increasing pressure to interact with devices will distract nurses and other health professionals from their focus on patient care, endangering patient safety (McBride, 2012). See Chapter 6 for additional information on legal and ethical issues related to the use of cell phones and other mobile devices.

TECHNOLOGY AND INTERPROFESSIONAL LEARNING

The virtual environment may provide an ideal platform for expanding the boundaries of interprofessional multidisciplinary education. The anonymity of virtual worlds may provide an opportunity to overcome barriers that promote segregated professional education. Many health professions-related concepts such as values and ethics, roles and responsibilities, communication, and teamwork, are generally applicable (Interprofessional Education Collaborative Expert Panel, 2011). Environments that focus on the elements of culturally competent educational design (activities, contexts, narratives, and characters) can be created to include designed experiences with interactions and activities representing different facets of situated relevance across disciplines.

REFLECTION AND EVALUATION

Technology can support learning concepts as well as developing specific competencies. Regardless of the technology used, careful integration of the activity into the curriculum helps assure a positive program-level learning outcome (Nielsen, Noone, Voss, & Mathews, 2013). One of the key strategies that Benner et al. (2009) described as an exemplar of good teaching in any setting is teaching for salience—helping learners reflect on practice to identify what is important in a given situation. Coaching for reflection requires active engagement of the teacher, while reflecting requires active engagement of the learner. Reflection on a technology-based learning activity could be prompted by a list of questions such as, "How do you know?" and "What are the reasons?" considered during a dialogue or in a writing activity such as journaling, blogging, or posting in an online discussion (Ennis, 2010). Extensive question sets for discussion can be developed as framed around the Universal Intellectual Standards (Elder & Paul, 2010). Ongoing learning can be encouraged by asking what questions still remain in the learner's mind after the discussion (Nilson, 2010).

Billings and Connors (2012) suggested seven areas of outcomes to evaluate after implementing online technology in the curriculum:

- Access
- Convenience
- Connectedness
- Preparation for real world work
- Socialization to the profession
- Satisfaction with web-based learning
- Proficiency with computer skills, use of learning management system tools

SUMMARY

Technology has blurred the boundaries between classroom and clinical teaching. Students expect technology to be integrated into their curricula. Access to online resources supports a change in the clinical teacher's role from the direct provider of information to a facilitator and co-learner.

Clinical teachers can serve as technology stewards in adopting effective tools for teaching and learning. A wealth of resources such as web-based technologies, publishers' supplementary materials, health information technology, LOs, MOOCs, virtual reality, game-based learning, and mobile or handheld devices support exploration and application of clinical concepts. Technology can also be used to support interprofessional learning.

Learners integrate their personal experiences of technology activities through reflection. Careful curricular integration and ongoing evaluation of technology-supported activities help promote positive learning outcomes.

Exhibit 10.3

CNE EXAMINATION TEST BLUEPRINT CORE COMPETENCIES

1. **Facilitate Learning**

   A. Implement a variety of teaching strategies appropriate to
      1. content
      2. setting
      3. learner needs
      4. learning style
      5. desired learner outcomes

   B. Use teaching strategies based on
      1. educational theory
      2. evidence-based practices related to education

   C. Modify teaching strategies and learning experiences based on consideration of learners'
      2. past clinical experiences
      3. past educational and life experiences
      4. generational groups (i.e., age)

   D. Use information technologies to support the teaching-learning process

   N. Use knowledge of evidence-based practice to instruct learners

2. **Facilitate Learner Development and Socialization**

   B. Provide resources for diverse learners to meet their individual learning needs

   D. Create learning environments that facilitate learners' self-reflection, personal goal-setting, and socialization to the role of the nurse

   E. Foster the development of learners in these areas
      1. cognitive domain
      2. psychomotor domain
      3. affective domain

6. **Engage in Scholarship, Service, and Leadership**

   A. Function as a change agent and leader
      5. Implement strategies for change within the nursing program
      7. Adapt to changes created by external factors

REFERENCES

Agency for Healthcare Research and Quality. (2013). *Guidelines and recommendations*. Retrieved from http://www.ahrq.gov/professionals/clinicians-providers/guidelines-recommendations/index.html

Benner, P., Sutphen, M., Leonard, V., & Day, L. (2009). *Educating nurses: A call for radical transformation*. San Francisco, CA: Jossey-Bass.

Benner, P., Tanner, C., & Chesla, C. (2009). *Expertise in nursing: Caring, clinical judgment, and ethics*. New York, NY: Springer Publishing.

Billings, D., & Connors, H. (2012). *Best practices in online learning*. Retrieved from http://www.electronicvision.com/nln/chapter02/index.htm

Campbell, S. H., & Daley, K. (Eds.). (2013). *Simulation scenarios for nurse educators: Making it real* (2nd ed.). New York, NY: Springer Publishing.

Centers for Disease Control and Prevention (2013). *Home page*. Retrieved from http://www.cdc.gov

Creasman, P. (2012). *IDEA paper # 52: Considerations in online course design*. Manhattan, KS: The IDEA Center. Retrieved from http://www.theideacenter.org/sites/default/files/idea_paper_52.pdf

Creative Commons. (2013). *About the licenses*. Retrieved from http://creativecommons.org/licenses

Danforth, L. (2011). Why game learning works. *Library Journal, 136*(7), 67.

De Natale, M. L., & Malloy, S. E. (2012). The use of position statements in teaching best practices in nursing. *Nursing Education Perspectives, 33*, 378–379.

Dykes, P. C., Carroll, D. L., Hurley, A. C., Benoit, A., Chang, F., Pozzar, R., & Caligtan, C. A. (2013). Building and testing a patient-centric electronic bedside communication center. *Journal of Gerontological Nursing, 39*(1), 15–19. doi:10.3928/00989134-20121204-03

Edwards, M., Perry, B., & Janzen, K. (2011). The making of an exemplary online educator. *Distance Education, 32*, 101–118.

Elder, L., & Paul, R. (2010). Critical thinking: Competency standards essential for the cultivation of intellectual skills, Part 1. *Journal of Developmental Education, 34*(2), 38–39.

Ennis, R. (2010). *A super-streamlined conception of critical thinking*. Retrieved from http://www.criticalthinking.net

Frith, K. H., & Clark, D. J. (2013). *Distance education in nursing* (3rd ed.). New York, NY: Springer Publishing.

Games, I., & Bauman, E. (2011). Virtual worlds: An environment for cultural sensitivity education in the health sciences. *International Journal of Web Based Communities, 7*, 189–205. doi:10.1504/IJWBC.2011.039510

Gee, J. P. (2003). *What video games have to teach us about learning literacy*. New York, NY: Palgrave Macmillan.

Gonzalez, L., & Fenske, C. L. (2012). Use of a virtual community to contextualize learning activities. *Journal of Nursing Education, 51*, 38–41.

Gould, J., & Bauman, E. (2012). Virtual reality in medical education. In S. Tsuda, D. J. Scott, & D. B. Jones (Eds.), *Textbook of simulation, surgical skills and team training*. Woodbury, CT: Cine-Med.

Hagler, D., Kastenbaum, B., Brooks, R., Morris, B., & Saewert, K. J. (2013). Leveraging the technology du jour for overt and covert faculty development. *Journal of Faculty Development, 27*(3), 22–29.

Henneman, P. L., Henneman, E. A., Marquard, J. L., Fisher, D. L., Bleil, J., Walsh, B., … Nathanson, B. H. (2012). Bar-code verification: Reducing but not eliminating medication errors. *The Journal of Nursing Administration, 42*, 562.

Higgins, A., & Hannan, M. M. (2013). Improved hand hygiene technique and compliance in healthcare workers using gaming technology. *The Journal of Hospital Infection, 84*, 32. doi:10.1016/j.jhin.2013.02.004

Interprofessional Education Collaborative Expert Panel. (2011). *Core competencies for interprofessional collaborative practice: Report of an expert panel.* Washington, DC: Interprofessional Education Collaborative.

Kastenbaum, B., Hagler, D., Brooks, R., & Ruiz, E. (2011). Simulation: Realistic cultural encounters. *Academic Exchange Quarterly, 15*(2), 27–32.

Kellogg, S. (2013). Online learning: How to make a MOOC. *Nature, 499*, 369–371.

Kopp, W., & Hanson, M. A. (2012). High-fidelity and gaming simulations enhance nursing education in end-of-life care. *Clinical Simulation in Nursing, 8*(3), e97–e102. doi:10.1016/j.ecns.2010.07.005

Krisik, K. M. (2013). Lessons learned: How to smooth your EHR implementation. *Health Management Technology, 34*(3), 8.

McBride, D. L. (2012). The distracted nurse. *Journal of Pediatric Nursing, 27*, 275. doi:10.1016/j.pedn.2012.02.002

MERLOT. (2013). *Search other libraries.* Retrieved from http://fedsearch.merlot.org/fedsearch/fedsearch.jsp

Nielsen, A. E., Noone, J., Voss, H., & Mathews, L. R. (2013). Preparing nursing students for the future: An innovative approach to clinical education. *Nurse Education in Practice, 13*, 301–309. doi: 10.1016/j.nepr.2013.03.015

Nilson, L. B. (2010). *Teaching at its best: A research-based resource for college instructors.* San Francisco, CA: Jossey-Bass.

Poon, E. G., Keohane, C. A., Yoon, C. S., Ditmore, M., Bane, A., Levtzion-Korach, O., … Gandhi, T. K. (2010). Effect of bar-code technology on the safety of medication administration. *New England Journal of Medicine, 362*, 1698–1707.

Rystedt, H., & Sjöblom, B. (2012). Realism, authenticity, and learning in healthcare simulations: Rules of relevance and irrelevance as interactive achievements. *Instructional Science, 40*, 785–798. doi: 10.1007/s11251-012-9213-x

Sanford, A. J., & Emmott, C. (2012). *Mind, brain and narrative.* Cambridge University Press. Retrieved from http://www.myilibrary.com?ID=418340

Walsh, M. (2011). Narrative pedagogy and simulation: Future directions for nursing education. *Nurse Education in Practice*, 216–219. doi: 10.1016/j.nepr.2010.10.006

Wenger, E., White, N., & Smith, J. D. (2009). *Digital habitats: Stewarding technology for communities.* Portland, OR: CPsquare.

Windle, R. J., McCormick, D., Dandrea, J., & Wharrad, H. (2011). The characteristics of reusable learning objects that enhance learning: A case-study in health-science education. *British Journal of Educational Technology, 42*, 811–823. doi:10.1111/j.1467-8535.2010.01108.x

CHAPTER 11

Case Method, Case Study, and Grand Rounds

Clinical practice provides opportunities for students to gain the knowledge and skills needed to care for patients; develop values important in professional practice; and develop cognitive skills for processing and analyzing data, deciding on problems and interventions, and evaluating their effectiveness. Ability to apply concepts and theories to clinical situations, solve clinical problems, arrive at carefully thought out decisions, and provide safe, quality care are essential competencies gained through clinical practice. Case method, case study, and grand rounds are teaching methods that help students meet these learning outcomes. Case method and case study describe a clinical situation developed around an actual or a hypothetical patient for student review and critique. In case method, the case provided for analysis is generally shorter and more specific than in case study. Case studies are more comprehensive in nature, thereby presenting a complete picture of the patient and clinical situation. Grand rounds involve the observation and often interview of a patient or several patients in the clinical setting, through a webcast of grand rounds conducted elsewhere or a multimedia program.

CASES AND GRAND ROUNDS FOR DEVELOPING COGNITIVE SKILLS

With cases and grand rounds, students can apply concepts and theories to clinical situations, identify patient and other types of problems, propose varied approaches for solving them, weigh them against the evidence, and choose the most appropriate approaches. These methods provide

237

experience for students in analyzing clinical situations and thinking through possible decisions.

Problem Solving

The nursing literature contains various perspectives on problem solving, decision making, critical thinking, and clinical judgment. In general, problem solving is the ability to solve clinical problems, some relating to the patient and others that arise from clinical practice. Problem solving begins with recognizing and defining the problem, gathering data to clarify it further, identifying possible approaches, weighing them against evidence, and choosing the best one considering patient needs and responses (Oermann & Gaberson, 2014).

Viewed as a cognitive skill, problem solving can be developed through experiences with patients, such as in grand rounds, or via simulated cases, such as case method and study. The student does not need to provide hands-on care to develop problem-solving skills. By observing and discussing patients during grand rounds and analyzing cases, students gain experience in understanding patient problems and the clinical situation and deciding on approaches to use. Cases and grand rounds expose students to clinical situations that they may not encounter in their own clinical practices.

In clinical practice, nurses make many important decisions when caring for patients, families, and communities. They decide on data to collect and what they mean, problems and their priority, interventions, resources, and effectiveness of interventions. Tanner (2006) referred to this cognitive process as clinical reasoning: the process of generating different alternatives, weighing them against evidence, and deciding on the most appropriate approach to use. With cases and rounds, students can practice these skills: they can generate possible alternatives, weigh them against evidence, consider the consequences of each, then arrive at a decision following this analysis.

Critical Thinking

Critical thinking enables the nurse to make reasoned and informed judgments in the practice setting and decide what to do in a given situation. It is purposeful and informed reasoning in clinical practice and in other settings (Alfaro-LeFevre, 2013). Critical thinking is a judgment process. Nurses and other clinicians decide what to believe or do in a particular situation based on available evidence and using the knowledge and skills they acquired through their education and practice; that process also involves weighing the likely consequences of different actions and evaluating their effectiveness (Facione & Facione, 2008).

Critical thinking development can be viewed as a process through which students progress. Elder and Paul (2010) described stages of critical thinking. These include the: (a) unreflective thinker, (b) challenged thinker, (c) beginning thinker, (d) practicing thinker, (e) advanced thinker, and (f) accomplished thinker (Elder & Paul, 2010). These stages were used by nursing faculty members to develop unfolding cases for simulation (West, Holmes, Zidek, & Edwards, 2013).

Critical thinking can also be viewed as reflective thinking about patient problems when the problem is not obvious or the nurse knows what is wrong but is unsure what to do. Through critical thinking, the learner:

- Considers multiple perspectives to care
- Critiques different approaches possible in a clinical situation
- Weighs approaches against evidence and patient responses
- Arrives at sound judgments
- Raises questions about issues to clarify them further
- Resolves issues with a well–thought out approach (Alfaro-LeFevre, 2013; Facione, 2011; Facione & Facione, 2008)

Clinical Judgment

Tanner (2006) developed a model of clinical judgment in nursing that incorporates concepts of problem solving, decision making, and critical thinking. In this model, clinical judgment involves interpreting a patient's needs and problems and deciding on actions and approaches, taking the patient's responses into consideration. The clinical judgment process includes four aspects: (a) noticing, grasping the situation; (b) interpreting, understanding the situation in order to respond; (c) responding, deciding on actions that are appropriate or that no actions are needed; and (d) reflecting, being attentive to how patients respond to the nurse's actions.

This model provides a framework for guiding students' reflections of how they think about clinical situations, interpret them, and arrive at decisions. In simulated cases, students can describe what they would expect to find in the clinical situation in the case (noticing), the meaning of the data in the case, and appropriate interventions or why they would take no action. In grand rounds, students can observe a patient's responses to actions and reflect on how they influence subsequent decisions. The model provides a framework for coaching students in how they think about clinical situations.

CASE METHOD AND STUDY

Case method and case study serve similar purposes in clinical teaching: they provide a simulated case for student review and critique. In case method, the case provided for analysis is generally shorter and more specific than in case study.

Case Method

In case method, short cases are developed around actual or hypothetical patients followed by open-ended questions to encourage students' thinking about the case. Short cases are used to avoid directing students' thinking in advance (Oermann, 2008). Depending on how the case is written, case method is effective for applying concepts and other types of knowledge to clinical practice and for promoting development of cognitive skills. With cases, students can analyze patient data, identify needs and problems, and decide on the best approaches in that situation after weighing the evidence. Cases also assist students in relating course content to clinical practice and integrating different concepts and theories in a particular clinical situation. Examples of case method are presented in Exhibit 11.1.

Exhibit 11.1

EXAMPLES OF CASE METHOD

Mrs. F has moderate dementia. She lets the nurse practitioner do a pelvic examination because she has a "woman's problem." The examination shows an anterior wall prolapse. While helping Mrs. F to get dressed, the nurse practitioner observes that, as soon as the patient stands up, urine begins leaking onto the floor. Mrs. F appears embarrassed.

1. List and prioritize Mrs. F's problems. Provide a rationale for how the problems are prioritized.
2. Develop a plan of care for Mrs. F.

Your patient is admitted from the emergency department with severe headache, right-sided weakness, and aphasia. Her temperature is normal, pulse 120, respirations 16, and blood pressure 180/120.

1. What are possible reasons for these symptoms? Provide an explanation for your answer.
2. What additional data would you collect on admission to your unit? Why is this information important to planning the patient's care?

Mrs. B, 29 years old, is seen for a prenatal checkup. She is in her 24th week of pregnancy. The nurse practitioner notes swelling of the ankles and around

(continued)

Mrs. B's eyes. Mrs. B has not been able to wear her rings for a week because of swelling. Her blood pressure is 144/96.

1. What are possible problems Mrs. B might be facing? List all possible problems given the above information.
2. What additional data should be collected at this time? Why?

You are working in a pediatrician's office. Mrs. C brings her son in for a check-up after a severe asthma attack a month ago that required emergency care. When you ask Mrs. C how her son is doing, she begins to cry softly. She tells you she is worried about his having another asthma attack and this time not recovering from it. When the pediatrician enters the examination room, Mrs. C is still crying. The physician says, "What's wrong? Look at him. He's doing great."

1. What would you say to Mrs. C, if anything, in this situation?
2. What would you say to the pediatrician, if anything?

You have a new patient, 81 years old, with congestive heart failure. The referral to your home health agency indicates that Mr. A has difficulty breathing, tires easily, and has edema in both legs, making it difficult for him to get around. He lives alone.

1. What are problems you anticipate for Mr. A? Include a rationale for each of these problems.

At your first home visit, you find Mr. A sitting in a chair with his feet on the floor. During your assessment, he gets short of breath talking with you and has to stop periodically to catch his breath.

1. Describe at least three different nursing interventions that could be used in Mr. A's care.
2. Specify outcome criteria for evaluating the effectiveness of the interventions you selected.
3. What would you teach Mr. A?
4. Select one of your interventions and review the evidence on its use. What are your conclusions about the effectiveness of the intervention?
5. Identify one published research study that relates to Mr. A's care. Critique the study and describe whether you could use the findings in caring for Mr. A and similar patients.

Mrs. M is a 42-year-old elementary school teacher with a history of inflammatory bowel disease. She calls the clinic for an appointment because of diarrhea that has lasted for 2 weeks. The nurse answering the phone tells Mrs. M to stop taking all of her medications until she is seen in the clinic.

1. Do you agree or disagree with the nurse's advice to Mrs. M? Why?

You have been working in the clinical agency for nearly 6 months. Recently you noticed a colleague having difficulty completing his assignments on time. He also has been late for work on at least three occasions. Today you see him move from one patient to the next without washing his hands.

1. What are your options in this situation?
2. Discuss possible consequences of each option.
3. What would you do? Why is this the best approach?

(continued)

As you record a patient's vital signs in the electronic medical records, she asks you to show the computer screen to her husband so he can read about the diagnoses they are ruling out.

1. What would you say to this patient?
2. What principles guide your decision? Provide a rationale for your response.

Mrs. J brings her 8-year-old daughter, Laura, into the office for her annual visit. In reviewing the immunization record, the nurse notices that Laura never received the second dose of the measles, mumps, rubella (MMR) vaccine. The nurse tells the mother not to worry; Laura can get the second dose when she is 11 or 12 years old.

1. Do you agree or disagree with the nurse's advice to the mother? Provide a rationale for your decision.

Read the following statements: One in three adults and one in five adolescents are overweight. Being overweight is prevalent among certain racial and ethnic groups.

1. What additional information do you need before identifying the implications of this statement for your community?
2. Why is this information important?

The heart failure clinic at your hospital has been effective in reducing the number of readmissions, but, to save costs, the hospital is closing it. As the nurse practitioner in that clinic, write a report about why the clinic should remain open, with data to support your position. To whom would you send that report and why? Then write a report from the perspective of the hospital administration supporting closure of the clinic.

Case Study

A case study provides an actual or hypothetical patient situation for students to analyze and arrive at varied decisions. Case studies typically are longer and more comprehensive than in case method, providing background data about the patient, family history, and other information for a more complete picture. For this reason, students can analyze case studies in greater depth than with case method and present a more detailed rationale for their analysis. In their critique of the case study, students can describe the concepts and theories that guided their analysis, how they used them in understanding the case, and the literature they reviewed. Examples of case studies are presented in Exhibit 11.2.

Using Case Method and Case Study in Clinical Courses

Short cases, as in case method, and longer case studies can be integrated in clinical courses throughout the curriculum to assist students in applying concepts and knowledge they are learning in their courses to clinical

Exhibit 11.2

EXAMPLE OF A CASE STUDY

Mary, 44 years old, is seen in the physician's office with hoarseness and a slight cough. During the assessment, Mary tells the nurse that she also has shortness of breath, particularly when walking fast and going up the stairs. Mary has never smoked. Her vital signs are: blood pressure 120/80; heart rate 88 beats per minute; respirations 32 per minute; and temperature 36.6° C (97.8° F).

Mary is married with two teenage daughters. She works part-time as a substitute teacher. Mary has always been health conscious, watching her weight and eating properly. She tells the nurse how worried she is because she has read about women getting lung cancer even if they never smoked.

1. The physician orders a combined PET/CT scan. What is a PET/CT scan, and why was it ordered for Mary?
2. What would you say to Mary prior to the scan to prepare her for it?
3. Identify a potential diagnosis for Mary and add data to the case consistent with that diagnosis. What types of problems would you anticipate for Mary? Describe nursing management for each of those problems.
4. Add data about Mary and her family to the case. Select a family theory and use it to analyze this family. What did you learn about the family, and how will this influence your care?
5. What resources are available in your community for Mary?

situations of increasing complexity. In beginning clinical courses, teachers can develop cases that present problems that are relatively easy to identify and require standard nursing interventions. At this level, students learn how to apply concepts to clinical situations and think through them. Students can work as a group to analyze cases; explore different perspectives of the case, what students noticed about it, and their interpretations; and discuss possible approaches to use.

In the beginning, the teacher should "think aloud," guiding students through the analysis, pointing out significant aspects of the case and his or her own expectations and interpretations. By thinking aloud, the teacher can model the clinical judgment process step by step through a case. As students progress through the curriculum, the cases can become more complex with varied problems and approaches that could be used in the situation.

Students can analyze cases in a postclinical conference, as an independent activity, or online either individually or in small groups. They can share resources they used to better understand the case. If cases are analyzed individually, further discussion about the case can occur with the clinical group as a whole, or students can post their thoughts and responses online for others to reflect and comment on.

Based on the questions asked about the case, cases can be used to meet many different learning outcomes of a clinical course. For example, if the goal of the case is to guide students in interpreting data, then questions might ask students to identify significant information in the situation and explain what the data mean. Cases are effective as an instructional method, and they can also be graded similar to essay items.

Complexity of Cases for Review

Cases may be of varying levels of complexity. Some cases are designed with the problems readily apparent. With these cases, the problem is described clearly, and sufficient information is included to guide decisions on how to intervene. Nitko and Brookhart (2011) called these cases well structured: They provide an opportunity for students to apply knowledge to a clinical situation and develop an understanding of how it is used in practice. Cases of this type link knowledge presented in class, online, and through readings to practice situations. With well-structured cases, there is usually one correct answer that students can identify based on what they are currently learning in the clinical course or learned in previous courses and experiences.

Well-structured cases are effective for students beginning a clinical course in which they have limited background and experience. These cases give students an opportunity to practice their thinking before caring for an actual patient.

Most patient care situations, however, are not that easily solved. In clinical practice, the problems are sometimes difficult to identify, or the nurse may be confident about the patient's problem but unsure how to intervene. These are problems in Schön's (1990) swampy lowland—ones that do not lend themselves to resolution by a technical and rational approach. These are cases that vary from the way the problems and solutions were presented in class and through readings. For such cases, the principles learned in class may not readily apply, and clinical judgment is required for analysis and resolution.

Nitko and Brookhart (2011) referred to these cases as ill structured, describing problems that reflect real-life clinical situations faced by students. With ill-structured cases, different problems may be possible; there may be an incomplete data set to interpret; or the need and problem may be clear, but multiple approaches may be possible. Exhibit 11.3 presents examples of a well-structured and an ill-structured case.

Developing Cases

Case method and study have two components: a case description and questions to answer about the case or its analysis. In case method, the situations

---

Exhibit 11.3

WELL-STRUCTURED AND ILL-STRUCTURED CASES

Well-Structured Case

Mrs. D, 53 years old, reports having bad headaches for the last month. The headaches occur about twice weekly usually in the late morning. Initially, the pain began as a throbbing at her right temple. Her headaches now affect either her right or left eye and temple. The pain is so severe that she usually goes to bed. Mrs. D reports that her neck hurts, and the nurse notes tenderness in the posterior neck on palpation.

1. What type or types of headache might Mrs. D be experiencing?
2. Describe additional data that should be collected from Mrs. D. Why is this information important to deciding what is wrong with Mrs. D?
3. Select two interventions that might be used for Mrs. D. Provide evidence for their use.

Ill-Structured Case

Ms. J, 35 years old, calls for an appointment because she fell yesterday at home. She has a few bruises from her fall and a tingling feeling in her legs. Ms. J had been at the eye doctor's office last week because of double vision.

1. What do you think about this patient?
2. What are possible problems that Ms. J might be experiencing?
3. Plan additional data to collect to better understand those problems and explain why that information is important.

---

described are typically short and geared to specific outcomes to be met. Case studies include background information about the patient, family history, and complete assessment data to provide a comprehensive description of the patient or clinical situation.

The case should provide enough information for analysis without directing the students' thinking in a particular direction. The case may be developed first, then the questions, or the teacher may draft the questions first, then develop the case to present the clinical situation. Once students have experience in analyzing cases, another strategy is for students to develop a case scenario based on data provided by the teacher. In this method, students need to think about what patient needs and problems might fit the data, which promotes their critical thinking.

The questions developed for the case are the key to its effective use. The questions should be geared to the outcomes to be met. For instance, if the intent of the case method or study is for students to analyze laboratory data, apply physiological principles, and use concepts of pathophysiology for the analysis, then the questions need to relate to each of these. Similarly, if the goal is to improve skill in responding to clinical situations, then the questions should ask about possible actions to take for the situation, including no immediate intervention, and evidence to consider in deciding on actions. With most cases, questions should be included that focus on the underlying thought process used to arrive at an answer rather than the answer alone.

Cases can be written for the development of specific cognitive skills. In designing cases to promote problem solving, the teacher should develop a case that asks students to:

- Identify patient and other problems apparent or expected in the case
- Suggest alternative problems that might be possible if more information were available and identify the information needed
- Identify relevant and irrelevant information in the case
- Interpret the information to enable a response
- Propose different approaches that might be used
- Weigh approaches against the evidence
- Select the best approaches for the case situation
- Provide a rationale for those approaches
- Identify gaps in the literature and evidence as related to the case
- Evaluate the effectiveness of interventions
- Plan alternative interventions based on analysis of the case

An example of a case for problem solving is:

Ms. G, a 56-year-old patient admitted for shortness of breath and chest pain, is scheduled for a cardiac catheterization. She has been crying on and off for the last hour. When the nurse attempts to talk to her, Ms. G says, "Don't worry about me. I'm just tired."

1. What is one problem in this situation that needs to be solved?
2. What assumptions about Ms. G did you make in identifying this problem?
3. What additional information would you collect from the patient and her medical records before intervening? Why is this information important?

Other cases can provide experience with making decisions about clinical situations. A case may present a clinical situation up to the point of a decision, then ask students to analyze the case and arrive at a decision. Or the case may describe a situation and decision, then ask whether students agree or disagree with it. For both of these types, the questions should lead the students through the decision-making process, and students should include a rationale for their responses.

For decision making, the teacher should develop a case that asks students to:

- Identify the decisions needed in the case
- Identify information in the case that is critical for arriving at a decision
- Specify additional data needed for a decision
- Examine alternative decisions possible and the consequences of each
- Arrive at a decision and provide a rationale for it

An example of a case intended for decision making is:

The charge nurse on the midnight shift in a large hospital assigns a nurse new to the unit to work with Ms. P, an experienced RN. Ms. P, however, is irate that she needs to orient a new nurse when she is so busy herself. Ms. P tells the new nurse that she is too busy to work with her tonight. When learning this, the charge nurse reassigns the new nurse to another RN.

1. Do you agree or disagree with the charge nurse's decision? Why?
2. Describe at least two strategies you could use in this situation. What are the advantages and disadvantages of each?
3. How would you handle this situation?

Case method and case study also meet critical thinking outcomes. There are a number of strategies that teachers can use when developing cases that are intended for critical thinking. These are listed in Exhibit 11.4.

An example of a case for critical thinking is:

You are a nurse practitioner working in a middle school. Ms. S, a 16-year-old, comes to your office for nausea and vomiting. She says she feels "bloated." She confides in you that she is pregnant and asks you not to tell her parents.

1. What are your options at this time?
2. What option would you choose to implement? Why?
3. Choose another option that you listed for question 1. What are the advantages and disadvantages of that approach over your first choice?

Exhibit 11.4

STRATEGIES FOR DEVELOPING CASE STUDIES FOR CRITICAL THINKING

Develop:	Ask students to:
Present an issue for analysis, a question to be answered that has multiple possibilities, or a complex problem to be solved.	Analyze the case and provide a rationale for the thinking process they used for the analysis. Examine the assumptions underlying their thinking. Describe the evidence on which their reasoning was based. Describe the concepts and theories they used for their analysis and *how* they applied to the case.
Have different and conflicting points of view.	Analyze the case from their own points of view and then analyze the case from a different point of view.
Present complex data for analysis.	Analyze the data and draw possible inferences given the data. Specify additional information needed and why it is important.
Present clinical situations that are unique and offer different perspectives.	Analyze the clinical situation, identify multiple perspectives possible, and examine assumptions made about the situation that influenced thinking.
Describe ethical issues and dilemmas.	Propose alternative approaches and consequences. Weigh alternatives and arrive at a decision. Critique an issue from a different point of view.

Cases can also be written with the intent to promote clinical judgment skills. Using Tanner's (2006) model of clinical judgment, cases can ask students to:

- Describe what they notice in the clinical situation that demands attention
- Explain the clinical situation based on their prior and current learning

- Interpret the meaning of the data
- Suggest possible courses of action, if any, that would be appropriate
- Provide a rationale for taking no action or to support the proposed actions
- Hypothesize how patients might respond to each of those actions
- Reflect on their own thinking and decisions

An example of a case for this purpose is:

You make a home visit to an 86-year-old patient who lives alone and is having problems concentrating, loss of memory, crying spells, and fatigue. You recommend a follow-up visit with the primary care physician. The patient is diagnosed with depression and treated with a selective serotonin reuptake inhibitor. Two weeks later, you visit the patient and learn she still has fatigue and now also has loss of appetite and difficulty sleeping.

1. What do you notice in this situation?
2. Provide alternative explanations for the patient's current symptoms of fatigue, loss of appetite, and difficulty sleeping.
3. Discuss the case with a peer and compare interpretations. Decide on next steps to be taken by the home health nurse.

Unfolding Cases

A variation of case study is unfolding cases in which the clinical situation changes, thereby creating a simulation for students to analyze. Ulrich and Glendon (2005) proposed writing three paragraphs. The first paragraph sets the context of the case, including background information about the patient and others, a description of the clinical situation, and questions for discussion by students. After the initial analysis of the case by the students, the next paragraph is revealed, changing the scenario in some way. Students then critique the new information and answer related questions. After reading the last paragraph, students complete a reflective writing exercise in which they project future learning needs and share individual feelings and reactions to the case.

Day (2011) described the development of unfolding cases for classroom instruction. In this process, the narrative, which is the patient's story, is central and provides the structure for the classroom discussion. With the case, students learn the concepts and content for providing care in that particular clinical situation. The teacher begins by identifying the goals of the class and understanding the learners and their needs; then the teacher specifies the content to be learned, which is taught through the case study as it unfolds. In the next phase the teacher develops the narrative (what should the case do) and decides on the patient situation to achieve the goals and learn the essential content. Unfolding cases are also used frequently in simulation. As the case unfolds in the simulation, students analyze the new information and make decisions about relevant actions to take.

GRAND ROUNDS

Grand rounds involve the observation and often interview of a patient or several patients in the clinical setting, a webcast of grand rounds conducted elsewhere, or a multimedia program of the grand rounds. Grand rounds provide an opportunity to observe a patient with a specific condition, discuss assessment and interpretation of data, and propose interventions and changes in the plan of care. Rounds are valuable for examining issues facing patients, families, and communities and for exposing students to situations they may not encounter in their clinical experiences. During rounds, students can examine best practices, connect classroom learning and clinical practice, and develop professional skills such as those related to leadership and communication (Lanham, 2011). Grand rounds may involve nursing students and staff members only or be interdisciplinary.

Nursing grand rounds can also be used for staff education. Grand rounds can be used to keep nurses up-to-date on new approaches to care, present best practices, and explore new evidence and how it might be used in a patient's care. Rounds can be presented live in the classroom, and then recorded for viewing via the intranet and Internet. Gormley, Costanzo, Lewis, Slone, and Savage (2012) found that nurses in both urban and rural hospitals were interested in nursing grand rounds offered as online recorded sessions. Grand rounds provide an opportunity for highlighting nurses' clinical expertise and promoting best practices. Odedra and Hitchcock (2012) implemented nursing grand rounds in their hospital with the goal of sharing clinical and professional expertise and promoting quality care. With the rounds, clinical nurse specialists were able to promote their role and teach care processes in their areas of expertise. Interdisciplinary team members attended the rounds.

Rather than conducting rounds in the clinical setting, faculty members may decide to use webcasts of grand rounds that are available. A number of organizations offer webinars of grand rounds that could be used for staff education and also in nursing education programs.

Grand rounds enable students to:

- Identify patient problems and issues in a clinical situation
- Evaluate the effectiveness of nursing and interdisciplinary interventions
- Share clinical knowledge with peers and identify gaps in their own understanding
- Develop new perspectives about the patient's care
- Gain insight into other ways of meeting patient needs
- Think critically about the nursing care they provide and that given by their peers
- Dialogue about patient care and changes in clinical practice with peers and experts participating in the rounds

Regardless of whether the rounds are conducted in the clinical setting or viewed on a webcast, the teacher should first identify the outcomes that students should meet at the end of the rounds. The outcomes guide the teacher in planning the rounds and their focus. Second, it should be clear why the particular patient or clinical situation was selected for grand rounds. Third, the questions asked after rounds should encourage students to think critically about the patient and care, compare this case to the textbook picture and other patients for whom students have cared, and explore alternative interventions and perspectives of the situation. The final area of discussion should focus on what students have learned from this experience and new insights they have gained about clinical practice. Students might write a short paper reflecting on their learning and new perspectives.

Grand rounds may be conducted by an advanced practice nurse, a staff nurse, the teacher, a student, or another health care professional. For student-led rounds, the teacher is responsible for confirming the plan with the patient. Patients should be assured of their right to refuse participation and should be comfortable to tell those involved in the rounds when they no longer want to continue with it.

For grand rounds in the clinical setting, activities at the patient's bedside should begin with an introduction of the patient to the students, emphasizing the patient's contribution to student learning. If possible, the person conducting the rounds should include the patient and family in the discussion, seeking their perspective of the health problem and input into care. The teacher's role is that of consultant, clarifying information and assisting the student in keeping the discussion on the goals set for the rounds. Students should direct any questions to the teacher prior to and after the grand rounds, and sensitive issues should be discussed when the rounds are completed and out of the patient's presence.

SUMMARY

Case method and case study describe a clinical situation developed around an actual or hypothetical patient for student review and analysis. In case method, the case is generally shorter and more specific than in case study. Case studies are more comprehensive in nature, thereby presenting a complete picture of the patient and clinical situation.

With these clinical teaching methods, students apply knowledge to practice situations, identify needs and problems, propose varied approaches for solving them considering evidence, decide on courses of action, and evaluate outcomes. As such, case method and study provide experience for students in thinking through different clinical situations.

Grand rounds involve the observation of a patient or several patients in the clinical setting, in a webcast, or in a multimedia program. Grand rounds may be conducted for nursing students and staff only or as an interdisciplinary activity. Rounds provide an opportunity to observe a patient with a specific condition, review assessment data, discuss interventions and their effectiveness, and make changes in the plan of care. Rounds are also valuable for examining issues facing patients and discussing ways of resolving them. Grand rounds, similar to case method and study, provide an opportunity for exploring patient problems and varied courses of action, analyzing care and proposing new interventions, and gaining insight into different clinical situations.

Exhibit 11.5

CNE EXAMINATION TEST BLUEPRINT CORE COMPETENCIES

1. **Facilitate Learning**

   A. Implement a variety of teaching strategies appropriate to
      1. content
      2. setting (i.e., clinical versus classroom)
      3. learner needs
      4. learning style
      5. desired learner outcomes

   B. Use teaching strategies based on
      1. educational theory
      2. evidence-based practices related to education

   D. Use information technologies to support the teaching–learning process
   G. Model reflective thinking practices, including critical thinking

   (continued)

> **H.** Create opportunities for learners to develop their own critical thinking skills
> **N.** Use knowledge of evidence-based practice to instruct learners
>
> 2. **Facilitate Learner Development and Socialization**
>
> > **E.** Foster the development of learners in these areas
> > 1. cognitive domain
> > 2. psychomotor domain
> > 3. affective domain
>
> 3. **Use Assessment and Evaluation Strategies**
>
> > **C.** Use a variety of strategies to assess and evaluate learning in these domains
> > 1. cognitive
> > 2. psychomotor
> > 3. affective

REFERENCES

Alfaro-LeFevre, R. (2013). *Critical thinking, clinical reasoning, and clinical judgment: A practical approach* (5th ed.). St. Louis, MO: Elsevier.

Day, L. (2011). Using unfolding case studies in a subject-centered classroom. *Journal of Nursing Education, 50,* 447–452. doi:10.3928/01484834-20110517-03

Elder, L., & Paul, R. (2010). *Critical thinking development: A state theory.* Retrieved from http://www.criticalthinking.org/pages/critical-thinking-development-a-stage-theory/48310.3928/01484834-20080301-02

Facione, N. C., & Facione, P. A. (Eds.). (2008). *Critical thinking and clinical reasoning in the health sciences: An international multidisciplinary teaching anthology.* Millbrae, CA: California Academic Press.

Facione, P. (2011). *Critical thinking: What it is and why it counts.* Retrieved from http://www.insightassessment.com/CT-Resources/Critical-Thinking-What-It-Is-and-Why-It-Counts

Gormley, D. K., Costanzo, A. J., Lewis, M. R., Slone, B., & Savage, C. L. (2012) Assessing nurses' continuing education preferences in rural community and urban academic settings. *Journal of Nurses in Staff Development, 28,* 279–284. doi:10.1097/NND.0b013e318272590c

Lanham, J. (2011). Nursing grand rounds as a clinical teaching strategy. *Journal of Nursing Education, 50,* 176. doi:10.3928/01484834-20110216-02

Nitko, A. J., & Brookhart, S. M. (2011). *Educational assessment of students* (6th ed.). Upper Saddle River, NJ: Pearson Education.

Odedra, K., & Hitchcock, J. (2012). Implementation of nursing grand rounds at a large acute hospital trust. *British Journal of Nursing, 21,* 182–185.

Oermann, M. H. (2008). Using short cases for teaching "thinking" in a nursing course. In N. C. Facione & P. A. Facione (Eds.), *Critical thinking and clinical reasoning in the health sciences: An international multidisciplinary teaching anthology* (pp. 123–129). Millbrae, CA: California Academic Press.

Oermann, M. H., & Gaberson, K. B. (2014). *Evaluation and testing in nursing education* (4th ed.). New York, NY: Springer.

Schön, D. A. (1990). *Educating the reflective practitioner*. San Francisco, CA: Jossey-Bass.

Tanner, C. A. (2006). Thinking like a nurse: A research-based model of clinical judgment in nursing. *Journal of Nursing Education, 45,* 204–211.

Ulrich, D. L., & Glendon, K. J. (2005). *Interactive group learning: Strategies for nurse educators* (2nd ed.). New York, NY: Springer.

West, E., Holmes, J., Zidek, C., & Edwards, T. (2013). Intraprofessional collaboration through an unfolding case and the just culture model. *Journal of Nursing Education, 52,* 470–474. doi:10.3928/01484834-20130719-04

CHAPTER 12

Discussion and Clinical Conference

Discussions with learners and clinical conferences provide a means of sharing information, developing critical thinking skills, and learning how to collaborate with others in a group. Discussion is an exchange of ideas for a specific purpose; clinical conference is a form of group discussion that focuses on some aspect of clinical practice. Teachers and students engage in many discussions in planning, carrying out, and evaluating clinical learning activities. Similarly, there are varied types of clinical conferences for use in teaching. Effective conferences and discussions require an understanding of their goals, the types of questions for encouraging exchange of ideas and higher level thinking, and the roles of the teacher and students.

DISCUSSION

Discussions between teacher and student, preceptor and orientee, and nurse manager and staff occur frequently but do not always promote learning. These discussions often involve the teacher telling the learner what to do or not to do for a patient. Discussions, though, should be an exchange of ideas through which the teacher, by asking open-ended questions and supporting learner responses, encourages students to arrive at their own decisions or to engage in self-assessment about clinical practice. Discussions are not intended to be an exchange of the teacher's ideas to the students. In a discussion, both teacher and student actively participate in sharing ideas and considering alternative perspectives.

Discussions give learners an opportunity to interact with one another, critique each other's ideas, and learn from others. For that reason, discussions are an effective method for promoting critical thinking. The teacher can ask open-ended and thought-provoking questions, which encourage higher-level thinking if students perceive that they are free to discuss their own ideas and those of others involved in the discussion. The teacher is a resource for students, giving immediate feedback and further instruction as needed. Discussions also provide a forum for students to explore feelings associated with their clinical practice and simulation experiences, clarify values and ethical dilemmas, and learn to interact in a group format. Those outcomes are not as easily met in a large group setting. Over a period of time, students learn to collaborate with peers in working toward solving clinical problems.

Creating a Climate for Discussion

An important role of the teacher is to develop a climate in which students are comfortable discussing concepts and issues without fear that the ideas expressed will affect the teacher's evaluation of their performance and subsequent clinical grade. Similarly, discussions between preceptor and orientee and between manager and staff should be carried out in an atmosphere in which nurses feel comfortable to express their own opinions and ideas and to question others' assumptions. Discussions are for formative, not summative, evaluation; they provide feedback to learners individually or in a small group to guide their learning and thinking. Without this climate for exchanging ideas, though, discussions cannot be carried out effectively, because students fear that their comments may influence their clinical evaluation and grade—or, for nurses, their performance ratings.

The teacher sets an atmosphere in which listening, respect for others' comments and ideas, and openness to new perspectives are valued. Learners need to be free to discuss their ideas with the teacher, who can guide their critical thinking through careful questioning. Without support from the teacher, students will not participate freely in the discussion nor will they be willing to examine controversial points of view, critique different perspectives of care and decisions, or share misunderstandings with the teacher and peers.

Studies on teacher effectiveness highlight the importance of this interpersonal relationship between teacher and students. Conveying confidence in students and their ability to perform in clinical practice, demonstrating respect for students, being honest and direct with them, and encouraging students to ask questions and participate freely in discussions are important characteristics of effective clinical teaching. Considering the many demands on students as they learn to care for patients, students need to view the teacher as someone who supports them in their learning. This is a critical role of clinical teachers and staff with whom they work.

Guidelines for Discussion

Discussions can be face to face in the clinical setting or conducted online. They can be carried out individually with learners or in a small group. The size of the group for a discussion can range from 2 to 10 people. A larger group makes it difficult for each person to participate.

The teacher is responsible for planning the discussion to meet the intended outcomes of the clinical course or specific goals to be achieved through the discussion. An effective teacher keeps the discussion focused; avoids talking too much, with students in a passive role; and avoids side-tracking. While the teacher may initiate the discussion, the interaction needs to revolve around the students, not the teacher. Rephrasing students' questions for them to answer suggests that the teacher has confidence in students' ability to arrive at answers and provides opportunities to develop critical thinking skills. Open-ended questions without one specific answer encourage critical thinking among both students and nurses. By using open-ended questions in a discussion the teacher can uncover the student's cognitive abilities, such as ability to integrate knowledge, problem solve, analyze situations, and propose innovative actions (Roberts, 2013).

The teacher should also be aware of the environment in which the discussion takes place. For discussions that are held face to face with students, chairs should be arranged in a configuration that encourages interaction, such as a circle, semicircle, or U shape. For some discussions, students may be divided into pairs or other small groups. Exhibit 12.1 summarizes the roles of the teacher and students in clinical discussions.

Exhibit 12.1

ROLES OF TEACHER AND STUDENT IN DISCUSSION

Teacher
- Plans discussion
- Presents problem, issue, case for analysis
- Develops questions for discussion
- Facilitates discussion with students as active participants
- Develops and maintains atmosphere for open discussion of ideas and issues
- Monitors time
- Avoids side-tracking
- Provides feedback

Student
- Prepares for discussion
- Participates actively in discussion
- Works collaboratively with group members to arrive at solutions and decisions
- Examines different points of view
- Is willing to modify own view and perspective to reach group consensus

(continued)

- Reflects on clinical experience and simulation
- Identifies implications for own practice and development

Teacher and Student
- Summarize outcomes of discussion and learning
- Identify implications of discussion for other clinical situations

Listed below are guidelines for planning a discussion and effectively using it with students in clinical practice:

- Identify the outcomes and goals to be achieved in the discussion considering the time frame.
- Plan questions for structured discussions ahead of time. They may be written for the teacher only or also for students. If not written, the teacher should think about the questions to ask, their order, and important content to discuss prior to beginning the interaction.
- Plan *how* the discussion will be carried out. Will all students in the clinical group participate, or will they be divided into smaller groups or pairs, then share the results of their individual discussions to the clinical group? Will the discussion be held in the clinical setting or conducted online?
- Sequence questions according to the desired outcomes of the discussion.
- Ask open-ended questions that encourage multiple perspectives and different lines of thinking.
- Think about how the questions are phrased before asking them.
- Ask questions to the group as a whole or ask for volunteers to respond. If questions are directed to a specific learner, be sensitive to his or her comfort in responding and do not create undue stress for the student. If this occurs, the teacher should provide prompts or cues for responding.
- Wait a few seconds between the question and request for students to answer it during face-to-face interactions.
- Give students time to answer the questions. If no one responds, the teacher should try rephrasing the question.
- Reinforce students' answers, indicating why they were or were not appropriate for the question.
- Give nonverbal and verbal feedback to encourage student participation without overusing it.
- Avoid interrupting the learner, even if errors are noted in the line of thinking or information.

- Correct students' errors in thinking when they are finished answering the question. It is critical that the teacher give feedback to students and correct their errors without belittling them. The goal is to focus on the answer and errors in reasoning, not on the student.
- Listen carefully to students' responses and make notes to remember points made in the discussion. The teacher should tell students ahead of time that any notes are for use only during the discussion, not for student evaluation or other purposes. The notes should be destroyed so students are assured of their freedom to respond in discussions.
- Assess own skill in directing discussions and identify areas for improvement.

Discussions may begin with questions raised by the teacher or by students, or discussions may be integrated with other instructional methods, such as case scenarios, simulations, games, role-play, and media clips. Case scenarios, for instance, may be critiqued and then discussed by students in a clinical conference, either as part of the clinical practicum or online at a later time. Or students may play a game and complete a role-play exercise, followed by discussion. Media clips provide an effective format for presenting a clinical situation for analysis and discussion.

These guidelines also apply to online discussions about clinical practice. With an online discussion or forum, following the clinical experience, students have time for reflection about the care they provided and their interactions with patients, families, and others with whom they interacted. Students also have time to gather literature and other resources to analyze their approaches and alternate possibilities, with supporting evidence, before participating in the discussion. Online discussions about clinical practice promote learning by allowing students to view and respond to the thinking of their peers, similar to postconference discussions. It is critical that no information is shared about patients and others in the clinical setting, and students need to be told this prior to beginning the course. An online discussion can refer to "a patient" or "a staff member with whom I interacted." Often these discussions are best carried out using generic phrases such as "a patient with heart failure" to avoid any chance of identifying a patient, provider, setting, or specific case. The teacher can post higher level questions to begin the discussion and specify when students need to post their answers. Similar to a face-to-face discussion, the teacher's role is to facilitate the discussion with prompts and responses to stimulate further thinking but not to dominate with own comments. Similar to any discussion forum, there needs to be a set time frame for the discussion, for example, 1 week. With online discussions the teacher can prepare questions to help students relate their learning from class and readings to clinical practice, reflect on their care and interactions, identify other perspectives and approaches, and seek further evidence that is relevant to their patient care. Online discussions may also promote affective learning because students may be more comfortable sharing their feelings and values online than in person. For students who are quiet and are hesitant to participate in face-to-face discussions, online ones may build their confidence.

Purposes of Discussion

In a discussion, the teacher has an opportunity to ask carefully selected questions about students' thinking and the rationale used for arriving at decisions and positions about issues. Discussions promote several types of learning depending on the goals and structure:

1. Development of problem-solving, critical thinking, and clinical judgment skills
2. Debriefing of clinical experiences and following simulations
3. Development of cooperative learning and group process skills
4. Assessment of own learning
5. Development of oral communication skills

Every discussion will not necessarily promote each of these learning outcomes. The teacher should be clear about the intent of the discussion so it may be geared to the particular outcomes to be achieved. For instance, discussions for critical thinking require carefully selected questions that examine alternative possibilities and "what if" types of questions. This same type of questioning, however, may not be necessary if the goal is to develop cooperative learning or group process skills.

Development of Cognitive Skills

An important purpose of discussion is to promote development of problem-solving, critical thinking, and clinical judgment skills. Discussions are effective because they provide an opportunity for the teacher to gear the questioning toward each of these skills. Not all discussions, though, lead to these higher levels of thinking. The key is the type of questions asked by the teacher or discussed among students—questions need to encourage students to examine alternative perspectives and points of view in a given situation and to provide a rationale for their thinking. Exhibit 12.2 presents strategies for directing discussions toward development of higher level cognitive skills.

In these discussions, students can be given a hypothetical or real clinical situation involving a patient, family, or community to critique and

---

Exhibit 12.2

DISCUSSIONS FOR COGNITIVE SKILL DEVELOPMENT

Ask students to:
- Identify problems and issues in a real or hypothetical clinical situation.
- Identify possible alternative problems.
- Assess the problem and clinical situation further.
- Differentiate relevant and irrelevant information for the problem or issue being discussed.
- Discuss their own point of view and others' points of view.
- Examine their own assumptions and those of other students.
- Identify different solutions, courses of action, and consequences of each.
- Consider both positive and negative consequences.
- Compare possible alternatives and defend the choice of one particular solution or action over another.
- Take a position about an issue and provide a rationale both for and against that position.
- Identify their own biases, values, and beliefs that influence their thinking.
- Identify obstacles to solving a problem.
- Evaluate the effectiveness of interventions and approaches to solving problems.

---

identify potential problems. Students can then discuss possible decisions in that situation, consequences of different options they considered as part of their decision making, and other points of view. Discussions are particularly valuable in helping students analyze ethical dilemmas, consider different points of view, and explore their own values and beliefs.

Debriefing of Clinical Experiences

Discussions provide an opportunity for students to report on their clinical learning activities; describe and analyze the care they provided to patients, families, and communities; and reflect on their practice. In these discussions, students receive feedback from peers and the teacher about their clinical decisions and other possible approaches they could use with their patient's care. Debriefing also provides an opportunity to share feelings about clinical practice and talk about experiences within available support systems (Williams, 2013). Issues related to patients, staff, and others may be examined by the group.

Debriefing clinical experiences allows students to share feelings and perceptions about their patients and clinical situations in a comfortable environment. In distance education courses, online discussions are critical to provide a way for students to share their experiences with peers, learn about resources from each other that they might use in their own patient care, and keep faculty members apprised of students' experiences (Roehm & Bonnel, 2009). Online discussions in traditional clinical courses can be used to meet these same goals.

Debriefing also occurs after a simulation and is a critical component of simulation. In the debriefing discussion, the teacher and students examine and reflect on the experience. Through this reflection, guided by the teacher, students develop their clinical reasoning and judgment skills (Dreifuerst, 2009, 2012; Dufrene & Young, 2013). However, for reflection to occur, it is important for teachers to consider the types of questions they ask in debriefing (Husebø, Dieckmann, Rystedt, Søreide, & Friberg, 2013). Typically, the educator focuses the debriefing discussions on the intended learning outcomes and goals of the simulation. Debriefing also enables the teacher to identify performance gaps and provide feedback, discussion, and instruction to close those gaps in learning and performance (Rudolph, Simon, Raemer, & Eppich, 2008).

Development of Cooperative Learning Skills

Group discussions are effective for promoting cooperative learning skills. In cooperative learning, students work in small groups to meet particular learning outcomes related to the course. Students are actively involved in their learning and foster the learning of others in the group.

Discussions using cooperative learning strategies begin with the teacher planning the discussion, presenting a task to be completed by the group or a problem to be solved, developing an environment for open discussion, and facilitating the discussion. Students work cooperatively in groups to propose solutions, complete the task, and present the results of their discussions to the rest of the students. Students can work in pairs or small groups to avoid too large a group for discussion. With small groups students can share and discuss their ideas in a safe learning environment (Kitchen, 2012).

Assessment of Own Learning

Discussions provide a means for students to assess their own learning, identify gaps in their understanding, and learn from others in a nonthreatening environment. Students can ask questions of the group and use the teacher and peers as resources for their learning. If the teacher is effective in developing an atmosphere for open discussion, students, in turn, will share their feelings, concerns, and questions as a beginning to their continued development.

Development of Oral Communication Skills

The ability to present ideas orally, as well as in written form, is an important outcome to be achieved by students in clinical courses. Discussions provide opportunities for students to present ideas to a group, explain concepts clearly, handle questions raised by others, and refine presentation style. Participation in a discussion requires formulating ideas and presenting them logically to the group.

Students may make formal presentations to the clinical group as a way of developing their oral communication skills. They may lead a discussion and present on a specific topic related to the outcomes of the clinical course. Discussion provides an opportunity for peers and the teacher to give feedback to students on how well students communicated their ideas to others and to improve their communication techniques.

Exhibit 12.3 presents an assessment form that students may use to rate the quality of presentations and provide feedback on ability to lead a group discussion. This form is not intended for summative or grading purposes, but instead is designed for giving feedback to students following a presentation to the clinical group.

Exhibit 12.3

EVALUATION FORM FOR RATING PRESENTATIONS IN CONFERENCES

Name _____

Title of presentation _____

Rate each of the behaviors listed below. Circle the appropriate number and give feedback to the presenter in the space provided.

	Rating				
Behavior	To a limited extent				To a great extent
Leadership Role in Conference					
1. Leads the group in discussion of ideas	1	2	3	4	5
2. Encourages active participation of peers in conference	1	2	3	4	5

(continued)

	Rating				
Behavior					
Leadership Role in Conference					
3. Encourages open discussion of ideas	1	2	3	4	5
4. Helps group synthesize ideas presented	1	2	3	4	5
Comments:					
Quality of Content Presented					
5. Prepares objectives for presentation that reflect clinical goals	1	2	3	4	5
6. Presents content that relates to objectives and is relevant for students' clinical practice	1	2	3	4	5
7. Presents content that is accurate and up to date	1	2	3	4	5
8. Presents content that reflects theory and research	1	2	3	4	5
Comments:					
Quality of Presentation					
9. Organizes and presents material logically	1	2	3	4	5
10. Explains ideas clearly	1	2	3	4	5
11. Plans presentation considering time demands, needs of clinical group, and type of conference (face to face vs. online)	1	2	3	4	5
12. Emphasizes key points	1	2	3	4	5
13. Encourages students to ask questions and reflect on responses	1	2	3	4	5
14. Answers students' questions accurately	1	2	3	4	5

(continued)

		Rating			
Quality of Presentation					
15. Supports alternative viewpoints and encourages their discussion	1	2	3	4	5
16. Is enthusiastic	1	2	3	4	5
Comments:					

Level of Questions

The level of questions asked in any discussion is the key to directing it toward the intended learning outcomes. In most clinical discussions, the goal is to avoid a predominance of factual questions and focus instead on higher level and open-ended questions. Teachers can use a framework such as Bloom's taxonomy to sequence questions in a discussion or can level those questions in a more general way, beginning with recall (low level) and progressing through clarifying to critical thinking (high level).

The taxonomy of the cognitive domain, related to knowledge and intellectual skills, was developed by Bloom Englehart, Furst, Hill, and Krathwohl (1956) many years ago but is still of value today for developing test items and for leveling questions. Learning in the cognitive domain includes the acquisition of facts and specific information, concepts and theories, and higher level cognitive skills (Oermann & Gaberson, 2014). The original cognitive taxonomy includes six levels that increase in complexity: knowledge, comprehension, application, analysis, synthesis, and evaluation. Because these levels are arranged in a hierarchy, recall of specific facts and information is the least complex level of learning, and evaluating clinical situations and making judgments is the most complex. This taxonomy was updated, and the names for the levels of learning were reworded as verbs (Anderson & Krathwohl, 2001). For example, the "knowledge" level was renamed "remember," and synthesis and evaluation were reordered. In the updated taxonomy, the highest level of learning is "create," which is the process of synthesizing elements to form a new product.

The cognitive taxonomy is useful in asking questions in a discussion or planning questions for student response, because it levels them along a continuum from ones requiring only recall of facts to higher-level questions requiring judgments and synthesis of knowledge. The teacher may begin by asking students factual questions and then progress to questions that are answered based on students understanding, applying knowledge to clinical practice, analyzing data and clinical situations, making judgments based on criteria and standards (evaluation), and synthesizing material from different sources to create a new plan or product.

A description and sample questions for each of the six levels of the updated cognitive taxonomy follow. Sample words for use in developing questions at each level are presented in Exhibit 12.4.

1. Remember: Recall of facts and specific information; memorization of facts.

    "Define the term percussion."
    "What is this type of dysrhythmia called?"

2. Understand: Interpreting; ability to describe and explain.

    "Tell me about your patient's shortness of breath."
    "What does this potassium level indicate?"

3. Apply: Use of information in a new or unfamiliar situation; ability to transfer knowledge to a new situation.

    "Why are these interventions the most effective ones for your patient?"
    "Tell me about your patient's problems and related pathophysiological changes. Why are each of these changes important for you to monitor?"

4. Analyze: Ability to break down material into component parts and identify the relationships among them.

    "What are possible reasons for the patient's adverse events following transfer from the neonatal intensive care unit?"
    "What assumptions did you make about this family that influenced your decisions? What are alternative approaches to consider?"

5. Evaluate: Making judgments about value based on criteria and standards; critiquing.

    "Take a position for or against closing the clinic and shifting patients to the other center. Provide a rationale for your position."
    "What is the impact on patients and families of providing one less home care visit?"

6. Create: Ability to develop new ideas and materials; combining elements to form a new product or pattern not there before.

"Tell me about your plan to improve prenatal care for the women who come to your clinic. Why is your plan better than the existing services?"

"Develop a discharge plan for patients after hip replacement."

Exhibit 12.4

QUESTION CLASSIFICATION

Level	Types of Questions	Sample Words for Questions
1. Remember (knowledge)	*Recall, recognition* Questions that can be answered by recall of facts and previously learned information	Define, identify, list, name, select
2. Understand (comprehension)	*Interpret, explain* Questions that can be answered by explaining and describing	Describe, differentiate, draw conclusions, explain, give examples of, interpret, tell me in your own words
3. Apply	*Use, implement* Questions that require use of information in new or unfamiliar situations	Apply, relate, use
4. Analyze	*Divide into component parts* Questions that ask student to break down material into its component parts, to analyze data and clinical situations	Analyze, compare, contrast, detect, identify reasons and assumptions, provide evidence to support conclusions, relate
5. Evaluate	*Make judgments based on criteria* Questions that require student to critique or make a judgment based on criteria and standards	Appraise, assess, compare, critique, evaluate, formulate, judge, plan, produce
6. Create (synthesis)	*Develop new ideas and products* Questions that ask students to develop new ideas, plans, products	Construct, create, design, develop, propose a plan, suggest a new approach

Questions for discussions should be sequenced from low to high level. The taxonomy provides a schema for asking progressively higher level questions (Profetto-McGrath, Smith, Day, & Yonge, 2004). These higher level questions cannot be answered by memory alone and often have more than one answer. Higher level questions ask students to apply information they have learned to patient care or a clinical scenario, analyze a complex clinical situation, evaluate options and alternatives, and create new plans and approaches.

An example of a progression of questions using the taxonomy follows:

Remember: "Define the gate control theory of chronic pain."

Understand: "Explain the physiological mechanisms underlying this theory of pain."

Apply: "Tell me about an intervention you are using for your patient and how its use and effectiveness may be explained by the gate control theory."

Analyze: "Your patient seems more agitated. What additional data have you collected? What are possible reasons for this response?"

Evaluate: "You indicated that your patient's pain continues to increase. What alternative pain interventions do you propose? Why would these interventions be more effective? Describe the evidence you reviewed on these new approaches you are considering for your patient."

Create: "Develop a pain management plan for your patient now and for his discharge home."

Research suggests that teachers by nature do not ask high-level questions of students. Typically, the questions asked in a discussion focus on recall and comprehension rather than higher levels of thinking (Hsu, 2007; Profetto-McGrath et al., 2004). Although the intent of clinical discussions may be to improve thinking and clinical reasoning, this goal will not be met with questions that are answered by memorization of facts and specific information.

CLINICAL CONFERENCES

Clinical conferences are discussions in which students share information about their clinical experiences, engage in thinking about and reflecting on clinical practice, lead others in discussions, and give formal presentations to the group. Some clinical conferences involve other disciplines and provide opportunities to work with other health care professionals in planning and evaluating patient care. Conferences serve the same goals as any discussion: develop problem-solving, critical thinking, and clinical judgment skills; reflect on clinical experiences; assess own learning; and develop oral communication skills. The teacher has an important role in clinical conferences in facilitating discussions that help students understand and search for meaning in their clinical experiences (Megel, Nelson, Black, Vogel, & Uphoff, 2013). Guidelines for conducting clinical conferences are the same as for discussion and therefore are not repeated here.

There are many types of clinical conferences. *Preclinical conferences* are small group discussions that precede clinical learning activities. In preclinical conferences, students ask questions about their clinical learning activities, seek clarification about their patients' care and other aspects of clinical practice, and share concerns with the teacher and with peers. Preclinical conferences assist students in identifying patient problems, setting priorities, and planning care; they prepare students for their clinical activities. An important role of the teacher in preclinical conferences is to ensure that students have the essential knowledge and competencies to complete their clinical activities. In many instances, the teacher needs to instruct students further and fill in the gaps in students' learning. Preclinical conferences may be conducted on a one-to-one basis with students or as a clinical group.

Postclinical conferences are held at the conclusion of clinical learning activities. Postclinical conferences provide a forum for analyzing patient care and exploring other options, thereby facilitating critical thinking. Postclinical conferences may be used for peer review and critiquing each other's work. They are not intended as substitutes for classroom instruction with the teacher lecturing and presenting new content to students. A similar problem often occurs with guest speakers who treat the conference as a class, lecturing to students about their area of expertise rather than encouraging group discussion.

Clinical conferences can also focus on ethical and professional issues associated with clinical practice. Conferences of this type encourage critical thinking about issues that students have encountered or may in the future. In these conferences, students can analyze events that occurred in the clinical setting, ones in which they were personally involved or learned about through their clinical experience. A student can present the situation to the group for analysis and discussion. The discussion should focus on varied approaches that might be used and how to decide on the best strategy. "What if" questions are effective for this type of conference.

Students and faculty members alike are often fatigued at the end of the clinical practicum. Rather than each student sharing what he or she did in clinical practice, discussions that focus on higher level learning and thinking and that involve each student may be more effective.

Debates provide a forum for analyzing problems and issues in depth, analyzing opposing viewpoints, and developing and defending a position to be taken. In a debate, students should provide a rationale for their decisions. Debates developed around clinical issues give students an opportunity to prepare an argument for or against a particular position and to take a stand on an issue.

Setting for Clinical Conferences

Clinical conferences can be face-to-face in the clinical or academic setting, or they can be conducted online. With online conferences after the clinical experience, students have time to reflect on their patient care and what they might have done or said differently. One disadvantage is that they might not remember important events to share with the group for discussion.

SUMMARY

Discussions are an exchange of ideas in a small group format. Discussions provide a forum for students to express ideas, explore feelings associated with their clinical practice, clarify values and ethical dilemmas, and learn to interact in a group format. Over a period of time, students learn to collaborate with peers in working toward solving clinical problems.

The teacher is a resource for students. By asking open-ended questions and supporting learner responses, the teacher encourages students to arrive at their own decisions and to engage in self-assessment about clinical practice. The teacher develops a climate in which students are comfortable discussing concepts and issues without fear that the ideas expressed will affect the teacher's evaluation of their performance and subsequent clinical grade.

Discussions promote several types of learning: developing higher-level thinking skills; debriefing clinical experiences; assessing own learning; and developing oral communication skills. Debriefing following simulation is a critical aspect of using simulation in nursing education. These discussions typically focus on the intended goals of the simulations and guide students' reflection of the experience.

The level of questions asked in any discussion is the key to directing it toward the intended learning outcomes. In most clinical discussions, the goal is to avoid a predominance of factual questions and focus instead on clarifying and higher level questions. Questions for student response may be leveled along a continuum from ones requiring only recall of facts to higher-level questions requiring evaluating and creating new products and patterns.

Clinical conferences are discussions in which students analyze patient care and clinical situations, lead others in discussions about clinical practice, present ideas in a group format, and give presentations to the group. Conferences serve the same goals as any discussion.

Exhibit 12.5

CNE EXAMINATION TEST BLUEPRINT CORE COMPETENCIES

1. **Facilitate Learning**

   A. Implement a variety of teaching strategies appropriate to
      1. content
      2. setting
      3. learner needs
      4. learning style
      5. desired learner outcomes
      6. method of delivery (e.g., face to face, remote, simulation)

   B. Use teaching strategies based on
      1. educational theory
      2. evidence-based practices related to education

   C. Modify teaching strategies and learning experiences based on consideration of learners
      1. cultural background
      2. past clinical experiences
      3. past educational and life experiences
      4. generational groups (i.e., age)

   E. Practice skilled oral and written (including electronic) communication that reflects an awareness of self and relationships with learners (e.g., evaluation, mentorship, and supervision)

   F. Communicate effectively orally and in writing with an ability to convey ideas in a variety of contexts

   G. Model reflective thinking practices, including critical thinking

   H. Create opportunities for learners to develop their own critical thinking skills

   I. Create a positive learning environment that fosters a free exchange of ideas

   N. Use knowledge of evidence-based practice to instruct learners

2. **Facilitate Learner Development and Socialization**

   D. Create learning environments that facilitate learners' self-reflection, personal goal setting, and socialization to the role of the nurse

(continued)

E. Foster the development of learners in these areas
1. cognitive domain
2. psychomotor domain
3. affective domain

F. Assist learners to engage in thoughtful and constructive self and peer evaluation

REFERENCES

Anderson, L. W., & Krathwohl, D. R. (Eds.). (2001). *A taxonomy for learning, teaching, and assessing: A revision of boom's taxonomy of educational objectives.* New York, NY: Longman.

Bloom, B. S., Englehart, M. D., Furst, E. J., Hill, W. H., & Krathwohl, D. R. (1956). *Taxonomy of educational objectives. The classification of educational goals. Handbook I: Cognitive domain.* White Plains, NY: Longman.

Dreifuerst, K. (2009). The essentials of debriefing in simulation learning: A concept analysis. *Nursing Education Perspectives, 30,* 109–114.

Dreifuerst, K. T. (2012). Using debriefing for meaningful learning to foster development of clinical reasoning in simulation. *Journal of Nursing Education, 51,* 326–333. doi:10.3928/01484834-20120409-02

Dufrene, C., & Young, A. (2013). Successful debriefing—Best methods to achieve positive learning outcomes: A literature review. *Nurse Education Today.* doi:10.1016/j.nedt.2013.06.026 [Epub ahead of print]

Hsu, L-L. (2007). Conducting clinical post-conference in clinical teaching: A qualitative study. *Journal of Clinical Nursing, 16,* 1525–1533.

Husebø, S. E., Dieckmann, P., Rystedt, H., Søreide, E., & Friberg, F. (2013). The relationship between facilitators' questions and the level of reflection in postsimulation debriefing. *Simulation in Health care, 8*(3), 135–142. doi:10.1097/SIH.0b013e31827cbb5c

Kitchen, M. (2012). Facilitating small groups: How to encourage student learning. *Clinical Teacher, 9*(1), 3–8. doi:10.1111/j.1743-498X.2011.00493.x

Megel, M. E., Nelson, A. E., Black, J., Vogel, J., & Uphoff, M. (2013). A comparison of student and faculty perceptions of clinical post-conference learning environment. *Nurse Education Today, 33,* 525–529. doi:10.1016/j.nedt.2011.11.021

Oermann, M. H., & Gaberson, K. B. (2014). *Evaluation and testing in nursing education* (4th ed.). New York, NY: Springer.

Profetto-McGrath, J., Smith, K. B., Day, R. A., & Yonge, O. (2004). The questioning skills of tutors and students in a context based baccalaureate nursing program. *Nurse Education Today, 24,* 363–372.

Roberts, D. (2013). The clinical viva: An assessment of clinical thinking. *Nurse Education Today, 33,* 402–406. doi:10.1016/j.nedt.2013.01.014

Roehm, S., & Bonnel, W. (2009). Engaging students for learning with online discussions. *Teaching & Learning in Nursing, 4,* 6–9.

Rudolph, J. W., Simon, R., Raemer, D. B., & Eppich, W. J. (2008). Debriefing as formative assessment: Closing performance gaps in medical education. *Academic Emergency Medicine, 15,* 1010–1016.

Williams, A. (2013). The strategies used to deal with emotion work in student paramedic practice. *Nurse Education in Practice, 13,* 207–212. doi:10.1016/j.nepr.2012.09.010

CHAPTER 13

Using Preceptors as Clinical Teachers and Coaches

As discussed earlier, the preceptor teaching model is an alternative to the traditional clinical teaching model. It is based on the assumption that a consistent one-to-one relationship between an experienced nurse and a nursing student or novice staff nurse is an effective way to provide individualized guidance in clinical learning as well as opportunities for professional socialization (Smedley & Penney, 2009). Preceptorships have been used extensively with senior nursing students, graduate students preparing for advanced practice roles, and new staff nurse orientees, but they have also been used effectively with beginning nursing students (Gardner & Suplee, 2010). This chapter discusses the effective use of preceptors as clinical teachers and coaches. The advantages and disadvantages of preceptorships are examined, and suggestions are made for selecting, preparing, evaluating, and rewarding preceptors.

PRECEPTORSHIP MODEL OF CLINICAL TEACHING

A preceptorship is a time-limited, one-to-one relationship between a learner and an experienced nurse who is employed by the health care agency in which the learning activities take place. The clinical teacher may not be physically present during the learning activities; the preceptor provides intensive, individualized learning opportunities that improve the learner's clinical competence and confidence. Regardless of learners' levels of education and experience, preceptorships provide opportunities for socialization into professional nursing roles. They also enhance the personal and professional development of the preceptors (Charleston & Happell, 2005; Smedley & Penney, 2009).

The preceptor model is collaborative. The teacher is a faculty member or educator who has overall responsibility for the quality of the clinical teaching and learning. The teacher provides the link between the educational program and the practice setting by selecting and preparing preceptors, assigning students to preceptors, providing guidance for the selection of appropriate learning activities, serving as a resource to the preceptor–student pair, and evaluating student and preceptor performance. The preceptor functions as a role model and provides individualized clinical instruction, coaching, support, and socialization for the learner. The preceptor also participates in evaluation of learner performance, although the teacher has ultimate responsibility for summative evaluation decisions (Gardner & Supplee, 2010; Smedley & Penney, 2009).

USE OF PRECEPTORSHIPS IN NURSING EDUCATION

In academic programs that prepare nurses for initial entry into practice, preceptorships are usually used for students in their last semester, but providing preceptors for beginning students may have even greater benefits. Beginning students may gain from the individual attention of the preceptor and from assignments that help them to expand their basic skills, develop independence, and improve their self-confidence.

Preceptorships are frequently used in graduate programs that prepare nurses for advanced clinical practice, administration, and education roles. At this level, a preceptorship involves well-defined learning objectives based on the student's past clinical, administrative, and teaching experience. The student observes and participates in learning activities that demonstrate functional role components, allowing rehearsal of role behaviors before actually assuming an advanced practice, administrative, or teaching role. The preceptor must be an expert practitioner who can model the role functions of advanced practice nurses, including decision making, problem solving, leadership, teaching, and scholarship.

In many health care organizations, preceptors participate in the orientation of newly hired staff nurses. Preceptors in these settings act as role models for new staff nurses and support them in their transition into professional practice or socialization into new roles. Preceptors work individually with new staff nurses, but there is wide variation in the scope of the preceptor role. In some settings, the preceptor is a more experienced peer who works side by side with the orientee; in other settings, the preceptor role is more formally that of clinical teacher.

Research findings on the effectiveness of the preceptor teaching model are varied. Generally, studies indicate positive outcomes of students and new staff nurses working with preceptors. Some early studies showed no difference in student performance between students assigned to preceptors and those who were taught according to a traditional clinical teaching model. Some investigators presented anecdotal evidence from preceptors, teachers, and students that preceptorships enhanced student performance. Students who are assigned to preceptors are generally satisfied with the experience because they develop their confidence and independence. However, students may also experience communication and interpersonal problems with their preceptors, and, if these conflicts are not resolved successfully, negative outcomes can result (Mamchur & Myrick, 2003). The decision to use preceptors for clinical teaching should be based on the perceived benefits to students, the educational program, and the clinical staff members after a careful evaluation of the potential advantages and disadvantages.

ADVANTAGES AND DISADVANTAGES OF USING PRECEPTORS

The use of preceptors in clinical teaching has both advantages and disadvantages for the involved parties. Effective collaboration is required to minimize the drawbacks and achieve advantages for the educational program, clinical agency, teachers, preceptors, and students.

Preceptorships hold many potential advantages for preceptors and the clinical agencies that employ them. The presence of students in the clinical environment tends to enhance the professional development, leadership, and teaching skills of preceptors. While preceptors enjoy sharing their clinical knowledge and skill, they also appreciate the stimulation of working with students who challenge the status quo and raise questions about clinical practice. The interest and enthusiasm of students is often rewarding to nurses who take on the additional responsibilities of the preceptor role (Smedley & Penney, 2009). Students may assist preceptors with research or teaching projects. In agencies that use a clinical ladder, serving as a preceptor may be a means of advancing professionally within the system. The preceptorship model also produces opportunities to recruit potential staff members for the agency from among students who work with preceptors.

The greatest drawback of preceptorships to agencies and preceptors is usually the expected time commitment. Some clinical agencies may not agree to provide preceptors because of increased patient acuity and decreased staff levels, or potential preceptors may decline to participate because of the perception that to do so would add to their workloads. Because of current economic conditions, health care agencies seeking to decrease costs and increase efficiency often make changes in nurses' working conditions, such as increased workloads, decreased number of work hours, decreasing numbers of full-time and increasing numbers of part-time and casual employees, and increased use of technology. These organizational changes do not often facilitate adding the preceptor role to a registered nurse's workload (Gardner & Suplee, 2010, p. 56; Smedley & Penney, 2009; Yonge, Myrick, Ferguson, & Lughana, 2005). Increased workload, the need to produce sufficient billable patient encounters, and concerns about liability issues and lack of preparation for teaching are some of the reasons for nurse practitioners' declining to precept graduate nursing students (Amella, Brown, Resnick, & McArthur, 2001; Wilson, Bodin, Hoffman, & Vincent, 2009).

Students who participate in preceptorships enjoy a number of benefits. They have the advantage of working one-on-one with experts who can coach them to increased clinical competence and performance. Preceptorships also provide opportunities for students to experience the realities of clinical practice, including scheduling learning activities on evening and night shifts and weekends in order to follow their preceptors' schedules (Gardner & Suplee, 2010, p. 69). However, following their preceptors' schedules often creates conflicts with students' academic, work, and family commitments. Additionally, a preceptor's patient assignment may not be always appropriate for a student's clinical learning objectives.

Preceptorships offer many advantages for the educational program in which they are used. The use of preceptors provides more clinical teachers for students and thus more intensive, individualized guidance of students' learning activities. Results of one study (Hendricks, Wallace, Narwold, Guy, & Wallace, 2013) comparing preceptored and traditional clinical learning placements for undergraduate prelicensure students showed significantly more clinical practice opportunities for teaching and counseling patients, receiving reports about patients, taking vital signs, documenting care, urinary catheterization, physical assessment, and administration of oral and intravenous medications. However, there were no differences in cognitive performance among students in the two groups. Working collaboratively with preceptors also helps faculty members to stay informed about the current realities of practice; up-to-date clinical information benefits ongoing curriculum development.

Several disadvantages related to the use of preceptors may affect educational programs. Contrary to a common belief, teachers' responsibilities do not decrease when students work with preceptors. Initial selection of preceptors, preparation of preceptors and students, and ongoing collaboration and communication with preceptors and students require as much time or more as the traditional clinical teaching model. The preceptorship model requires considerable indirect teaching time for the development of relationships with agencies and preceptors and the evaluation of preceptors and students. When preceptors are used as clinical teachers, faculty members may be responsible for more students in several clinical agencies and feel uncertain whether students are learning the application of theory and research findings to practice.

SELECTING PRECEPTORS

The success of preceptorships largely depends on the selection of appropriate preceptors; such selection is one of the teacher's most important responsibilities. Most faculty members consider the educational preparation of the preceptor to be important; most academic programs require the preceptor to have at least the degree for which the student is preparing, although insistence on this level of educational preparation does not guarantee that learners will be exposed only to professional role models.

The desire to teach and willingness to serve as a preceptor are important qualities of potential preceptors. Nurses who feel obligated to enact this role do not usually do not make enthusiastic, effective preceptors. Additional attributes of effective preceptors, according to Gardner and Suplee (2010), include:

- *Clinical expertise or proficiency, depending on the level of the learner.* Preceptors should be able to demonstrate expert psychomotor, problem-solving, critical thinking, clinical reasoning, and decision-making skills in their clinical practice. Nursing students and new staff nurses need preceptors who are at least proficient clinicians; graduate students need preceptors who are expert clinicians, administrators, or educators, depending on the goals of the preceptorship.
- *Leadership abilities.* Good preceptors are change agents in the health care organizations in which they are employed. They demonstrate effective communication skills and are trusted and respected by their peers.
- *Teaching skill.* Preceptors must understand and use principles of adult learning. They should be able to communicate ideas effectively to learners and give descriptive positive and negative feedback.
- *Professional role behaviors and attitudes.* Because preceptors act as role models for learners, they must demonstrate behaviors that represent important professional values. They are accountable for their actions and accept responsibility for their decisions. Good preceptors demonstrate maturity and self-confidence; their approach to learners is nonthreatening and nonjudgmental. They welcome questions from learners and do not interpret them as criticisms or

judgments about the practice setting or care approach. Flexibility, open-mindedness, enthusiasm about working with students, willingness to work with a diverse population of learners, and a sense of humor are additional attributes of effective preceptors.

The selection of preceptor and setting should also take into account the learner's interest in a specific clinical specialty as well as the need for development of particular skills. The teacher may collaborate with nurse managers to select appropriate preceptors. It is wise not to choose preceptors from newly established units or those with recent high staff turnover.

Potential preceptors for nursing students may be found in any clinical setting that meets the requirements of the nursing education program. The staff development or education department is a good first contact with an agency; some agencies ask that all requests for preceptors for nursing students be directed to a specified staff member who can suggest appropriate matches. Students may be able to suggest good potential preceptors from their work experience as nursing assistants or other unlicensed assistive personnel or from their contacts with nursing staff members in their previous clinical learning experiences. Alumni of the nursing education program are a rich source of potential preceptors; many of them would like to give back to their alma mater and are flattered to be asked to preceptor students. They can be recruited at alumni association gatherings, by telephone or e-mail, or through an alumni newsletter (Gardner & Suplee, 2010, p. 70). Offering appropriate incentives and rewards to preceptors acknowledges the value of their time and effort and can be an effective recruiting tool at a time when employee benefits may be diminishing. A more complete discussion of rewards for preceptors is included later in this chapter.

PREPARING THE PARTICIPANTS

Thorough preparation of preceptors and students for their roles is key to the success of preceptorships. Teachers are responsible for initial orientation and continuing support of all participants; preparation can be formal or informal.

Preceptor Preparation

Preparation of preceptors may begin with a general orientation, possibly for groups of potential preceptors at the selected agency or for all preceptors working with students from one nursing education program. A preceptorship preparation program acknowledges the need for and commitment to the notion of collaboration in nursing education and supports the learning needs of preceptors to enable them to enact their role effectively and confidently (Smedley & Penney, 2009).

Content of a preceptorship preparation program may include the following information:

- Benefits and challenges of precepting
- Characteristics of a good preceptor
- Principles of adult learning
- Assessment of learner needs
- Clinical teaching methods, including motivating and challenging learners, dealing with difficult learning situations, and when to use coaching techniques
- Evaluation of learning, including how to give effective feedback and use of clinical evaluation tools
- The preceptor's role in developing and implementing an individualized learning contract, if used
- The academic program curriculum structure, framework, and goals (Gardner & Suplee, 2010, p. 70; Smedley & Penney, 2009)

After preceptors have been selected, they need a specific orientation to their responsibilities. This orientation may take the form of a face-to-face or telephone conference with the teacher; written guidelines may be used to supplement the conference. Exhibit 13.1 is an example of written guidelines for preceptors of graduate nursing students. The conference and written guidelines may include information such as:

- *The educational level and previous experience of the student.* Graduate students need learning activities that build on their previous learning and experience in order to produce advanced practice outcomes. Beginning students may not have developed the knowledge and skill to participate in all of the preceptor's activities. Nurses who have served as preceptors for new staff nurses may have expectations for nursing student performance that are unrealistically high (Di Leonardi & Oermann, 2010).
- *How to choose specific learning activities based on learning objectives.* The teacher may share samples of learning contracts or lists of learning activities to guide the preceptor's selection of appropriate activities for the student.
- *Scheduling of clinical learning activities.* A common feature of preceptorships is the scheduling of the student's learning activities according to the preceptor's work schedule. Preceptors should be

---

Exhibit 13.1

SAMPLE GUIDELINES FOR A PRECEPTOR OF A GRADUATE NURSING STUDENT

The preceptor is expected to:

- Facilitate the student's entry into the health care organization
- Provide the student with an orientation to the organization
- After receiving the student's goals for the practicum, provide suggestions for how these goals can be accomplished
- Assist the student with identifying a project that is consistent with organizational needs and the student's interests, abilities, and learning needs
- Meet with the student at regular intervals to discuss progress on project and achievement of individual and course objectives
- Provide the student with regular feedback regarding his or her performance
- Communicate regularly with the faculty member regarding the student's progress

At the end of the preceptorship, provide a written evaluation of the student's performance related to goal achievement, clinical knowledge and skill, problem-solving and decision-making skills, communication and presentation skills, and interpersonal skills.

---

advised of dates on which students and teachers may not be available because of school holidays, examinations, and other course requirements.
- How and under what circumstances to contact the course faculty member (Gardner & Suplee, 2010).

New preceptors have learning needs much like those of students and new staff nurses; supportive role models and coaching are essential to success. In fact, the teacher needs to "precept the preceptor" (Mamchur & Myrick, 2003, p. 194). Preceptor programs for newly hired staff nurses may hold regular meetings of preceptors with staff development instructors and nurse managers to review material such as adult learning principles, teaching and evaluation strategies, and conflict resolution.

Student Preparation

Learners also need to understand the purposes and process of the preceptorship. They need an orientation to the process of planning individual learning activities, an explanation of teacher and preceptor roles, and a review of unit policies specific to student practice. At the beginning of the preceptorship, teachers should clarify evaluation responsibilities and expectations such as dates for learning contract approval, site visits, and conferences with faculty members.

IMPLEMENTATION

Successful implementation of preceptorships depends on mutual under-standing of the roles and responsibilities of the participants. The teacher, student, and preceptor collaborate to plan and implement learning activi-ties that will facilitate the student's goal attainment. Key to these pro-cesses is frequent, clear, effective communication among the participants (Gardner & Suplee, 2010).

Roles and Responsibilities of Participants

Preceptors

Preceptors are responsible for patient care in addition to clinical teaching of the student. The preceptor is expected to be a positive role model and a resource person for the student. The clinical teaching responsibilities of the preceptor include creating a positive learning climate, including the student in activities that relate to learning goals, and providing feedback to the student and teacher.

Role-model behaviors important for preceptors to demonstrate can be classified into four categories:

- Technical and technology skills—demonstrates nursing care proce-dures; operation of equipment unique to that clinical setting; use of the electronic health record, and evidence based, current nursing practices
- Interpersonal skills—uses effective communication techniques with patients and family members; interacts with physicians in a collegial, confident manner; displays appropriate use of humor; demonstrates caring attitude toward patients; gives positive feedback; gives con-structive negative feedback
- Critical thinking—listens carefully during change-of-shift reports and patient hand-overs and asks pertinent questions about patients' conditions; demonstrates proficient problem solving, decision mak-ing, critical thinking, and clinical reasoning
- Professional role behaviors—identifies self to patients at first con-tact, keeps patient information confidential, encourages discussion

of ethical issues, demonstrates enthusiasm about nursing, demonstrates accountability for own actions

Sometimes preceptors experience conflict between the educator and evaluator roles, especially when precepting new staff members. If the learner is unable to perform according to expectations, the faculty member or staff development instructor must be notified so that a plan for correcting the deficiencies may be established. In one study, preceptors were found to experience conflict in the preceptor–student relationship when they perceived a lack of competency on the part of the learner related to the learner's knowledge and skill level (Mamchur & Myrick, 2003). In some cases, the conflict is related to unrealistic expectations of the preceptor for student performance (Gardner & Suplee, 2010, p. 75).

When preceptors perceive that a student is unable to perform patient care tasks appropriately, they are often tempted to step in and take over by demonstrating the proper technique to the learner. This inclination may be due to the preceptor's concurrent responsibility of a patient care assignment and a genuine desire to share clinical knowledge and skill with the student. However, doing so interferes with both the student's and the patient's perceptions of the student as an "authentic care provider" (Gardner & Suplee, 2010, p. 89). To support students as they learn to care for patients, preceptors should use a coaching process. In sports, coaches stand on the sidelines; they do not participate in or interfere with the game unless there is a risk of injury (e.g., the soccer coach who sees lightening on the horizon interrupts the game by getting the referee's attention to stop play and clear the field). A good preceptor, using coaching techniques, allows the learner to be in control of the patient situation and stands nearby, monitoring the unfolding situation, offering verbal cues when needed, asking questions to guide the student's problem solving, offering encouragement (e.g., "that's right," "keep going"), and then giving immediate feedback for the student to reflect on. The coach's expression of belief in the student's capacity to succeed "helps the student develop self-efficacy and self-confidence." Thus, effective coaching can help students feel more confident in their clinical abilities and see themselves as authentic care providers. However, if a student "freezes" because of overwhelming anxiety, an error, inadequate preparation, or an unexpected occurrence, the preceptor may need to intervene if this places the patient at risk. The preceptor may need to temporarily assume responsibility for the task the student was attempting to perform, beginning or taking the next step of the task, and then encouraging the student to continue while continuing to coach from the sidelines (Gardner & Suplee, 2010).

Students

The student is expected to be an adult learner, actively participating in planning his or her own learning activities (Gardner & Suplee, 2010, p. 71). Planning may take the form of a learning contract that specifies individualized objectives and clinical learning activities. Because the teacher is not always present during learning activities, the student must communicate frequently with the teacher; communication may take the form of a reflective journal that is shared with teacher on a regular basis. The student must notify the teacher immediately of any problems encountered in the implementation of the preceptorship. In one study of conflict in preceptorships, Mamchur and Myrick (2003) found that 20% of students experienced conflict in their preceptorships but did not acknowledge or report it. Students may not report conflict for several reasons:

- They perceive that they are expected to fit in to the practice setting with minimal disruption.
- They feel powerless and dependent upon the preceptor's evaluation to complete the clinical practicum successfully.
- They fear receiving an unfavorable reference from the preceptor for future employment in that clinical agency (Mamchur & Myrick, 2003).
- Important aspects of the preceptor's workplace culture and work conditions did not provide a positive, supportive, caring learning environment (Smedley & Penney, 2009).

The student's responsibilities also include self-evaluation and evaluation of the preceptor's teaching effectiveness, as will be discussed later in this chapter.

Teachers

As previously discussed, the teacher is responsible for making preceptor selections, pairing students with preceptors, and orienting preceptors and students. The teacher is an important resource to preceptors and students to assist in problem solving. The teacher must be alert to any sign of conflict in the student–preceptor relationship and promptly take a proactive role in resolving it. If a conflict cannot be resolved to the satisfaction of student, preceptor, and faculty member, the student's well-being should take precedence, and, if necessary, the student should be reassigned (Mamchur & Myrick, 2003).

Teacher availability is particularly important if a problem arises at the clinical site that the preceptor and student cannot resolve. The teacher must make arrangements for consultation via telephone, e-mail, or pager. The teacher also arranges individual and group conferences with students and preceptors and visits the clinical sites as needed or requested by any of the participants. If students submit reflective journal entries, the teacher responds to them with feedback that helps students to evaluate their progress. Teachers have responsibility for the final evaluation of learner performance with input from preceptors, and they evaluate the effectiveness of preceptors with input from students.

Planning and Implementing Learning Activities

A common strategy for planning and implementing students' learning activities in the preceptorship model of clinical teaching is the use of an individualized learning contract. A learning contract is an explicit agreement between a teacher and student that clarifies expectations of each participant in the teaching–learning process. It specifies the learning goals that have been established, the learning activities selected to meet the objectives, and the expected outcomes and criteria by which they will be evaluated. In a preceptorship, the learning contract is negotiated among the teacher, student, and preceptor and guides the planning and implementation of the student's learning activities. Exhibit 13.2 is an example of a learning contract format that could be adapted for any level of learner.

As discussed previously, effective communication among the preceptor, student, and teacher is critical to the success of the preceptorship. Communication between teacher and student may be facilitated by the student keeping a reflective journal and sharing it with the teacher on a regular basis. In the journal, the student describes and analyzes learning activities that relate to the objective, reflecting on the meaning and value of the experiences. The journal entries may be recorded in a computer file, on paper, on audiotape, or posted to an online discussion board; the teacher responds via the same medium. Additionally, the student and teacher have telephone, e-mail, or face-to-face contact as necessary for the teacher to give consultation and guidance. Similarly, the teacher and preceptor should have regular contact by telephone, e-mail, text messaging, or face-to-face meetings so that the teacher receives feedback about learner performance and offers guidance and consultation as needed. Results of one study of clinicians who precepted nurse practitioner graduate students from one university (Brooks & Niederhauser, 2010) showed that the majority of preceptors expected two site visits from the students' teachers per semester

Exhibit 13.2

LEARNING CONTRACT TEMPLATE

Student Information
    Name and credentials:
    Address:
    Home phone number:
    Mobile phone number:
    e-mail address:

Teacher Information
    Name and credentials:
    Address:
    Office phone number:
    Mobile phone number:
    e-mail address:

Preceptor Information
    Name and credentials:
    Address:
    Office phone number:
    Mobile phone number:
    e-mail address:

Clinical Learning Objectives	Learning Activities and Resources	Evaluation Evidence, Responsibility, and Time Frame

Start date: Completion date:
    Student Signature _____   Date _____
    Preceptor Signature _____   Date _____
    Teacher Signature _____   Date _____

and that the first site visit should occur in the first 4 weeks of the semester. Preceptors also expected teachers to observe at least two patient encounters per student, suggesting that they wanted the site visits to be more substantive than social.

The realities of clinical and academic cultures present challenges to effective communication among teacher, preceptor, and student. Preceptors often work a variety of shifts, students often have complicated academic and work schedules, and teachers have multiple responsibilities in addition to clinical teaching. Flexibility and commitment to establishing and maintaining communication are essential to overcome these challenges.

EVALUATING THE OUTCOMES

Students, teachers, and preceptors share responsibility for monitoring the progress of learning and for evaluating outcomes of the preceptorship. Student performance may be evaluated according to the terms specified in the learning contract or through the clinical evaluation methods used by the educational program. If a learning contract is used, student self-evaluation is usually an important strategy for assessing outcomes. As discussed earlier, preceptors are expected to give feedback to the learner and to the teacher, but the teacher has the responsibility for the summative evaluation of learner performance.

An important aspect of evaluation concerns the teaching effectiveness of preceptors. Students are an important source of information about the quality of their preceptors' clinical teaching, but the teacher should also assess the degree to which preceptors were able to effectively guide the students' learning. A modified form of a teaching effectiveness tool used to evaluate clinical teachers may be used to collect data from students regarding their preceptors (Gardner & Suplee, 2010). Exhibit 13.3 is an example of a form for student evaluation of preceptor teaching effectiveness. Because each preceptor is typically assigned to one student at a time, it is usually impossible to maintain anonymity of student evaluations. Therefore, teachers may wish to share a summary of the student's evaluation, instead of the raw data, with the preceptor.

REWARDING PRECEPTORS

Preceptors make valuable contributions to nursing education programs, and they should receive appropriate rewards and incentives for their participation. At minimum, every preceptor should receive an individualized thank-you letter, specifying some of the benefits that the student received from the preceptorship. A copy of the letter may be sent to the preceptor's supervisor or manager to be used as evidence of clinical excellence at the time of the preceptor's next performance evaluation.

Other formal and informal ways of acknowledging the contributions of preceptors for nursing students are:

- A name badge that identifies the nurse as a preceptor
- A certificate of appreciation, signed by the administrator of the nursing education program or the staff development program
- An annual preceptor recognition event, including refreshments and an inspirational speaker

Exhibit 13.3

SAMPLE TOOL FOR STUDENT EVALUATION OF PRECEPTOR TEACHING EFFECTIVENESS

Directions: Rate the extent to which each statement describes your preceptor's teaching behaviors by circling a number following each item, using the following scale:

4 = to a large extent
3 = to a moderate extent
2 = to a small extent
1 = not at all

1. The preceptor was an excellent professional role model.	4	3	2	1
2. The preceptor guided my clinical problem solving.	4	3	2	1
3. The preceptor helped me to apply theory to clinical practice.	4	3	2	1
4. The preceptor was responsive to my individual learning needs.	4	3	2	1
5. The preceptor provided constructive feedback about my performance.	4	3	2	1
6. The preceptor communicated clearly and effectively.	4	3	2	1
7. The preceptor encouraged my independence.	4	3	2	1
8. The preceptor was flexible and open-minded.	4	3	2	1
9. Overall, the preceptor was an excellent clinical teacher.	4	3	2	1
10. I would recommend this preceptor for other students.	4	3	2	1

- Free or reduced-price registration for continuing education programs offered by the nursing education program or clinical facility (Smedley & Penney, 2009)
- Travel expenses and registration fees to attend professional development conferences off site
- Verification of contact hours for certification (Campbell & Hawkins, 2007)
- Free or reduced-rate tuition for one or more academic courses (Smedley & Penney, 2009)

- Free or reduced admission price to campus events such as athletic games, public lectures, and concerts (Campbell & Hawkins, 2007)
- Bookstore gift certificates
- Adjunct or affiliate faculty appointment
- Differential pay or adjustment of work schedule (e.g., exemption from weekend shifts) for preceptors who work with new staff members, nomination of preceptors for awards, providing letters of reference, editing manuscripts, and collaborating on research projects (Campbell & Hawkins, 2007)
- A gift such as a fruit basket or plant

SUMMARY

The use of preceptors is an alternative to the traditional clinical teaching model based on the assumption that a consistent relationship between an experienced nurse and a nursing student or novice staff nurse is an effective way to provide individualized guidance in clinical learning and professional socialization. Preceptorships have been used extensively with senior nursing students, graduate students preparing for advanced practice roles, and new staff nurse orientees.

A preceptorship is a time-limited, one-to-one relationship between a learner and an experienced nurse. The teacher may not be physically present during the learning activities; the preceptor provides intensive, individualized learning opportunities that improve the learner's clinical competence and confidence. The teacher has overall responsibility for the quality of the clinical teaching and learning and provides the link between the educational program and the practice setting. The preceptor functions as a role model and provides individualized clinical instruction, coaching, support, and socialization for the learner.

Preceptorships are frequently used for students in their last semester of academic preparation for entry into practice and for graduate students preparing for advanced clinical practice, administration, and education roles.

The use of preceptors in clinical teaching has both advantages and disadvantages for the educational program, clinical agency, teachers, preceptors, and students. Benefits for preceptors and their employers include the stimulation of working with learners who raise questions about clinical practice, assistance from students with research or teaching projects, rewards through a clinical ladder system for participation as a preceptor, and opportunities to recruit potential staff members for the agency from among students who work with preceptors. The greatest drawback of preceptorships to agencies and preceptors is usually the expected time commitment.

Students experience the benefits of working one-on-one with clinical experts who can coach them to improved performance as well as opportunities to experience the realities of clinical practice. However, following their preceptors' schedules often creates conflicts with students' academic, work, and family commitments.

Preceptorships offer many advantages to teachers and educational programs. The use of preceptors provides more clinical teachers for students and thus more intensive guidance of students' learning activities. Working collaboratively with preceptors also helps teachers to stay informed about the current realities of practice. Disadvantages include the amount of indirect teaching time required to select, prepare, and communicate with preceptors and students.

Selection of appropriate preceptors is important to the success of preceptorships. Most academic programs require the preceptor to have at least the degree for which the student is preparing. Desire to teach and willingness to serve as a preceptor are very important qualities of potential preceptors. Additional attributes of effective preceptors include clinical expertise or proficiency, leadership abilities, teaching skill, and professional role behaviors and attitudes.

Teachers are responsible for the initial orientation and continuing support of all participants; preparation can be formal or informal. A general orientation for potential preceptors may include information about benefits and challenges of precepting, characteristics of a good preceptor, principles of adult learning, clinical teaching and coaching techniques, evaluation methods, and the structure and goals of the nursing education program. After preceptors have been selected, they need a specific orientation to their responsibilities, including information about the student's educational level and previous experience, choosing specific learning activities based on learning objectives, and scheduling of clinical learning activities. Learners also need an orientation that includes information about the purposes of the preceptorship, the process of planning individual learning activities, and an explanation of teacher and preceptor roles.

Successful implementation of preceptorships depends on mutual understanding of the roles and responsibilities of the participants. The preceptor is expected to be a positive role model and a resource person for the student. The responsibilities of the preceptor include creating a positive learning climate, including the student in activities that relate to learning goals, and providing feedback to the student and teacher. The student usually arranges the schedule of clinical learning activities to coincide with the preceptor's work schedule and is expected to participate actively in planning learning activities. Because the teacher is not always present during learning activities, the student must keep the teacher informed about progress through frequent communication. In addition to making preceptor selections and orienting preceptors and students, the teacher is an important resource to preceptors and students to assist in problem solving. Teachers must make adequate arrangements for communication with other participants.

A common strategy for planning and implementing students' learning activities is the use of an individualized learning contract—an explicit agreement between the teacher, student, and preceptor that specifies the learning goals, learning activities selected to meet the objectives, and the expected outcomes and criteria by which they will be evaluated. The learning contract guides the planning and implementation of the student's learning activities.

Students, teachers, and preceptors share responsibility for monitoring the progress of learning and for evaluating outcomes of the preceptorship. Student performance is assessed according to the terms specified in the learning contract or through the clinical evaluation methods used by the educational program, through self-evaluation, and through feedback from preceptors. The teacher is responsible for the summative evaluation of learner performance. Students are an important source of information about their preceptors' clinical teaching effectiveness, but the teacher should also assess the degree to which preceptors were able to effectively guide students' learning.

Preceptors should receive appropriate rewards and incentives for the contributions they make to the educational program. At minimum, every preceptor should receive an individualized thank-you letter, specifying some of the benefits that the student received from the preceptorship. Other formal and informal ways of acknowledging the contributions of preceptors were discussed.

Exhibit 13.4

CNE EXAMINATION TEST BLUEPRINT CORE COMPETENCIES

1. **Facilitate Learning**

   A. Implement a variety of teaching strategies appropriate to
      1. content
      2. setting
      3. learner needs
      5. desired learner outcomes

   B. Use teaching strategies based on
      1. educational theory
      2. evidence-based practices related to education

(continued)

E. Practice skilled oral and written (including electronic) communication that reflects an awareness of self and relationships with learners (e.g., evaluation, mentorship, and supervision)

F. Communicate effectively orally and in writing with an ability to convey ideas in a variety of contexts

H. Create opportunities for learners to develop their own critical thinking skills

I. Create a positive learning environment that fosters a free exchange of ideas

N. Use knowledge of evidence-based practice to instruct learners

2. **Facilitate Learner Development and Socialization**

   E. Foster the development of learners in these areas
      1. cognitive domain
      2. psychomotor domain
      3. affective domain

   F. Assist learners to engage in thoughtful and constructive self and peer evaluation

3. **Use Assessment and Evaluation Strategies**

   E. Use a variety of strategies to assess and evaluate learning in these domains
      1. cognitive
      2. psychomotor
      3. affective

   J. Use assessment and evaluation data to enhance the teaching–learning process
   K. Advise learners regarding assessment and evaluation criteria
   L. Provide timely, constructive, and thoughtful feedback

REFERENCES

Amella, E. J., Brown, L., Resnick, B., & McArthur, D. B. (2001). Partners for NP education: The 1999 AANP preceptor and faculty survey. *Journal of the American Academy of Nurse Practitioners, 13*, 517–523.

Brooks, M. V., & Niederhauser, V. P. (2010). Preceptor expectations and issues with nurse practitioner clinical rotations. *Journal of the American Academy of Nurse Practitioners, 22*, 573–579. doi:10.1111/j.1745–7599.2010.00560.x

Campbell, S. H., & Hawkins, J. W. (2007). Preceptor rewards: How to say thank you for mentoring the next generation of nurse practitioners. *Journal of the American Academy of Nurse Practitioners, 19*, 24–29. doi:10.1111/j.1745-7599.2006.00186.x

Charleston, R., & Happell, B. (2005). Preceptorship in psychiatric nursing: An impact evaluation from an Australian perspective. *Nurse Education in Practice, 5*, 129–135.

Di Leonardi, B. H., & Oermann, M. H. (2010). Teaching in a clinical setting. In L. Caputi (Ed.), *Teaching nursing: The art and science* (pp. 126–177). Glen Ellyn, IL: College of DuPage Press.

Gardner, M. R., & Suplee, P. D. (2010). *Handbook of clinical teaching.* Sudbury, MA: Jones and Bartlett.

Hendricks, S. M., Wallace, L. S., Narwold, L., Guy, G., & Wallace, D. (2013). Comparing the effectiveness, practice opportunities, and satisfaction of the preceptored clinical and the traditional clinical for nursing students. *Nursing Education Perspectives, 34,* 310–314.

Mamchur, C., & Myrick, F. (2003). Preceptorship and interpersonal conflict: A multi-disciplinary study. *Journal of Advanced Nursing, 43,* 188–196.

Smedley, A., & Penney, D. (2009). A partnership approach to the preparation of preceptors. *Nursing Education Perspectives, 30,* 31–36.

Wilson, L. L., Bodin, M. B., Hoffman, J., & Vincent, J. (2009). Supporting and retaining preceptors for NNP programs: Results from a survey of NNP preceptors and program directors. *Journal of Perinatal & Neonatal Nursing, 23,* 284–292. doi:10.1097/JPN.0b013e3181b3075d

Yonge, O., Myrick, F., Ferguson, L., & Lughana, F. (2005). Promoting effective preceptorship experiences. *Journal of Wound, Ostomy, and Continence Nursing, 32,* 407–412.

Evaluation Strategies in Clinical Teaching

CHAPTER 14

Written Assignments

Written assignments enable students to learn about concepts relevant to clinical practice, develop higher level thinking skills, and examine values and beliefs that may affect patient care. Written assignments about clinical practice combined with feedback from the teacher provide an effective means of developing students' writing abilities. Although writing assignments may vary with each clinical course, depending on the outcomes of the course, assignments may be carefully sequenced across courses for students to develop their writing skills as they progress through the nursing program. The teacher is responsible for choosing written assignments that support the learning outcomes of the course and meet other curriculum goals.

PURPOSES OF WRITTEN ASSIGNMENTS

Written assignments for clinical learning have four main purposes: (1) assist students in understanding concepts, theories, and other content that relate to care of patients; (2) develop higher level thinking skills; (3) examine their own feelings, beliefs, and values generated from their clinical learning experiences; and (4) develop writing skills.

In choosing written assignments for clinical courses, the teacher should first consider the outcomes to be met through the assignments and the competencies that students need to develop in the course and nursing program. Writing assignments should build on one another to progressively develop students' skills. Another consideration is the number of assignments to be completed. How many assignments are needed to demonstrate mastery? It may be that one assignment well done is sufficient for meeting the outcomes of the clinical course, and students may then progress to other learning activities. Teachers should avoid using the same written assignments repeatedly throughout a clinical course and should instead choose assignments for specific learning outcomes.

Promote Understanding

In written assignments, students can describe concepts, theories, and other information relevant to the care of their patients and can explain how that knowledge guides their clinical decisions and judgments. Assignments for this purpose need a clear focus to prevent students from merely summarizing and reporting what they read. Shorter assignments that direct students to apply particular concepts to clinical practice may be of greater value in achieving this purpose than longer assignments for which students summarize readings they completed without any analysis of the meaning of those readings for their particular patients (Oermann, 2006).

Examples of written assignments to promote understanding of concepts, theories, and other information related to clinical practice are:

■ Compare, in no more than three pages, two interventions appropriate for your patient in terms of their rationale and evidence. How will you evaluate their effectiveness?
■ Read a research article related to care of one of your patients, critique the article, report on the analysis, and explain why the research findings are or are not applicable to the patient's care.
■ Compare data collected from your patient with the description of that condition in your textbook. What are similarities and differences? Why?
■ Select a family theory and complete an assessment of a family using this theory.
■ Investigate systems in your clinical setting for preventing medication errors. Write a summary report with recommendations.

Develop Higher Level Thinking Skills

Written assignments provide an opportunity for students to analyze patient and other problems they have encountered in clinical practice, evaluate their interventions, and propose new approaches. In writing assignments, students can analyze data and clinical situations, identify additional assessment data needed for decision making, identify patient needs and problems, propose approaches, compare interventions based on evidence, and evaluate the effectiveness of care. Writing assignments are particularly valuable for learning about evidence-based practice (EBP). Students can search for and examine the evidence underlying different interventions and make decisions about the best approaches to use with their patients. Students can identify assumptions they made about patients' responses that influenced their clinical decisions, critique arguments, take a stand about an issue and develop a rationale to support it, and draw generalizations about patient care from different clinical experiences.

Assignments geared to critical thinking should give students freedom to develop their ideas and consider alternative perspectives. If the assignment is too restrictive, students are inhibited in their thinking and ways of approaching the problem.

Written assignments for developing higher level thinking skills can be short, ranging from one to two paragraphs to a few pages. In developing these assignments, the teacher should avoid activities in which students merely report on the ideas and thinking of others. Instead, the assignment should ask students to consider an alternative point of view or a different way of approaching an issue. Short assignments also provide an opportunity for teachers to give prompt feedback to students on alternative ways of thinking about the clinical situation (Oermann, 2006).

The writing assignment should focus on meeting a particular learning outcome and should have specific directions to guide students' writing. For example, students may be asked to prepare a one-page paper comparing the physiological processes of asthma and bronchitis. Rather than writing on everything they read about asthma and bronchitis, students focus their papers on the physiology of these two conditions.

Examples of written assignments for developing higher level cognitive skills follow:

- Describe in one paragraph significant information you collected from your patient and why it is important to your decisions about approaches to use with that patient.
- Select one need or problem you identified for your patient and provide a rationale for it. What is one alternative need or problem you might also consider and why? Complete this assignment in two typed pages.
- Identify a near miss (close call) or an unsafe practice that you experienced or observed in your clinical setting. Analyze what went wrong and practices that should have been used. Prepare a response integrating the concept of just culture.
- Identify an issue affecting your patient, family, or community. Analyze that issue from two different points of view. Provide a

rationale for actions to be taken from both perspectives. How would you approach this issue and why?

- Identify a procedure you performed in your clinical setting. Find the written policy. Was your performance consistent with that policy? Why or why not? Are there deviations or workarounds you observed on the unit with that procedure? Write a report about what you learned.

Examine Feelings, Beliefs, and Values

Written assignments help learners examine feelings generated from caring for patients and reflect on their beliefs and values that might influence that care. Journals, for instance, provide a way for students to record their feelings about a patient or clinical activity and later reflect on these feelings. Assignments may be developed for students to identify their own beliefs and values and analyze how they affect their interactions with patients, families, and staff. Value-based statements may be given to students for written critique, or students may be asked to analyze an ethical issue, propose alternative courses of actions, and take a stand on the issue.

Examples of writing assignments that help students explore their feelings, beliefs, and values are:

- Identify an issue that affects patient care. Read about the issue, identify a journal that publishes articles in that area of clinical practice, and write an editorial that describes how you would address the issue either as a nurse manager or in the role of a staff nurse.
- In your journal, write about your feelings about caring for your patient and other patients in this setting. In what way do those feelings influence your care?
- A peer tells you she forgot to give her patient the scheduled pain medications but is not telling her faculty member because the patient never complained of pain. What would you say to this individual? Why did you choose this approach?
- Think about the community in which you are currently practicing. How do your values, beliefs, and personal goals influence your practice in that community?

Develop Writing Skills

An important outcome of writing assignments is the development of skill in communicating ideas in written form. Assignments help students learn how to organize thoughts and present them clearly. This clarity in writing develops through planned writing activities integrated in the nursing program. As a skill, writing ability requires practice, and students need to complete writing assignments across clinical courses. All too often, writing assignments are not sequenced progressively across courses or levels in the program; students, then, do not have the benefit of building writing skills sequentially.

Learning to write effectively is the responsibility of the entire faculty and requires more than taking an English course or writing one term paper in a clinical nursing course. Students need an opportunity to write about nursing in varied contexts. Through writing assignments in nursing courses, students learn to disseminate their ideas and inform, explain, direct, and persuade (Oermann, 2013). This is referred to as writing in the discipline (Writing Across the Curriculum [WAC] Clearinghouse, 2013a). By writing multiple types of papers with feedback from the teacher, students learn the writing style and conventions of the field. For example, in a prelicensure clinical course students might write a brief evidence summary to support a nursing intervention, whereas at the graduate level the writing assignment may be a systematic review of the evidence. Through writing in the discipline students begin to think like a nurse and communicate clearly within the field. Generally these papers are formal papers that adhere to the format and style of the field (WAC Clearinghouse, 2013b). These assignments should be sequenced across the nursing curriculum to improve students' writing skills. Luthy, Peterson, Lassetter, and Callister (2009) described an extensive program they developed to integrate writing competencies in a baccalaureate nursing program. Examples of written assignments include integrated literature reviews, analyses of ethical dilemmas, preparation of resumes, and others. In this program, some of the writing assignments, such as the literature reviews, are divided into smaller activities that then build on one another. With writing assignments incorporated throughout the curriculum, peer critique, and teacher feedback on writing, students develop their writing skills over time (Luthy et al., 2009). Students can begin with short assignments related to the clinical course, such as summarizing data they collected on a patient or preparing a report on how their assessment or nursing care related to their textbook and other readings. In later assignments, students can complete literature reviews, EBP papers, critiques of research studies related to clinical practice, analyses of quality and safety problems on the unit, and term papers. In this way, the writing assignments become more complex and require advanced writing skills; they also provide variety for students.

A benefit of this planned approach to teaching writing is faculty feedback, provided through drafts and rewrites of papers. Drafts are essential to foster development of writing skill. Drafts should be critiqued by faculty members for accuracy of content, development of ideas, organization, clarity of expression, and writing skills such as sentence structure, punctuation, and spelling (Oermann & Hays, 2010).

Small group critique of each others' writing is appropriate particularly for formative purposes. Small group critique provides a basis for subsequent revisions and gives feedback to students about both content and writing style. Although students may not identify every error in sentence structure and punctuation, they can provide valuable feedback on content, organization, how the ideas are developed, and clarity of writing. In a study with graduate students, peer review of the draft of the final assignment was an effective strategy to improve the quality of the paper and student understanding of the content (Schlisselberg & Moscou, 2013). Peer review should be used for giving feedback only, not for determining a grade for the assignment.

TYPES OF WRITING ASSIGNMENTS FOR CLINICAL LEARNING

Many types of writing assignments are appropriate for enhancing clinical learning. Some assignments help students learn the content they are writing about but do not necessarily improve writing skill, and other assignments also promote competency in writing. For example, structured assignments such as care plans provide minimal opportunity for freedom of expression, originality, and creativity. Other assignments, though, such as term papers on clinical topics, promote understanding of new content and its use in clinical practice as well as writing ability.

Types of written assignments for clinical learning include concept map, concept analysis paper, short written assignments, nursing care plan, case method and study, EBP papers, teaching plan, journal, group writing, and portfolio.

Concept Map

A concept map is a graphic or pictorial arrangement of key concepts related to a patient's care, which shows the interrelationships of those concepts. By developing a concept map, students can visualize how signs and symptoms, other assessment data, problems, interventions, medications, and other aspects of a patient's care relate to one another. Concept maps are also useful for teaching in the classroom and online courses. Students can develop a concept map for organizing ideas, brainstorming, taking notes, and learning collaboratively (Spencer, Anderson, & Ellis, 2013). They can also be used to teach concepts rather than focusing on content. Hunter Revell (2012) found that weekly concept map building increased students' engagement and their theoretical thinking. The concept maps also promoted application of theory to practice.

Concept maps have many uses in clinical learning. First, students may complete a concept map from their readings to assist them in linking new information to their patients. The readings that students complete for clinical practice, and in nursing courses overall, contain vast amounts of facts and specific information; concept maps help students process this information in a meaningful way, linking new and existing ideas.

Second, concept maps are useful in helping students prepare for clinical practice. They can be developed prior to a clinical experience as a way of organizing assessment information, relating it to the patient's needs and problems, and planning nursing care. In preclinical conferences, students can present the maps for feedback from the teacher and from peers. Students can modify the maps as they provide care for patients.

Third, concept maps may be developed collaboratively by students in clinical conferences. For this purpose, students may present a patient for whom they have provided care, and the clinical group then develops a concept map about that patient's care. Or the clinical group may develop a concept map about conditions or community problems they are learning about in the course. As another strategy, students can present the concept maps they developed for their patients, and the group can analyze and discuss them. Critiquing each others' concept maps enhances critical thinking, learning from one another, and group process; it also allows for feedback from the teacher and peers.

Concept maps are organized with specific concepts written under more general ones. Students first identify relevant concepts for their patients' care and then link these concepts. Different types of lines can be used to illustrate the relationships among the concepts. Figure 14.1 provides an example of a concept map. Concept maps are most appropriately used for formative evaluation, although students could write papers or present on the concepts in the maps, their interrelationships, and rationale, which could then be graded by faculty members.

Concept Analysis Paper

Concept analysis papers help students understand difficult concepts and how they are applied in patient care. For these papers, students identify and define a concept related to clinical practice, such as family-centered care or a problem such as pain. They then explore characteristics of the concept

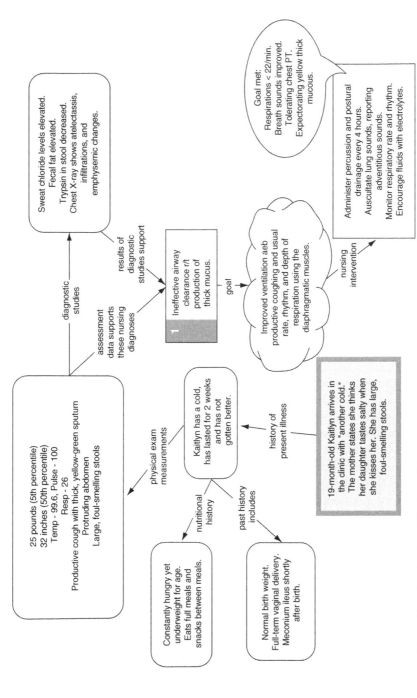

Sweat chloride levels elevated.
Fecal fat elevated.
Trypsin in stool decreased.
Chest X-ray shows atelectasis, infiltrations, and emphysemic changes.

Goal met:
Respirations < 22/min.
Breath sounds improved.
Tolerating chest PT.
Expectorating yellow thick mucous.

Administer percussion and postural drainage every 4 hours.
Auscultate lung sounds, reporting adventitious sounds.
Monitor respiratory rate and rhythm.
Encourage fluids with electrolytes.

results of diagnostic studies support

diagnostic studies

assessment data supports these nursing diagnoses

1 Ineffective airway clearance r/t production of thick mucus.

goal

Improved ventilation aeb productive coughing and usual rate, rhythm, and depth of respiration using the diaphragmatic muscles.

nursing intervention

25 pounds (5th percentile)
32 inches (50th percentile)
Temp - 99.6, Pulse - 100
Resp - 26
Productive cough with thick, yellow-green sputum
Protruding abdomen
Large, foul-smelling stools

physical exam measurements

Kaitlyn has a cold, has lasted for 2 weeks and has not gotten better.

history of present illness

19-month-old Kaitlyn arrives in the clinic with "another cold." The mother states she thinks her daughter tastes salty when she kisses her. She has large, foul-smelling stools.

nutritional history

past history includes

Constantly hungry yet underweight for age.
Eats full meals and snacks between meals.

Normal birth weight.
Full-term vaginal delivery.
Meconium ileus shortly after birth.

aeb, as evidenced by; r/t, related to; PT, physical therapy

Figure 14.1 This concept map depicts the plan of care for a 19-month-old who has been diagnosed with cystic fibrosis. Developed by Deanne Blach, MSN, RN. Reprinted by permission Deanne Blach.

and how that concept would be seen in clinical practice. Students can write papers about the concept and can develop a model case or scenario that exemplifies its various characteristics. These papers can be used as term papers, because students need to review the literature as the basis for their analysis. As an example, an assignment might be to:

> Identify a concept related to long-term care. Review the literature and provide a summary of the review. Define the characteristics of the concept—that is, how the concept would be seen in clinical practice, an organization, or the health care system. What are the issues you learned about this concept? Discuss implications for nursing practice related to your concept.

Short Written Assignments

Short written assignments in clinical courses are valuable for promoting critical thinking and analysis. Short assignments avoid students' summarizing what others have written without thinking about the content themselves (Oermann, 2006). With a short assignment, students can analyze patient needs and problems, compare interventions with their evidence, explore decisions that might be made in a clinical situation, analyze an issue and approaches, and analyze a case scenario. Sample assignments are found in Exhibit 14.1.

Exhibit 14.1

EXAMPLES OF SHORT WRITTEN ASSIGNMENTS FOR CLINICAL COURSES

- The unit secretary is slow about notifying nursing staff when patients use their call bells. It appears that only the assigned staff will answer the call bells; other nurses and aides who happen to be close by the patient's room will not respond. Develop a quality improvement project to address this issue.
- Select an intervention or treatment you used in patient care. Search for evidence related to that intervention or treatment. What were your sources of evidence? Summarize the strength of the evidence and discuss what it means for patient care.
- Read the article on loneliness. In no more than one page, explain how you would use that concept in an assessment.
- Describe the concept of patient-centered care and its use in a community setting.

(continued)

- In what ways did your patient's needs and problems compare to the description in your textbook?
- Your patient had a knee replacement and reports too much pain to go to physical therapy. Two hours ago, the prior nurse recorded in the medical record that the patient "had no pain and walked twice around the room." What are two different ways of approaching this situation? What would you do and why?
- Your patient is readmitted with congestive heart failure. He is agitated, and his respiratory rate is increasing rapidly. He is receiving oxygen by nasal cannula at 2 L/min. What additional data would you collect? What would you do next? Provide a rationale for your answer.
- Identify a decision you made in clinical practice involving either patients or staff. Describe the situation and why you responded that way. Propose another approach that could have been used.
- Describe the process on your unit for handoff at the end of the shift. What changes would you propose in that process and why?

Nursing Care Plan

Nursing care plans enable students to analyze patients' health problems and design plans of care. With care plans, students can record assessment data, identify patient needs and problems, select evidence-based interventions, and identify outcomes to be measured. Care plans should be usable—they should guide students' planning of their patients' care, be realistic, and be able to be implemented in the health care setting.

Completing a written care plan may help the student identify nursing and other interventions for specific problems, but whether that same care plan promotes problem-solving learning and higher-level thinking is questionable. Often students develop care plans from their textbook or the literature without thinking about the content. Even if the care plan is an appropriate written assignment for the course outcomes, the question remains as to how many care plans students need to complete in a clinical course to meet the learning goals. Once the goals have been achieved, then other written assignments may be more effective for clinical learning.

Case Method and Case Study

Case method and case study describe a clinical situation developed around an actual or a hypothetical patient for student review and critique. In case method, the case provided for analysis is generally shorter and more specific than in case study. Case studies are more comprehensive, thereby presenting a complete picture of the patient and clinical situation. After analyzing the case, students complete written questions about it; questions may be answered individually or by small groups of students. Case method and case study are discussed in detail in Chapter 11.

EBP Papers

Assignments in clinical courses can guide students' learning about EBP and its use in patient care. Studies continue to reveal the limited understanding of nurses about EBP, barriers to EBP, and nurses' reliance on colleagues for guidance with clinical decisions rather than on research and other sources of evidence (Chan et al., 2011; Dogherty, Harrison, Graham, Vandyk, & Keeping-Burke, 2013; Gale & Schaffer, 2009; Spenceley, O'Leary, Chizawsky, Ross, & Estabrooks, 2008; Strickland & O'Leary-Kelley, 2009). Clinical assignments that are integrated in courses throughout the nursing program foster students' knowledge about EBP and prepare students with the skills they need to search for and use evidence in their future practice.

Melnyk, Fineout-Overholt, Stillwell, and Williamson (2010) identified seven steps in the EBP process. These steps can be used as a framework for planning learning activities for students and assignments in clinical courses in the nursing education program. By using a framework such as this one or another EBP model, teachers can plan assignments for each clinical course in the curriculum, assisting students in integrating EBP into their practice. Exhibit 14.2 provides sample clinical assignments for learning about EBP and steps in the process.

Teaching Plan

Teaching plans enable students to apply concepts of learning and teaching to patients, families, and communities. This is another type of written assignment that may be completed individually or in small groups. After developing the teaching plan, students may use it as a basis for their teaching. There are many formats for teaching plans, but typically the assignment would include objectives, content, teaching strategies, and evaluation strategies.

Clinical Journals

Journal writing assists students in relating theory to clinical practice, linking their classroom and online instruction to care of patients, and reflecting on their clinical learning activities. When students reexamine their clinical decisions and propose alternative actions, journaling also encourages the development of higher level thinking skills and clinical judgment.

Exhibit 14.2

SAMPLE CLINICAL ASSIGNMENTS FOR LEARNING ABOUT EBP

Develop Questions About Clinical Practice

Write a clinical question using PICOT (patient, intervention, comparison, outcome, and time) format.

Think about a patient for whom you cared this week. Identify a question you had about that patient's care and write the question in PICOT format. List two sources of information you could consult to answer that question with a rationale for why these are appropriate. Discuss your question with a peer during postclinical conference. Is your question specific enough to guide a search? If not, revise it.

Identify a change in practice needed on your unit. Why is it needed? What led you to this decision? Write a short paper (no more than one page).

Search for Evidence

Conduct a search using your PICOT question. Identify key words or terms to search for an answer. Go to the Cumulative Index to Nursing and Allied Health Literature (CINAHL) and modify your key words as needed. Complete the search in CINAHL, mapping out your search strategy. Summarize your findings. What would you do differently with this search the next time? Write a two- to three-page paper on this search and what you found.

Conduct the same search in PubMed (MEDLINE). What are the differences, if any, in the results of your search? What did you learn about these two databases? Present in clinical conference.

Conduct a search using your PICOT question. For this search, start with PubMed Clinical Queries and describe your search strategy and results. Then continue your search in CINAHL. What evidence did you find related to your PICOT question?

Identify a bibliographic database other than CINAHL or PubMed that you might use in your clinical practice—for example, PsycINFO. Identify a clinical question that could be answered by searching in that database. Conduct the search and summarize your results. How could you use these results in clinical practice? What did you learn about this database? Present in the discussion board.

Critically Appraise the Evidence

Identify a PICOT question or a change in practice that might be indicated. Search for evidence and record your search strategy and results. What studies are relevant for inclusion in your review and why? Critique the evidence (consider validity, relevance, and applicability). Summarize your findings and develop a written proposal for use of this evidence to guide practice or why a practice change is not indicated.

(continued)

Review clinical research studies in an area of nursing practice related to the course. Critically appraise those studies and synthesize findings. What are issues in implementing those findings in your clinical setting? What would you propose to facilitate implementation? Prepare a paper on your review and analysis.

Discuss how you can use the Cochrane Database of Systematic Reviews in your patient care. Select a nursing intervention and locate information about this intervention in Cochrane. Write a three- to four-page report on your findings.

Select one of your PICOT questions and searches. Critique the evidence you found in that search. Use an established evidence hierarchy and rate the strength of the evidence. Discuss the implications of the evidence for nursing practice.

Use the Evidence in Clinical Practice

How do the nurse's clinical expertise and the patient's preferences and values interface with EBP? Should the evidence be weighed more heavily in decisions than patient preferences? Lead a discussion on this topic in the discussion board.

List interventions for one of your patients. What is the evidence base for each of these? Provide a rationale for their use based on the strength of the evidence. Include the sources of information you used to determine the evidence base. What evidence is missing, and what do you propose?

Review your patient's care. Select one problem not adequately met with current practices. Search for evidence to suggest a change in practice, evaluate the evidence, and write a paper about how you would change practice based on your review. What would you do differently the next time you care for that patient or patients with similar problems?

Select an intervention and find evidence using resources from the Joanna Briggs Institute. Describe the evidence you located. Did it help you make a decision about the effectiveness of the intervention? Why or why not? How would you use this information in your clinical practice? Prepare a short paper.

Evaluate Outcomes of Practice Decisions

For a practice change or evidence-based intervention you proposed in an earlier assignment, plan how you would evaluate its effect on patient outcomes. Present in online discussion forum.

Identify a question you had about your patient's care. Go to the National Guideline Clearinghouse. What EBP guidelines are relevant for this patient? If you implemented one of these guidelines in your clinical setting, what outcomes would you measure?

Implement one evidence-based intervention in patient care and evaluate its outcomes. Write a short (no more than two pages) report on your findings.

Assignments in which students write in journals about their clinical practice can achieve many outcomes; some of these are listed in Exhibit 14.3.

Journals are also a good strategy for examining one's own thoughts and actions in clinical practice and developing reflective practice (Adamshick &

Exhibit 14.3

USES OF CLINICAL JOURNALS

- Reflect on clinical practice experiences and their meaning.
- Document feelings related to clinical practice and reflect on their meaning personally and professionally.
- Describe perceptions of patients, families, communities, and experiences with other providers.
- Develop values and affective skills.
- Analyze ethical issues and dilemmas.
- Assess one's own knowledge and performance.
- Identify gaps in learning and how to improve performance.
- Analyze one's own actions and decisions following a clinical experience.
- Record accomplishments in clinical practice.
- Communicate with the clinical teacher, preceptor, and others involved in learning experience.

August-Brady, 2012; Davies, Reitmaier, Smith, & Mangan-Danckwart, 2013; Langley & Brown, 2010; Schuessler, Wilder, & Byrd, 2012; Zori, Kohn, Gallo, & Friedman, 2013). In a journal, students can reflect on their clinical experiences and reexamine them, improving their awareness of their own behaviors and responses within the context of the clinical environment. Callister, Luthy, Thompson, and Memmott (2009) found from an analysis of undergraduate students' reflective journals that the journals enabled students to explore their caring beliefs and how they implemented them with patients. Langley and Brown (2010) studied the use of reflective journals in an online graduate nursing course. Positive outcomes included integrating theory and practice, recognizing personal strengths and weaknesses, and exploring new ideas.

Through a reflective journal, students can:

- Find meaning in their clinical experiences
- Integrate theory and practice
- Examine their own values and develop values for professional practice
- Develop effective communication skills
- Learn about the perspectives of others, including patients, families, communities, nurses, and interprofessional team members
- Reflect on one's own role and the roles and responsibilities of others, including interprofessional teams in the health care setting
- Develop thinking and clinical reasoning skills

There are different ways of structuring journals, and the decision should be based on the intended outcomes of using the journal in the clinical course. The first step for the teacher is to identify the learning outcomes to be met through journal writing, such as reflecting on clinical decisions or describing feelings in caring for a patient, and then how journal entries should be made. Students should understand what learning outcomes are being achieved through journaling so they can gear their entries to those goals. Journals can be done electronically with course management systems, e-mail, blogs, and by using software for this purpose. Electronic journaling makes it easier for teachers to provide prompt feedback, dialogue with students, and store the journals.

Journals are not typically graded but provide an opportunity for giving feedback to learners and developing a dialogue with them. Students have greater freedom in recording feelings, ideas, and responses when the journal is used only for feedback. Faculty members are responsible for providing thoughtful and prompt feedback similar to any written assignment.

Group Writing

Not all writing assignments need to be done by students individually. There is much to be gained with group writing exercises as long as the groups are small and the exercises are carefully focused. Short written assignments, such as analyzing an issue and reporting in writing the outcomes of the analysis or developing a protocol as a group, may be completed in clinical conferences or done online in small groups. These group assignments provide opportunities for students to express their ideas to others in the group and work collaboratively to communicate the results of their thinking as a group in written form.

Portfolio

A portfolio provides an opportunity for students to present projects they completed in their clinical courses over a period of time. Portfolios may include evidence of student learning for a series of clinical learning activities over the duration of a clinical course or for documenting competencies in terms of overall course or program outcomes (Oermann & Gaberson, 2014).

There are two types of portfolios: best-work and growth and learning progress (Nitko & Brookhart, 2011). Best-work portfolios include materials and products developed by students in clinical practice that demonstrate their learning and achievements. These portfolios reflect the best work of the students in the clinical course. In contrast, growth and learning progress portfolios include materials and products in the process of being developed. These portfolios serve as a way of monitoring students' progress in clinical practice (Oermann & Gaberson, 2014). With both types of portfolios, the teacher reviews them periodically and provides feedback on the materials and products in the portfolio.

The content of the portfolio depends on the goals to be achieved. Students may include in their portfolios any materials they developed individually or in a group that provide evidence of their achieving the outcomes of the clinical course or demonstrating the clinical competencies. Examples of these materials are:

- Documents that students developed for patient care
- Teaching plans and materials
- Papers written about clinical practice
- Selected journal entries
- Reports of group work and products
- Reports and observations made in the clinical setting
- A self-assessment
- Reflections of their patient care experiences and meaning to them
- Other products that demonstrate their clinical competencies and what they learned in the course

Exhibit 14.4 presents a process for developing a portfolio for a clinical course.

Exhibit 14.4

DEVELOPING A PORTFOLIO FOR CLINICAL LEARNING

Step 1: Identify the purpose of the portfolio.

- Why is a portfolio useful in the course? What goals will it serve?
- Will the portfolio serve as a means of assessing students' development of clinical competencies, focusing predominantly on the growth of the students? Will the portfolio provide evidence of the students' best work in clinical practice, including products that reflect their learning over a period of time? Or, will the portfolio meet both demands, enabling the teacher to give continual feedback to students on the process of learning and projects on which they are working, as well as providing evidence of their accomplishments and achievements in clinical practice?
- Will the portfolio be used for formative or summative evaluation? Or both?
- Will the portfolio provide assessment data for use in a clinical course? Or, will it be used for curriculum and program evaluation?
- Will the portfolio serve as a means of assessing prior learning and therefore have an impact on the types of learning activities or courses that students

(continued)

complete, for instance, for assessing the prior learning of registered nurses entering a higher degree program or for licensed practical nurses entering an associate degree program?

- What is the role of the students, if any, in defining the focus and content of the portfolio?

Step 2: Identify the type of entries and content to be included in the portfolio.

- What types of entries are required in the portfolio, for example, products developed by students, descriptions of projects with which the students are involved, descriptions of clinical learning activities and reflections about them, observations made in clinical practice and analysis of them, and papers completed by the students, among others?
- In addition to required entries, what other types of content and entries might be included in the portfolio?
- Who determines the content of the portfolio and the types of entries? Teacher only? Student only? Or both?
- Will the entries be the same for all students or individualized by the student?
- What is the minimum number of entries to be considered satisfactory?
- How should the entries in the portfolio be organized, or will the students choose how to organize them?
- Are there required times for entries to be made in the portfolio, and when should the portfolio be submitted to the teacher for review and feedback?
- Will teacher and student meet in a conference to discuss the portfolio?

Step 3: Decide on the evaluation of the portfolio entries, including criteria for evaluation of individual entries and the portfolio overall.

- How will the portfolio be integrated within the clinical evaluation grade and course grade, if at all?
- What criteria will be used to evaluate, and perhaps score, each type of entry and the portfolio as a whole?
- Will only the teacher evaluate the portfolio and its entries? Will only the students evaluate their own progress and work? Or, will the evaluation be a collaborative effort?
- Should a rubric be developed for scoring the portfolio and individual entries? Is there one available in the nursing education program that could be used? If not, who will develop the rubric?

Note. From Oermann, M. H., & Gaberson, K. B. (2014). *Evaluation and testing in nursing education* (4th ed., pp. 290–292). New York, NY: Springer. Copyright ©2014 by Springer. Reprinted with permission.

EVALUATING WRITTEN ASSIGNMENTS

Written assignments may be evaluated formatively or summatively. Formative evaluation provides feedback to students for their continued learning but not for grading purposes. Periodic assessment of drafts of papers and work in progress is formative in nature and is not intended for arriving at a grade. Summative evaluation of completed writing assignments is designed for grading the assignment, not for giving feedback to the student.

For written assignments that are not graded, the teacher's role is to give prompt and sufficient feedback for students to learn from the assignment. If the assignment will be graded at a later time, however, then criteria for grading should be established and communicated to the learner. Any assignment that will eventually be graded should have clear, specific, and measurable criteria for evaluation. Some writing assignments, such as journals, do not lend themselves to grading and instead are best used for formative evaluation only.

Drafts

If drafts of written assignments are to be submitted, the teacher should inform students of each required due date. All written assignments benefit from prompt and specific feedback from the teacher. Feedback should be given on the quality of the content, as reflected in the criteria for evaluation, and on writing style if appropriate for the assignment. Students need specific suggestions about revisions, not general statements such as "unclear objectives in teaching plan." Instead, tell students exactly what needs to be changed; for instance, "Objective #1 in teaching plan is not measurable. Revise the verb; content is clear and relevant." Drafts of written assignments are important because they serve as a means of improving writing and thinking about the content. Prompt, clear, and specific feedback about revisions is essential to meet this purpose. Feedback is typically provided in written form but can also be given via audio recordings (Bourgault, Mundy, & Joshua, 2013). Drafts in most instances are used for feedback and are therefore not graded.

Criteria for Evaluation

The criteria for evaluation should relate to the learning outcomes to be met with the assignment. For example, if students write a short paper to meet the objective, "Compare interventions for nausea associated with chemotherapy," criteria should relate to the appropriateness and evidence for the interventions selected for critique, how effectively the student compared them, the rationale developed for the analysis, and the like.

General criteria for evaluating written assignments in clinical courses are presented in Exhibit 14.5. These criteria need to be adapted based on the type of assignment and its intent. For assignments that are graded, students should have the criteria for evaluation and scoring protocol or rubric before they begin writing so they are clear about how the assignment will be assessed.

Exhibit 14.5

GENERAL CRITERIA FOR EVALUATING PAPERS IN CLINICAL COURSES

Content

Content is relevant to patient or clinical situation.
Content is accurate.
Significant concepts and theories are presented.
Concepts and theories are used appropriately for analysis.
Content is comprehensive.
Content reflects current research and evidence.
Hypotheses, conclusions, and decisions are supported.

Organization

Content is organized logically.
Ideas are presented in logical sequence.
Paragraph structure is appropriate.
Headings are used appropriately to indicate new content areas.

Process

Process used to arrive at approaches, decisions, judgments, and so forth is adequate.
Consequences of decisions are considered and weighed.
Sound rationale is provided based on theory and research as appropriate.
For papers analyzing issues, rationale supports position taken.
Multiple perspectives and new approaches are considered.

Writing Style

Ideas are described clearly.
Sentence structure is clear.
There are no grammatical errors.
There are no spelling errors.
Appropriate punctuation is used.
Writing does not reveal bias related to gender, sexual orientation, racial or ethnic identity, age, or disabilities.
Length of paper is consistent with requirements.
References are cited appropriately throughout paper.
References are cited accurately according to required format.

Grading Assignments

In grading written assignments, a scoring protocol should be developed based on the criteria established for evaluation. The protocol should include the elements to be evaluated and points allotted for each one. The scoring protocol must be used in the same way for all students. This is an important principle in grading written assignments to assure consistency across papers and to focus the evaluation on the specific criteria. Some teachers tend to be more lenient, and others tend to be more critical in their review of papers. A scoring protocol helps the teacher base the grade on the established criteria rather than some other standard. Teachers will be more consistent in grading papers if they first establish specific criteria for evaluation, then develop a scoring protocol based on these criteria, and then use that scoring protocol in the same way for each student.

For some papers, a scoring rubric can be developed to guide the evaluation. A rubric lists the criteria to be met in the paper or characteristics of the paper and the points given for their evaluation. Exhibit 14.6 shows an example of how a rubric for scoring papers is developed using the general

Exhibit 14.6

SAMPLE SCORING RUBRIC FOR PAPERS IN CLINICAL COURSES

Content

Content relevant to patient or clinical situation, comprehensive, and in-depth	Content relevant to patient or clinical situation with critical information included	Some content not relevant to patient or clinical situation, critical information missing, lacks depth
5	4 3	2 1
Content accurate	Most of content accurate	Major errors in content
5	4 3	2 1
Sound background developed from peer-reviewed articles and wide range of information sources	Textbook and websites predominant sources of information for developing background	Background not developed, limited support for ideas
5	4 3	2 1
Current research and evidence synthesized and integrated effectively	Current research and evidence summarized	Limited research and evidence in paper, not used to support ideas
10–7	6–4	3–1

Organization

Purpose of paper well developed and clearly stated	Purpose apparent but not developed sufficiently	Purpose poorly developed, not clear
3	2	1

(continued)

Content well organized and logically presented, organization supports arguments and development of ideas	Clear organization of main points and ideas	Poorly organized, content not developed adequately
10–7	6–4	3–1
Effective conclusions based on analysis	Conclusions based on summary of content, limited analysis	Poor conclusions, not based on content in paper
3	2	1

Writing Style and Format

Sentence structure clear, smooth transitions, correct grammar and punctuation, no spelling errors	Adequate sentence structure and transitions; few grammar, punctuation, and spelling errors	Poor sentence structure and transitions; errors in grammar, punctuation, and spelling
10–7	6–4	3–1
Professional appearance of paper, all parts included, length consistent with requirements	Paper legible, some parts missing or too short or too long considering requirements	Unprofessional appearance, missing sections, paper too short or too long considering requirements
3	2	1
References used appropriately, references current, no errors in references, correct use of APA style	References used appropriately but limited, most references current, some citations or references with errors or some errors in APA style	Few references and limited breadth, old references (not classic), errors in references, errors in APA style
6 5	4 3	2 1

Total score _____ (sum points for total score; maximum score 60)

criteria in Exhibit 14.5. There are different types of rubrics. With a holistic rubric, the teacher scores the paper as a whole without assessing individual parts of the paper. An analytic rubric guides the assessment of separate parts of the paper and then sums them for a total score. For short written assignments in clinical courses, a protocol for scoring them is sufficient. However, for term papers or longer assignments, the teacher can develop a more detailed rubric for use in evaluating them.

Written assignments that are graded should be read anonymously if at all possible. This is sometimes difficult with small groups of students. Nevertheless, students can record on their papers their student numbers rather than their names. There is a tendency in evaluating papers and other written assignments, similar to essay items, for the teacher to be influenced by a general impression of the student. This is called the halo effect. The teacher may have positive or negative feelings about the student or other biases that may influence evaluating and grading the assignment.

Another reason to read papers anonymously is to avoid a carryover effect, in which the teacher carries an impression of the quality of one written assignment to the next one that the student completes. If the student develops an outstanding paper, the teacher may be influenced to score subsequent written assignments at a similarly high level; the same situation may occur with a poor paper. The teacher therefore carries the impression of the student from one written assignment to the next. If there are multiple questions that students answered as part of a written assignment, the previous scores should be covered to avoid being biased about the quality of the next answer. In addition, the teacher should evaluate all students' answers to one question before proceeding to the next question (Oermann, 2013; Oermann & Gaberson, 2014).

All written assignments should be read twice before scoring. In the first reading, it is important to note errors in content, omission of major content areas, problems with organization, problems with the process used for approaching the issue, and problems with writing style. Comments can be recorded on the student's paper with suggestions for revision. After reading through all of the papers, then the teacher should begin a second reading for scoring purposes. Reading the papers twice gives the teacher a sense of how students approached the assignment. This is important because, in some cases, the scoring protocol may need to be revised.

Papers and other types of written assignments should be read in random order. After the first reading, the teacher can shuffle the papers so they are read in a random order the second time. Papers read early may be scored higher than those read near the end (Oermann & Gaberson, 2014). Teacher fatigue may also set in and influence the grading of papers. Although this section discusses grading written assignments, the teacher should remember that many writing assignments will not be graded.

SUMMARY

Written assignments for clinical learning have four main purposes: to learn about concepts, theories, and other content related to clinical practice; develop thinking skills; examine values and beliefs that may affect patient care; and develop writing skills. Not all writing assignments achieve each of these outcomes. The teacher decides first on the outcomes to be met, then plans the writing assignment with these outcomes in mind.

Short written assignments can be used in clinical courses to encourage students' independent thinking and avoid their summarizing what others have written. In developing these assignments, the teacher should not ask students to merely report on the ideas of others; instead, the assignment should ask students to consider an alternative point of view or a different way of approaching an issue. Short assignments also provide an opportunity for faculty members to give prompt feedback to students.

Written assignments help learners examine feelings generated from caring for patients and reflect on their beliefs and values that might influence that care. They also help students learn how to organize thoughts and present them clearly. Some faculty members have developed writing-to-learn programs in which written assignments are sequenced across the nursing curriculum.

Many types of written assignments can be used for clinical learning. Concept map, concept analysis paper, short written assignments, nursing care plan, case method and study, EBP papers, teaching plan, journal, group writing, and portfolio were presented in this chapter.

Written assignments may be evaluated formatively or summatively. Formative evaluation provides feedback to students for their continued learning but not for grading purposes. Periodic assessment of drafts of papers and work in progress is formative in nature and is not intended for arriving at a grade. Summative evaluation of completed writing assignments is designed for grading the assignment, not for giving feedback to the student.

In grading written assignments, a scoring protocol or rubric should be developed based on the criteria established for evaluation. The scoring protocol and rubric are used in the same way for all students. Many written assignments, though, are best if assessed formatively and not graded.

Exhibit 14.7

CNE EXAMINATION TEST BLUEPRINT CORE COMPETENCIES

1. **Facilitate Learning**

   A. Implement a variety of teaching strategies appropriate to
      1. content
      2. setting
      3. learner needs
      4. learning style
      5. desired learner outcomes
      6. method of delivery

(continued)

B. Use teaching strategies based on
   1. educational theory
   2. EBPs related to education
E. Practice skilled oral and written (including electronic) communication that reflects an awareness of self and relationships with learners (e.g., evaluation, mentorship, and supervision)
F. Communicate effectively orally and in writing with an ability to convey ideas in a variety of contexts
G. Model reflective thinking practices, including critical thinking
H. Create opportunities for learners to develop their own critical thinking skills
I. Create a positive learning environment that fosters a free exchange of ideas
N. Use knowledge of EBP to instruct learners

2. **Facilitate Learner Development and Socialization**

A. Foster the development of learners in these areas
   1. cognitive domain
   2. psychomotor domain
   3. affective domain
F. Assist learners to engage in thoughtful and constructive self and peer evaluation

3. **Use Assessment and Evaluation Strategies**

C. Use a variety of strategies to assess and evaluate learning in these domains
   1. cognitive
   2. psychomotor
   3. affective
J. Use assessment and evaluation data to enhance the teaching-learning process
K. Advise learners regarding assessment and evaluation criteria
L. Provide timely, constructive, and thoughtful feedback

REFERENCES

Adamshick, P., & August-Brady, M. (2012). Reclaiming the essence of nursing: The meaning of an immersion experience in Honduras for RN to bachelor of science students. *Journal of Professional Nursing, 28*, 190–198. doi:10.1016/j.profnurs.2011.11.011

Bourgault, A. M., Mundy, C., & Joshua, T. (2013). Comparison of audio vs. written feedback on clinical assignments of nursing students. *Nursing Education Perspectives, 34*, 43–46.

Callister, L., Luthy, K., Thompson, P., & Memmott, R. (2009). Ethical reasoning in baccalaureate nursing students. *Nursing Ethics, 16*, 499–510.

Chan, G. K., Barnason, S., Dakin, C. L., Gillespie, G., Kamienski, M. C., Stapleton, S., . . . Li, S. (2011). Barriers and perceived needs for understanding and using research among emergency nurses. *Journal of Emergency Nursing, 37*(1), 24–31. doi:10.1016/j. jen.2009.11.016

Davies, S. M., Reitmaier, A. B., Smith, L. R., & Mangan-Danckwart, D. (2013). Capturing intergenerativity: The use of student reflective journals to identify learning within an undergraduate course in gerontological nursing. *Journal of Nursing Education, 52,* 139–149. doi:10.3928/01484834-20120213-01

Dogherty, E. J., Harrison, M. B., Graham, I. D., Vandyk, A. D., & Keeping-Burke, L. (2013). Turning knowledge into action at the point-of-care: The collective experience of nurses facilitating the implementation of evidence-based practice. *Worldviews on Evidence Based Nursing, 10*(3), 129–139. doi:10.1111/wvn.12009

Gale, B., & Schaffer, M. (2009). Organizational readiness for evidence-based practice. *Journal of Nursing Administration, 39,* 91–97.

Hunter Revell, S. M. (2012). Concept maps and nursing theory: A pedagogical approach. *Nurse Educator, 37,* 131–135. doi:10.1097/NNE.0b013e31825041ba

Langley, M. E., & Brown, S. T. (2010). Perceptions of the use of reflective learning journals in online graduate nursing education. *Nursing Education Perspectives, 31,* 12–17.

Luthy, K., Peterson, N., Lassetter, J., & Callister, L. (2009). Successfully incorporating writing across the curriculum with advanced writing in nursing. *Journal of Nursing Education, 48,* 54–59.

Melnyk, B. M., Fineout-Overholt, E., Stillwell, S. B., & Williamson, K. M. (2010). Evidence-based practice: Step by step: The seven steps of evidence-based practice. *American Journal of Nursing, 110*(1), 51–63. doi:10.1097/01.NAJ.0000366056.06605.d2

Nitko, A. J., & Brookhart, S. M. (2011). *Educational assessment of students* (6th ed.). Upper Saddle River, NJ: Pearson Education.

Oermann, M. H. (2006). Short written assignments for clinical nursing courses. *Nurse Educator, 31,* 228–231.

Oermann, M. H. (2013). Enhancing writing in online education. In K. H. Frith & D. J. Clark (Eds.), *Distance education in nursing* (3rd ed., pp. 145–162). New York, NY: Springer Publishing.

Oermann, M. H., & Gaberson, K. B. (2014). *Evaluation and testing in nursing education* (4th ed.). New York, NY: Springer Publishing.

Oermann, M. H., & Hays, J. (2010). *Writing for publication in nursing* (2nd ed.). New York, NY: Springer Publishing.

Schlisselberg, G., & Moscou, S. (2013). Peer review as an educational strategy to improve academic work: An interdisciplinary collaboration between communication disorders and nursing. *Work, 44,* 355–360. doi:10.3233/WOR-121512

Schuessler, J. B., Wilder, B., & Byrd, L. W. (2012). Reflective journaling and development of cultural humility in students. *Nursing Education Perspectives, 33,* 96–99.

Spenceley, S. M., O'Leary, K. A., Chizawsky, L. L., Ross, A. J., & Estabrooks, C. A. (2008). Sources of information used by nurses to inform practice: An integrative review. *International Journal of Nursing Studies, 45,* 954–970.

Spencer, J. R., Anderson, K. M., & Ellis, K. K. (2013). Radiant thinking and the use of the mind map in nurse practitioner education. *Journal of Nursing Education, 52,* 291–293. doi:10.3928/01484834-20130328-03s

Strickland, R. J., & O'Leary-Kelley, C. (2009). Clinical nurse educators' perceptions of research utilization: Barriers and facilitators to change. *Journal for Nurses in Staff Development, 25*(4), 164–171. doi:10.1097/NND.0b013e3181ae142b

Writing Across the Curriculum Clearinghouse. (2013a). *Basic principles of WAC.* Retrieved from http://wac.colostate.edu/intro/pop3a.cfm

Writing Across the Curriculum Clearinghouse. (2013b). *What is writing in the disciplines?* Retrieved from http://wac.colostate.edu/intro/pop2e.cfm

Zori, S., Kohn, N., Gallo, K., & Friedman, M. I. (2013). Critical thinking of registered nurses in a fellowship program. *Journal of Continuing Education in Nursing, 44,* 374–380. doi:10.3928/00220124-20130603-03

CHAPTER 15

Clinical Evaluation and Grading

Nursing practice requires the development of higher-level cognitive skills, values, psychomotor and technological skills, and other competencies for care of patients across settings. Through clinical evaluation, the teacher arrives at judgments about students' competencies—their performance in practice. After establishing a framework for evaluating students in clinical practice and exploring one's own values, attitudes, and biases that may influence evaluation, the teacher identifies a variety of methods for collecting data on student performance. Clinical evaluation methods are strategies for assessing learning outcomes in clinical practice. Some evaluation methods are most appropriate for use by faculty members or preceptors who are onsite with students and can observe their performance; other evaluation methods assess students' knowledge, cognitive skills, and other competencies but do not involve direct observation of their performance. This chapter describes the process of clinical evaluation in nursing, methods for evaluating clinical performance, and how to grade students in clinical courses.

CONCEPT OF CLINICAL EVALUATION

Clinical evaluation is a process by which judgments are made about learners' competencies in practice. This practice may involve care of patients, families, and communities; other types of learning activities in the clinical setting; simulation activities; performance of varied skills in learning laboratories; or activities using multimedia. Most frequently, clinical evaluation involves observing performance and arriving at judgments about the student's competence. Judgments influence the data collected—that is, the specific types of observations made to evaluate the student's performance—and the inferences and conclusions drawn from the data about the quality of that performance. Teachers may collect different data to evaluate the same outcomes, and when presented with a series of observations about a student's performance in clinical practice, there may be minimal consistency in their judgments about how well that student performed.

Clinical evaluation is not an objective process; it involves subjective judgments of the teacher and others involved in the process. The teacher's values influence evaluation. This is most apparent in clinical evaluation, where teachers' values influence the observations they make of students and the judgments they make about the quality of their performance. Thus, it is important for teachers to be aware of their own values that might bias their judgments of students. For example, if the teacher prefers students who initiate discussions and participate actively in conferences, this value should not influence the assessment of students' competencies in other areas. The teacher needs to be aware of this preference to avoid an unfair evaluation of other dimensions of the students' clinical performance. Or, if the teacher is used to the fast pace of most acute care settings, when working with beginning students or someone who moves slowly, the teacher should be cautious not to let this prior experience influence expectations of performance. Faculty members and preceptors should examine their values, attitudes, and beliefs so that they are aware of them as they teach and assess students' performance in practice settings.

Clinical Evaluation Versus Grading

Clinical evaluation is not the same as grading. In evaluation, the teacher makes observations of performance and collects other types of data, then compares this information to a set of standards to arrive at a judgment. From this assessment, a quantitative symbol or grade may be applied to reflect the evaluation data and judgments made about performance. The clinical grade, such as pass–fail or A through F, is the symbol to represent the evaluation. Clinical performance may be evaluated and not graded, such as with formative evaluation or feedback to the learner, or it may be graded. Grades, however, should not be assigned without sufficient data about clinical performance.

Norm- and Criterion-Referenced Clinical Evaluation

Clinical evaluation may be norm- or criterion-referenced. In norm-referenced evaluation, the student's clinical performance is compared with that of other students, indicating that the performance is better than, worse than, or equivalent to that of others in the comparison group or that the student has more or less knowledge, skill, or ability than the other students. Rating students' clinical competencies in relation to others in the clinical group—for example, indicating that the student was "average"—is a norm-referenced interpretation.

In contrast, criterion-referenced clinical evaluation involves comparing the student's clinical performance to predetermined criteria, not to the performance of other students in the group. In this type of clinical evaluation, the criteria are known in advance and used as the basis for evaluation. Indicating that the student has met the clinical outcomes or achieved the clinical competencies, regardless of how other students performed, represents a criterion-referenced interpretation.

Formative and Summative Clinical Evaluation

Clinical evaluation may be formative or summative. Formative evaluation in clinical practice provides feedback to learners about their progress in meeting the outcomes of the clinical course or in developing the clinical competencies. The purposes of formative evaluation are to enable students to develop further their clinical knowledge, skills, and values; indicate areas in which learning and practice are needed; and provide a basis for suggesting additional instruction to improve performance. With this type of evaluation, after identifying the learning needs, instruction is provided to move students forward in their learning. Formative evaluation, therefore, is diagnostic; it should not be graded (Nitko & Brookhart, 2011). For example, the clinical teacher or preceptor might observe a student perform wound care and give feedback on changes to make with the technique. The goal of this assessment is to improve subsequent performance, not to grade how well the student carried out the procedure.

Summative clinical evaluation, however, is designed for determining clinical grades because it summarizes competencies the student has developed in clinical practice. Summative evaluation is done at the end of a period of time—for example, at midterm or at the end of the clinical practicum—to assess the extent to which learners have achieved the clinical outcomes or competencies. Summative evaluation is not diagnostic; it summarizes the performance of students at a particular point in time. For much of clinical practice in a nursing education program, summative evaluation comes too late for students to have an opportunity to improve performance. At the end of a course involving care of mothers and children, for instance, there may be many behaviors the student would not have an opportunity to practice in subsequent courses.

Any protocol for clinical evaluation should include extensive formative evaluation and periodic summative evaluation. Formative evaluation is essential to provide feedback to improve performance while practice experiences are still available.

FAIRNESS IN CLINICAL EVALUATION

Considering that clinical evaluation is not objective, the goal is to establish a fair evaluation system. Fairness requires that:

1. The teacher identify his or her own values, attitudes, beliefs, and biases that may influence the evaluation process.
2. Clinical evaluation be based on predetermined outcomes or competencies.
3. The teacher develop a supportive clinical learning environment.

Identify One's Own Values

Teachers need to be aware of their personal values, attitudes, beliefs, and biases that may influence the evaluation process. These can affect both the data collected about students and the inferences made. In addition, students have their own sets of values and attitudes that influence their self-evaluations of performance and their responses to the teacher's evaluations and feedback. Students' acceptance of the teacher's guidance in clinical practice and information provided to them for improving performance is affected by their past experiences in clinical courses with other faculty members. Students may have had problems in prior clinical courses, receiving only negative feedback and limited support from the teacher, staff members, and others. In situations in which student responses inhibit learning, the teacher may need to intervene to guide students in more self-awareness of their own values and the effect they are having on their learning.

Base Clinical Evaluation on Outcomes or Competencies

Clinical evaluation should be based on preset outcomes, clinical objectives, or competencies that are then used to guide the evaluation process. Without these, neither the teacher nor the student has any basis for evaluating clinical performance. What are the outcomes of the clinical course (or, in some nursing education programs, the clinical objectives) to be met? What clinical competencies should the student develop? These outcomes or competencies provide a framework for faculty members to use in observing performance and for arriving at judgments about achievement in clinical practice. For example, if the competencies relate to developing communication skills, then the learning activities—whether in the patient care setting, as part of a simulation, or in the learning laboratory—should assist students in learning how to communicate. The teacher's observations and subsequent assessment should focus on communication behaviors, not on other competencies unrelated to the learning activities.

Develop a Supportive Learning Environment

It is up to the teacher to develop a supportive learning environment in which students view the teacher as someone who will facilitate their learning and development of clinical competencies. Students need to be comfortable asking faculty and staff members questions and seeking their guidance rather than avoiding them in the clinical setting. A supportive environment is critical for effective assessment, because students need to recognize that the teacher's feedback is intended to help them improve performance.

Many factors influence the development of a supportive learning environment. The clinical setting needs to provide experiences that foster student learning and development. Staff members need to be supportive of students and work collaboratively with them and with the faculty member. Most of all, there has to be trust and respect between the teacher and students.

FEEDBACK IN CLINICAL EVALUATION

For clinical evaluation to be effective, the teacher should provide continuous feedback to students about their performance and how they can improve it. Feedback is the communication of information to students, based on the teacher's assessment, that enables students to reflect on their performance, identify continued learning needs, and decide how to meet them (Bonnel, 2008). Feedback may be verbal, by describing observations of performance and explaining what to do differently, or visual, by demonstrating correct performance.

Feedback should be accompanied by further instruction from the teacher or by working with students to identify appropriate learning activities. The ultimate goal is for students to progress to a point at which they can judge their own performance, identify resources for their learning, and use those resources to further develop competencies. Bonnel (2008) emphasized that, for feedback to be useful, students need to reflect on the information communicated to them and take an active role (p. 290).

Students must have an underlying knowledge base and beginning skills to judge their own performance. Nitko and Brookhart (2011) suggested that feedback on performance also identifies the possible causes or reasons why the student has not mastered the learning outcomes. Sometimes the reason is that the student does not have the prerequisite knowledge and skills for developing the new competencies. As such, it is critical for faculty members and preceptors to begin their clinical instruction by assessing whether students have learned the necessary concepts and skills and, if not, to start there.

Principles of Providing Feedback as Part of Clinical Evaluation

There are five principles for providing feedback to students as part of the clinical evaluation process. First, the feedback should be precise and specific. General information about performance, such as, "You need to work on your assessment" or "You need more practice in the simulation laboratory," does not indicate what behaviors need improvement or how to develop them. Instead of using general statements, the teacher should indicate what specific areas of knowledge are lacking, where there are problems in critical thinking and clinical judgments, and what particular competencies need more development. Rather than saying to a student, "You need to work on your assessment," the student would be better served if the teacher identified the specific areas of data collection omitted and the physical examination techniques that need improvement. Specific feedback is more valuable to learners than a general description of their behavior.

Second, for procedures, use of technologies, and any psychomotor skills, the teacher should provide both verbal and visual feedback to students. This means that the teacher should explain first, either orally or in writing, where the errors were made in performance and then demonstrate the correct procedure or skill. This should be followed by student practice of the skill with the teacher guiding performance. By allowing immediate practice, with the teacher available to correct problems, students can more easily use the feedback to further develop their skills.

Third, feedback about performance should be given to students at the time of learning or immediately following it. Giving prompt feedback is one of the seven core principles for effective teaching in undergraduate programs (Chickering & Gamson, 1987). Providing prompt and rich feedback is equally important when teaching graduate students, nurses, and other learners regardless of their educational level. The longer the period of time between performance and feedback from the teacher, the less effective is the feedback. As time passes, neither student nor teacher may remember specific areas of clinical practice to be improved. This principle holds true whether the performance relates to cognitive learning, a procedure or technical skill, or an attitude or value expressed by the student, among other areas.

Whether working with a group of students in a clinical setting, communicating with preceptors about students, or teaching an online course, the teacher needs to develop a strategy for giving focused and immediate feedback to students and following up with further discussion as needed. Recording short notes on paper or with some technology for later discussion with individual students helps the teacher remember important points about performance.

Fourth, students need different amounts of feedback and positive reinforcement. In beginning practice and with clinical situations that are new to learners, most students will need frequent and extensive feedback. As students progress through the program and become more competent, they should be able to assess their own performance and identify personal learning needs. Some students will require more feedback and direction from the teacher than others.

One final principle is that feedback should be diagnostic. After identifying areas in which further learning is needed, the teacher's responsibility is to guide students so that they can improve their performance. The process is cyclical—the teacher observes and assesses performance, gives students feedback about that performance, and then guides their learning and practice so they can become more competent.

RELATIONSHIP OF EVALUATION TO CLINICAL OUTCOMES AND COMPETENCIES

There are different ways of specifying the outcomes to be achieved in clinical practice, which in turn provide the basis for clinical evaluation. These may be stated in the form of outcomes to be met or as competencies to be demonstrated in clinical practice. The faculties of some nursing education programs specify the outcomes in the form of clinical objectives. Regardless of how these are stated, they represent what is evaluated in clinical practice.

The outcomes of clinical practice in Exhibit 5.1 can be used for developing specific outcomes or competencies for a clinical course. Not all clinical courses will have outcomes in each of these areas, and, in some courses, there may be other types of competencies unique to practice in that clinical specialty. In some nursing programs there are general outcomes that each clinical course addresses. For example, with this model, each course would have an outcome on communication. In a beginning clinical course, the outcome might be, "Identifies verbal and nonverbal techniques for communicating with patients." In a later course in the curriculum, the communication outcome might focus on the family and working with caregivers—for example, "Develops interpersonal relationships with families and caregivers." Then, in a community health course, the outcome might be, "Collaborates with other health care providers in care of patients in the community and the community as client."

As another approach, some teachers state the outcomes broadly and then indicate specific behaviors students should demonstrate to meet those outcomes in a particular course. For example, the outcome on communication might be stated as, "Communicates effectively with patients and others in the health system." Examples of behaviors that indicate achievement of this outcome in a course on care of children include, "Uses appropriate verbal and nonverbal communication based on the child's age, developmental status, and health condition" and "Interacts effectively with parents, caregivers, and others." Generally, the outcomes or competencies are then used for developing the clinical evaluation tool or form, which is discussed later in the chapter.

Regardless of how the outcomes are stated for a clinical course, they need to be specific enough to guide the evaluation of students in clinical practice. An outcome such as, "Use the nursing process in care of children" is too broad to guide evaluation. More specific outcomes such as, "Carries out a systematic assessment of children reflecting their developmental stage," "Evaluates the impact of health problems on the child and family," and "Identifies resources for managing the child's care at home" make clear to students what is expected of them in clinical practice.

Competencies are the abilities to be demonstrated by the learner in clinical practice. Boland (2009) viewed competencies as the knowledge, skills, and attitudes that students need to develop. For nurses in practice, these competencies reflect the proficiencies for performing a particular task or carrying out their defined role in the health care setting. Competencies for nurses are assessed as part of the initial employment and orientation to the health care setting and on an ongoing basis.

Caution should be exercised in developing clinical outcomes and competencies to avoid having too many for evaluation, considering the number of learners for whom the teacher is responsible, types of clinical learning opportunities available, and time allotted for clinical learning activities. In preparing outcomes or competencies for a clinical course, teachers should keep in mind that they need to collect sufficient data about students' performance of each outcome or competency specified for that course. The clinical outcomes or competencies need to be realistic and useful for guiding the assessment.

CLINICAL EVALUATION METHODS

There are many evaluation methods for use in nursing education. Some methods, such as journals, are most appropriate for formative evaluation, while others are useful for either formative or summative evaluation.

Selecting Clinical Evaluation Methods

There are several factors to consider when selecting clinical evaluation methods to use in a course. First, the evaluation methods should provide information on student performance of the clinical competencies associated with the course. With the evaluation methods, the teacher collects data on performance to judge whether students are developing the clinical competencies or have achieved them by the end of the course. For many outcomes of a course, different strategies can be used, thereby providing flexibility in choosing methods for evaluation. Most evaluation methods provide data on multiple clinical outcomes. For example, a written assignment in which students compare two data sets might relate to outcomes on assessment, analysis, and writing. In planning the evaluation for a clinical course, the teacher reviews the outcomes or competencies to be developed and decides which evaluation methods will be used for assessing them, recognizing that most methods provide information on more than one outcome or competency.

Second, there are many different clinical evaluation strategies that might be used to assess performance. Varying the methods maintains student interest and takes into account learners' individual needs, abilities, and characteristics. Some students may be more proficient in methods that depend on writing, while others prefer strategies such as conferences and other discussions. Using multiple evaluation methods in clinical courses takes into consideration these differences among students. It also avoids relying on one method, such as a rating scale, for determining the entire clinical grade.

Third, the teacher should select evaluation methods that are realistic considering the number of students to be evaluated, available practice or simulation activities, and constraints such as the teacher's or preceptor's time. Planning for an evaluation method that depends on patients with specific health problems or particular clinical situations is not realistic considering the types of experiences with actual or simulated patients available to students. Some methods are not appropriate because of the number of students who would need to use them within the time frame of the course. Others may be too costly or require resources not available in the nursing education program or health care setting.

Fourth, evaluation methods can be used for formative or summative evaluation. In the process of deciding how to evaluate students' clinical performance, the teacher should identify whether the methods will be used to provide feedback to learners (formative) or for grading (summative). With formative clinical evaluation, the focus is on the progression of students in meeting the learning goals (Clynes & Raftery, 2008; Gigante, Dell, & Sharkey, 2011). At the end of the rotation, course, or semester, summative evaluation establishes whether the student met those goals and is competent (Bourke & Ihrke, 2009). In clinical practice, students should know ahead of time whether the assessment by the teacher is for formative or summative purposes. Some of the methods designed for clinical evaluation provide feedback to students on areas for improvement and should not be graded. Other methods, such as rating scales and written assignments, can be used for summative purposes and can therefore be computed as part of the course or clinical grade.

Fifth, before finalizing the protocol for evaluating clinical performance in a course, the teacher should review the purpose and number required of each assignment completed by students in clinical practice. What are the purposes of these assignments, and how many are needed to demonstrate competency? In some clinical courses, students complete an excessive number of written assignments. Students benefit from continuous feedback from the teacher, not from repetitive assignments that contribute little to their development of clinical knowledge and skills. Instead of daily or weekly care plans or other assignments, which may not even be consistent with current practice, once students develop the competencies, they can progress to other, more relevant learning activities.

Sixth, in deciding how to evaluate clinical performance, the teacher should consider the time needed to complete the evaluation, provide feedback, and grade the assignment. Instead of requiring a series of written assignments in a clinical course, the same outcomes might be met through discussions with students, cases analyzed by students in clinical conferences, group writing activities, and other methods requiring less teacher time and accomplishing the same purposes. Considering the demands on nursing faculty members, it is important to consider one's own time when planning how to evaluate students' performance in clinical practice.

Observation

The main strategy for evaluating clinical performance is observing students in clinical practice, simulation and learning laboratories, and other settings. In a survey of 1,573 faculty members representing all types of prelicensure nursing programs (diploma, 128; associate degree, 866; baccalaureate, 563; and entry-level master's, 8), observation of student performance was the predominant strategy used across programs (n = 1,289, 93%; Oermann, Yarbrough, Ard, Saewert, & Charasika, 2009).

Although observation is widely used, there are threats to its validity and reliability. First, observations of students may be influenced by the teacher's values, attitudes, and biases, as discussed earlier. There may also be overreliance on first impressions, which might change as the teacher or preceptor observes the student over a period of time and in different situations. In any performance assessment, there needs to be a series of observations made before drawing conclusions about performance.

Second, in observing performance, there are many aspects of performance on which the teacher may focus attention. For example, while observing a student administer an intravenous medication, the teacher may focus mainly on the technique used for its administration, ask limited questions about the purpose of the medication, and make no observations of how the student interacts with the patient. Another teacher observing this same student may focus on other aspects.

Third, the teacher may arrive at incorrect judgments about the observation, such as inferring that a student is inattentive during conference when, in fact, the student is thinking about the comments made by others in the group. It is important to discuss observations with students, obtain their perceptions of their behavior, and be willing to modify one's own inferences when new data are presented. In discussing observations and impressions with students, the teacher can learn about their perceptions of performance; this, in turn, may provide additional information that influences the teacher's judgment about competencies (Oermann, 2008).

Fourth, every observation in the clinical setting reflects only a sampling of the learner's performance during a clinical activity. An observation of the same student at another time may reveal a different level of performance.

Finally, similar to other clinical evaluation methods, the outcomes or competencies guide the teacher on what to observe. They help the teacher focus the observations of performance. However, all observed behaviors should be shared with the students.

Notes About Performance

It is difficult, if not impossible, to remember the observations made of each student for each clinical activity. For this reason, teachers need a device to help them remember their observations and the context in which the performance occurred. There are several ways of recording observations of students in clinical settings, simulation and learning laboratories, and other settings: narrative notes about performance, checklists, and rating scales.

The teacher can make notes that describe the observations made of students in the clinical setting; these are sometimes called anecdotal notes. In a study by Hall (2013), 92.4% of faculty members reported using anecdotal notes for record keeping about students' performance. Some teachers include only a description of the observations and then, after a series of observations, review the pattern of the performance and draw conclusions about it. Other teachers record their observations and include a judgment about how well the student performed (Di Leonardi & Oermann, 2010). Notes about the student's performance should be recorded as close to the time of the observation as possible; otherwise, it is difficult to remember what was observed and the context (e.g., patient and clinical situation) of that observation. In the clinical setting, notes can be handwritten or recorded using some technology.

Notes about the observations made in clinical practice and the quality of the student's performance should be shared with students frequently; otherwise, they are not effective for feedback. Considering the issues associated with observations of clinical performance, the teacher should discuss observations with the students and be willing to incorporate their own judgments about the performance. These notes are also useful in conferences with students—for example, at midterm and at the end of term—for reviewing a pattern of performance over time.

Checklists

A checklist contains specific behaviors or activities to be observed with a place for marking whether they were present during the performance (Nitko & Brookhart, 2011). A checklist often lists the steps to be followed in performing a procedure or demonstrating a skill. Some checklists also include errors in performance that are commonly made. Checklists not only facilitate the teacher's observation of procedures and behaviors performed by students and nurses learning new technologies and procedures, but they also provide a way for learners to assess their own performance. With checklists, learners can review and evaluate their performance prior to assessment by the teacher.

For common procedures and skills, teachers can often find checklists already prepared that can be used for evaluation, and some nursing textbooks have accompanying skills checklists. When these resources are not available, teachers can develop their own checklists but should avoid including every possible step, which makes the checklist too cumbersome. Instead, the focus should be on critical behaviors and where they fit into the sequence.

Rating Scales

Rating scales, also referred to as clinical evaluation tools or instruments, provide a means of recording judgments about the observed performance of students in clinical practice. A rating scale has two parts: (a) a list of outcomes or competencies the student is to demonstrate in clinical practice and (b) a scale for rating their performance of them.

Rating scales are most useful for summative evaluation of performance; after observing students over a period of time, the teacher draws conclusions about performance, rating it according to the scale provided with the instrument. Rating scales may also be used to evaluate specific activities that students complete in clinical practice—for example, rating a student's presentation of a case in clinical conference or the quality of discharge teaching provided to a patient. Other uses of rating scales are to: (a) help students focus their attention on critical behaviors to be performed in clinical practice; (b) give specific feedback to students about their performance; and (c) demonstrate growth in clinical competencies over a designated time period if the same rating scale is used.

The same rating scale can be used for multiple purposes. Exhibit 15.1 shows sample competencies from a rating scale that is used midway through a course; in Exhibit 15.2, the same competencies are used for the final evaluation, but the performance is rated as satisfactory or unsatisfactory as a summative rating.

Types of Rating Scales

Many types of rating scales are used for evaluating clinical performance. The scales may have multiple levels for rating performance, such as 1 to 5 or exceptional to below average, or have two levels, such as pass–fail. Types of scales with multiple levels for rating performance include:

- Letters: A, B, C, D, E or A, B, C, D, F
- Numbers: 1, 2, 3, 4, 5
- Qualitative labels: excellent, very good, good, fair, poor; exceptional, above average, average, below average
- Frequency labels: always, usually, frequently, sometimes, never

Exhibit 15.3 provides an example of a rating scale for clinical evaluation that has multiple levels for rating performance.

A short description included with the letters, numbers, and labels for each of the outcomes or competencies rated improves objectivity and consistency (Nitko & Brookhart, 2011). For example, if teachers use a scale of exceptional, above average, average, and below average or a scale based on the numbers 4, 3, 2, and 1, short descriptions of each level in the scale could be written to clarify the performance expected at each level. For the clinical outcome "Collects relevant data from patient," the descriptors might be:

Exhibit 15.1

SAMPLE COMPETENCIES FROM RATING SCALE FOR FORMATIVE EVALUATION

Maternal–Newborn Nursing
Midterm Progress Report

Name _____   Date _____

Objective	Yes	No	Not Obs.
1. Provides patient-centered care to mothers and newborns			
A. Assesses the individual needs of mothers and newborns			
B. Plans care to meet the patient's needs			
C. Implements nursing interventions based on evidence			
D. Evaluates the outcomes of care			
E. Includes the family in planning and implementing care for the mother and newborn			
2. Participates in health teaching for maternal-newborn patients and families			
A. Identifies learning needs of mothers and families			
B. Uses opportunities to do health teaching when giving nursing care			

Note: Not Obs., not observed.

Exhibit 15.2

SAMPLE COMPETENCIES FROM SAME RATING SCALE FOR FINAL EVALUATION

Maternal–Newborn Nursing
Clinical Performance Evaluation

Name _____ Date _____

Objective	S	U
1. Provides patient-centered care to mothers and newborns		
A. Assesses the individual needs of mothers and newborns		
B. Plans care to meet the patient's needs		
C. Implements nursing interventions based on evidence		
D. Evaluates the outcomes of care		
E. Includes the family in planning and implementing care for the mother and newborn		
2. Participates in health teaching for maternal-newborn patients and families		
A. Identifies learning needs of mothers and families		
B. Uses opportunities to do health teaching when giving nursing care		

Note: S, satisfactory; U, unsatisfactory.

Exceptional (or 4): Differentiates relevant from irrelevant data, analyzes multiple sources of data, establishes comprehensive database, identifies data needed for evaluating all possible nursing diagnoses and patient problems.

Above average (or 3): Collects significant data from patients, uses multiple sources of data as part of assessment, identifies possible nursing diagnoses and patient problems based on the data.

Average (or 2): Collects significant data from patients, uses data to develop main nursing diagnoses and patient problems.

Below average (or 1): Does not collect significant data and misses important cues in data; unable to explain relevance of data for nursing diagnoses and patient problems.

Exhibit 15.3

CLINICAL EVALUATION TOOL WITH MULTIPLE LEVELS FOR RATING PERFORMANCE

Community Health Nursing (RN section)
CLINICAL EVALUATION FORM

Total Raw Score: _____   Student Name: _____

Mean Score: _____   Faculty Name: _____

Letter Grade: _____   Agency: _____

Uses a theoretical framework in care of individuals, families, and groups in the community	4	3	2	1	NO
A. Applies concepts and theories in the practice of community health nursing					
B. Examines multicultural concepts of care as they apply to the community					
C. Analyzes family theory as a basis for care of clients in a community setting					
D. Examines relationships of family members in a community setting					
E. Examines the community as a client through ongoing assessment					
F. Evaluates health care delivery systems in a community setting					
Uses the nursing process for care of individuals, families, and groups in the community and the community as client					
A. Adapts assessment skills in the collection of data from individuals, families, and groups in a community setting					
B. Uses relevant resources in the collection of data in the community					
*C. Analyzes client and community data					
D. Develops nursing diagnoses for individuals, families, and groups in the community and the community as client					
E. Develops measurable outcome criteria and plan of action					

(continued)

Uses a theoretical framework in care of individuals, families, and groups in the community	4	3	2	1	NO
F. Uses outcome criteria for evaluating plans and effectiveness of interventions					
***G.** Assumes accountability for own practice in the community					
H. Uses research findings and standards for community-based care					
***I.** Accepts differences among clients and communities					
Is responsible for identifying and meeting own learning needs					
***A.** Evaluates own development as a professional					
***B.** Meets own learning needs in community practice					
Collaborates with others in providing community care					
A. Interacts effectively with clients and others in the community					
B. Effectively uses community resources					
FACULTY–STUDENT NARRATIVE Faculty Comments: Signature: _____ Date: _____ Student Comments: Signature: _____ Date: _____					

Note: 4 = consistently excels in performance of behavior, independent; 3 = is competent in performance, independent; 2 = performs behavior safely, needs assistance; 1 = unable to perform behavior, requires guidance all the time. NO, not observed.

*Critical behaviors must be rated at or above 2.0 to pass clinical practicum.

Tool developed by Judith M. Fouladbakhsh, PhD, RN, APRN, BC, AHN-BC, CHTP. Adapted by permission of J. Fouladbakhsh, 2013.

Rating scales for clinical evaluation may also have two levels, such as pass–fail and satisfactory–unsatisfactory. A survey of nursing faculty members from all types of programs indicated that most faculty members (*n* = 1,116, 83%) used pass–fail in their clinical courses (Oermann et al., 2009). Exhibit 15.4 is an example of a clinical evaluation tool that has two levels for rating performance: satisfactory–unsatisfactory. This tool is based on the

Exhibit 15.4

CLINICAL EVALUATION TOOL WITH TWO LEVELS FOR RATING PERFORMANCE (BASED ON QSEN COMPETENCIES)

NICHOLLS STATE UNIVERSITY
DEPARTMENT OF NURSING
BSN PROGRAM

Clinical Performance Evaluation Tool
NURS 225 Level I

Self Evaluation _____
Faculty Evaluation _____

Student Name _____

Faculty _____   Course: NURS 225   Semester _____

Fill in appropriate fields to the right & below:

Student must obtain a Satisfactory "S" grade in all competencies at the Final Evaluation to pass the Course.

Core Competencies	Midterm			Final	
	S	NI	U	S	U
Focusing on wellness, health promotion, illness and disease management across the lifespan in a variety of settings while recognizing the diverse uniqueness of individuals, providing directed care to individuals with well-defined health alterations, the student at the end of N225, should be able to:					
I. Patient-Centered Care					
a. Develop an individualized plan of care with a focus on assessment and planning utilizing the nursing process					
b. Demonstrate caring behaviors					
c. Conduct a comprehensive assessment while eliciting patient values, preferences and needs					
d. Respect diversity of individuals					
e. Assess the presence and extent of pain and suffering					
f. Demonstrate beginning competency in skills					

(continued)

Core Competencies	Midterm			Final	
	S	NI	U	S	U
II. Teamwork and Collaboration					
a. Develop effective communication skills (orally and through charting) with patients, team members, and family					
b. Identify relevant data for communication in pre and post conferences					
c. Identify intra- and inter-professional team member roles and scopes of practice					
d. Establish appropriate relationships with team members					
e. Identify need for help when appropriate to situation					
III. Evidence-Based Practice					
a. Locate evidence-based literature related to clinical practice and guideline activities					
b Reference clinical related activities with evidence-based literature					
c Value the concept of evidence-based practice in determining best clinical practice					
IV. Quality Improvement					
a. Deliver care in timely and cost effective manner					
b. Seek information about processes/projects to improve care (QI)					
c. Value the significance of variance reporting					
V. Safety					
a. Demonstrate effective use of technology and standardized practices that support safety and quality					
b. Implement strategies to reduce risk of harm to self or others					
c. Demonstrate appropriate clinical decision making					

(continued)

Core Competencies	Midterm			Final	
	S	NI	U	S	U
d. Identify national patient safety goals and quality measures					
e. Use appropriate strategies to reduce reliance on memory					
f. Communicate observations or concerns related to hazards and errors to patient, families, and the health care team					
g. Organize multiple responsibilities and provide care in a timely manner					
VI. Informatics					
a. Navigate the electronic health record for patient information where appropriate for clinical setting					
b. Document clear and concise responses to care in the electronic health record, where appropriate for clinical setting					
c. Identify information and clinical technology using critical thinking to collect, process, and communicate data					
d. Manage data, information, and knowledge of technology in an ethical manner					
e. Protect confidentiality of electronic health records					
VII. Professionalism					
a. Demonstrate core professional values (caring, altruism, autonomy, integrity, human dignity, and social justice)					
b. Maintain professional behavior and appearance					
c. Comply with the Code of Ethics, Standards of Practice, and policies and procedures of Nicholls State University, Department of Nursing, and clinical agencies					
d. Accept constructive criticism and develop plan of action for improvement					

(continued)

Core Competencies	Midterm			Final	
	S	NI	U	S	U
e. Maintain a positive attitude and interact with inter-professional team members, faculty, and fellow students in a positive, professional manner					
f. Provide evidence of preparation for clinical learning experiences					
g. Arrive to clinical experiences at assigned times					
h. Demonstrate expected behaviors and complete tasks in a timely manner					
i. Accept individual responsibility and accountability for nursing interventions, outcomes, and other actions					
j. Engage in self evaluation					
k. Assume responsibility for learning					

Midterm Comments (Address strengths and weaknesses)

Faculty

Student

Student Signature _____ **Date** _____

Faculty Signature _____ **Date** _____

Final Comments (Address strengths and weaknesses)

Faculty

Student

Student Signature _____ **Date** _____

Faculty Signature _____ **Date** _____

(*continued*)

Mid-Clinical Evaluation: faculty and student *must* complete documentation for remediation of unsatisfactory areas. CPR Tool[a] must be initiated for any unsatisfactory areas.

Unsatisfactory Area	Remediation Strategy

Student Signature _____   Date _____

Faculty Signature _____   Date _____

Developed collaboratively by Nicholls State University Nursing Faculty. Reprinted by permission, 2012.

Two copies on file – 1 for student self evaluation; 1 for clinical faculty
*Content based upon QSEN Competencies and KSA's.
[a] **Clinical Performance Remediation tool.**

S = Satisfactory
NI = Needs Improvement
U = Unsatisfactory

©2012 Nicholls State University Department of Nursing, Thibodaux, LA.

Quality and Safety Education for Nurses (QSEN) competencies (QSEN, 2013). Competencies on this form could also be rated as pass–fail.

Issues With Rating Scales

One problem in using rating scales is apparent by a review of the sample scale descriptors. What are the differences between above average and average or between a 2 and a 1? Is there consensus among faculty members using the rating scale about what constitutes different levels of performance for each outcome, competency, or behavior evaluated? This problem exists even when descriptions are provided for each level of the rating scale. Teachers may differ in their judgments of whether the student collected relevant data, whether multiple sources of data were used, whether the database was comprehensive, if all possible nursing diagnoses were considered, and so forth.

Scales based on frequency labels are often difficult to implement because of limited experiences for students to practice and demonstrate a level of skill rated as "always, usually, frequently, sometimes, and never." How should teachers rate students' performance in situations in which they practiced the skill perhaps once or twice? Even two-dimensional scales such as pass–fail present room for variability among educators.

Nitko and Brookhart (2011) identified eight common errors that can occur with rating scales applicable to rating clinical performance. The first three errors can occur with tools that have multiple points on the scale for rating performance, such as 1 to 5 or below average to exceptional. The other errors can occur with any type of clinical performance rating scale.

1. Leniency error results when the teacher tends to rate all students toward the high end of the scale.
2. Severity error is the opposite of leniency, tending to rate all students toward the low end of the scale.
3. Central tendency error is hesitancy to mark either end of the rating scale and instead use only the midpoint of the scale.
4. Halo effect is a judgment based on a general impression of the student. With this error, the teacher lets an overall impression of the student influence the ratings of specific aspects of the student's performance. This impression affects the teacher's ability to objectively evaluate and rate specific competencies or behaviors on the tool. The halo may be positive, giving the student a higher rating than is deserved, or negative, letting a general negative impression of the student result in lower ratings of specific aspects of the performance.
5. Personal bias occurs when the teacher's biases influence ratings such as favoring nursing students who do not work while attending school over those who are employed while attending school.
6. Logical error results when similar ratings are given for items on the scale that are logically related to one another. This is a problem with rating scales in nursing that are too long and often too detailed. For example, there may be multiple behaviors on communication skills to be rated. The teacher observes some of these behaviors but not all of them. In completing the clinical evaluation form, the teacher gives the same rating to all communication behaviors on the tool. When this occurs, some of the behaviors on the rating scale can often be combined.
7. Rater drift occurs when teachers redefine the performance behaviors to be observed and assessed. Initially, in developing a clinical evaluation form, teachers agree on the competencies or behaviors to be rated and the scale to be used. However, over time, educators may interpret them differently, drifting away from the original intent. For this reason, faculty members in a course should discuss as a group each competency or behavior on the clinical evaluation form at the beginning and mid-point

in the course. This discussion should include the meaning of the competency or behavior and what a student's performance would look like at each rating level in the tool.

8. Reliability decay is a similar issue. Nitko and Brookhart (2011) indicated that, immediately following training on using a rating tool, educators tend to use the tool consistently across students and with each other. As the course continues, though, faculty members may become less consistent in their ratings. Discussion of the clinical evaluation tool among course faculty, as indicated earlier, may improve consistency in the use of the tool.

Although there are issues with rating scales, they allow teachers, preceptors, and others to rate performance over time and to note patterns of performance. Exhibit 15.5 provides guidelines for using rating scales for clinical evaluation in nursing.

Simulations for Clinical Evaluation

Simulations are not only effective for instruction in nursing, but they are also useful for clinical evaluation. Students can demonstrate procedures and technologies, conduct assessments, analyze clinical scenarios and make decisions about problems and actions to take, carry out nursing interventions, and evaluate the effects of their decisions. Each of these outcomes can be evaluated for feedback to students or for summative grading.

Many nursing education programs have simulation laboratories with human patient simulators, clinically equipped examination rooms, manikins and models for skill practice and assessment, areas for standardized patients, and a wide range of multimedia that facilitate performance evaluations. The rooms can be equipped with two-way mirrors, video cameras, microphones, and other media for observing and rating performance by faculty members and others. Videoconferencing technology can be used to conduct clinical evaluations of students in settings at a distance from the nursing education program, effectively replacing onsite performance evaluations by faculty members.

Incorporating Simulations Into Clinical Evaluation Protocol

The same principles for evaluating student performance in the clinical setting apply to using simulations. The first task is to identify which clinical outcomes will be assessed with a simulation. This decision should be made during the course planning phase as part of the protocol developed for clinical evaluation in the course. It is important to remember when deciding on evaluation methods that assessment can be done for feedback to students and thus remain ungraded, or it can be used for grading purposes.

Exhibit 15.5

GUIDELINES FOR USING RATING SCALES FOR CLINICAL EVALUATION

1. Be alert to the possible influence of your own values, attitudes, beliefs, and biases in observing performance and drawing conclusions about it.

2. Use the clinical outcomes or competencies to focus your observations. Give students feedback on other observations made about their performance.

3. Collect sufficient data on students' performance before drawing conclusions about it.

4. Observe the student more than one time before rating performance. Rating scales, when used for clinical evaluation, should represent a pattern of the students' performance over time.

5. If possible, observe students' performance in different clinical situations, either in the patient care or simulated setting. When not possible, develop additional strategies for evaluation so that performance is evaluated with different methods and at different times.

6. Do not rely on first impressions; they may not be accurate.

7. Always discuss observations with students, obtain their perceptions of performance, and be willing to modify judgments and ratings when new data are presented.

8. Review the available clinical learning activities and opportunities in the simulation and learning laboratories. Do they provide sufficient data for completing the rating scale? If not, new learning activities may need to be developed, or the behaviors on the tool may need to be modified to be more realistic considering the clinical teaching circumstances.

9. Avoid using rating scales as the only source of data about a student's performance—use multiple evaluation methods for clinical practice.

10. Rate each outcome or competency individually based on the observations made of performance and conclusions drawn. If you have insufficient information about achievement of a particular competency, do not rate it—leave it blank.

11. Do not rate all students high, low, or in the middle; similarly, do not let your general impression of the student or personal biases influence the ratings.

12. If the rating form is ineffective for judging student performance, then revise and reevaluate it. Consider these questions: Does the form yield data that can be used to make valid decisions about students' competence? Does the form yield reliable, stable data? Is it easy to use? Is it appropriate considering the types of learning activities that students have in their clinical settings?

13. Discuss as a group (with other educators and preceptors involved in the evaluation) each competency or behavior on the rating scale. Come to agreement about the meaning of the competencies and what a student's performance would look like at each rating level in the tool. Share examples of performance, how you would rate them, and your rationale. As a group exercise, observe a video clip or other simulation of a student's performance, rate it with the tool, and come to agreement about the rating. Such exercises and discussions should be held before the course begins and periodically during it to ensure reliability across teachers and settings.

Once the outcomes or clinical competencies to be evaluated with simulations are identified, the teacher can plan the specifics of the evaluation. Some questions to guide teachers in using simulations for clinical evaluation are:

- What are the specific clinical outcomes or competencies to be evaluated using simulations? These should be designated in the plan or protocol for clinical evaluation in a course.
- What types of simulations are needed to assess the designated outcomes—for example, simulations to demonstrate psychomotor and technological skills; ability to identify problems, treatments, and interventions; and pharmacological management?
- Do the simulations need to be developed, or are they already available in the nursing education program?
- If the simulations need to be developed, who will be responsible for their development? Who will manage their implementation?
- Are the simulations for formative evaluation only? If so, how many practice sessions should be planned? What is the extent of teacher and expert guidance needed? Who will provide that supervision and guidance?
- Are the simulations for summative evaluation (i.e., for grading purposes)? If used for summative clinical evaluation, then faculty members need to determine the process for rating performance and how those ratings will be incorporated into the clinical grade, whether pass–fail or another system for grading.
- Who will develop or obtain checklists or other methods for rating performance in the simulations?
- When will the simulations be implemented in the course?
- How will the effectiveness of the simulations be evaluated, and who will be responsible?

These are only a few of the questions for faculty members to consider when planning to use simulations for clinical evaluation.

Standardized Patients

One type of simulation for clinical evaluation uses standardized patients—individuals who have been trained to accurately portray the role of a patient with a specific diagnosis or condition. With simulations using standardized patients, students can be evaluated on a history and physical examination, related skills and procedures, and communication techniques, among other outcomes. Standardized patients are effective for evaluation, because the actors are trained to re-create the same patient condition and clinical situation each time they are with a student, providing for consistency in the performance evaluation.

When standardized patients are used for formative evaluation, they provide feedback to the students on their performance, an important aid to their learning. Standardized patients are trained to provide both written and oral feedback to students and evaluate their performance (McWilliam & Botwinski, 2012).

Objective Structured Clinical Examination

An Objective Structured Clinical Examination (OSCE) provides a means of evaluating performance in a simulation laboratory rather than in the clinical setting. In an OSCE, students rotate through a series of stations; at each station, they complete an activity or perform a task, which is then evaluated. Some stations assess the student's ability to take a patient's history, perform a physical examination, and implement other interventions while being observed by the teacher or an examiner. The student's performance can then be rated using a rating scale or checklist. At other stations, students might be tested on their knowledge and cognitive skills—they might be asked to analyze data, select interventions and treatments, and manage the patient's condition. OSCEs are typically used for summative clinical evaluation; however, they can also be used formatively to assess performance and provide feedback to students.

Different types of stations can be used in an OSCE. At one type of station the student may interact with a standardized patient as if interviewing or examining the patient (Hawkins & Boulet, 2008). At these stations the teacher or examiner can evaluate students' understanding of varied patient conditions and management of them and can rate the students' performance. At other stations students may demonstrate skills, perform procedures, use technologies, and demonstrate other technical competencies. Performance at those stations is often assessed with checklists. There may also be postencounter stations to facilitate the evaluation of cognitive skills such as interpreting lab results and other data, developing management plans, and making other types of decisions about patient care. Students may be asked to document their findings with the standardized patient, answer questions, and provide evidence for their decisions, among other competencies (Hawkins & Boulet, 2008).

Media Clips

Media clips—short segments of a digital recording, a DVD, a video from YouTube, and other forms of multimedia—may be viewed by students as a basis for discussions in postclinical conferences, on discussion boards, and for other online activities; for small group activities; and for critique and write-up as an assignment. Media clips are often more effective than written descriptions of a scenario, because they allow the student to visualize the patient and clinical situation.

Media clips are appropriate for assessing whether students can apply concepts and content being learned in class to the clinical situation depicted in the media clip, observe and collect data, identify possible problems, identify priority actions and interventions, and evaluate outcomes. Students can answer questions about the media clips as part of a graded learning activity in clinical courses. Media clips are also valuable for formative evaluation, particularly in a group format in which students discuss their ideas and receive feedback from the teacher and peers.

Written Assignments

Written assignments accompanying the clinical experience are effective methods for assessing students' critical thinking and higher-level learning, understanding of content relevant to clinical practice, and ability to express ideas in writing. Many types of written assignments for clinical courses were described in Chapter 14: concept map, concept analysis paper, short written assignments, nursing care plan, case method and study, evidence-based practice papers, teaching plan, clinical journal, group writing, and portfolio. Chapter 11 provided further information about assessing case scenarios. Written assignments can be included as part of the clinical evaluation. Some will be evaluated formatively, such as journals, while others can be graded.

Conferences

The ability to present ideas orally is an important outcome of clinical practice. Sharing information about a patient, leading others in discussions about clinical practice, presenting ideas in a group format, and giving presentations are skills that students need to develop in a nursing program. Working with nursing staff members and the interprofessional team requires the ability to communicate effectively. Conferences provide a method for developing oral communication skills and for evaluating competency in this area. Discussions also lead to problem solving and higher level thinking if questions are open ended and geared to those outcomes, as discussed in Chapter 12.

Criteria for assessing conferences include the ability of students to:

- Present ideas clearly and in a logical sequence to the group
- Participate actively in the group discussion
- Offer ideas relevant to the topic
- Demonstrate knowledge of the content discussed in the conference
- Offer different perspectives on the topic, engaging the group in critical thinking
- Assume a leadership role, if relevant, in promoting group discussion and arriving at group decisions

Most conferences are evaluated for formative purposes, with the teacher giving feedback to students as a group or to the individual who led the group discussion. When conferences are evaluated as a portion of the clinical or course grade, the teacher should have specific criteria to guide the evaluation and should use a scoring rubric. Exhibit 15.6 provides a sample form that can be used to evaluate how well a student leads a clinical conference or to assess student participation in a conference.

Group Projects

Most of the clinical evaluation methods presented in this chapter focus on individual student performance, but group projects also can be assessed as part of the clinical evaluation in a course. Some group work is short term—only for the time it takes to develop a product, such as a teaching plan or group presentation. Other groups may be formed for the purpose of cooperative learning, with students working in small groups or teams in clinical practice over a longer period of time. With any of these group formats, both the products developed by the group and the ability of the students to work cooperatively can be assessed.

There are different approaches for grading group projects. The same grade can be given to every student in the group (i.e., a group grade), although this does not take into consideration individual student effort and contribution to the group product. Another approach is for the students to indicate in the finished product the parts to which they contributed, providing a way of assigning individual student grades, with or without a group grade. Students can also provide a self-assessment of how much they contributed to the group project, which can then be integrated into their grade. Alternatively, students can prepare both a group and an individual product.

Rubrics should be used for assessing group projects and should be geared specifically to the project. To assess students' participation and collaboration in the group, the rubric also needs to reflect the goals of group

Exhibit 15.6

EVALUATION OF PARTICIPATION IN A CLINICAL CONFERENCE

Student's name _____

Conference topic _____

Date _____

Rate the behaviors listed below by circling the appropriate number. Some behaviors will not be applicable depending on the student's role in the conference; mark those as not applicable (na).

Behaviors	Poor				Excellent	
States goals of conference	1	2	3	4	5	na
Leads group in discussion	1	2	3	4	5	na
Asks thought-provoking questions	1	2	3	4	5	na
Uses strategies that encourage all students to participate	1	2	3	4	5	na
Participates actively in discussion	1	2	3	4	5	na
Includes important content	1	2	3	4	5	na
Includes evidence for practice	1	2	3	4	5	na
Offers new perspectives to group	1	2	3	4	5	na
Considers different points of view	1	2	3	4	5	na
Assists group members in recognizing biases and values	1	2	3	4	5	na
Is enthusiastic about topic	1	2	3	4	5	na
Is well prepared for discussion	1	2	3	4	5	na
If leading group, monitors time	1	2	3	4	5	na
Develops quality materials to support discussion	1	2	3	4	5	na
Summarizes major points at end of conference	1	2	3	4	5	na

work. With small groups, the teacher can observe and rate individual student cooperation and contributions to the group. However, this is often difficult because the teacher is not a member of the group, and the group dynamics change when the teacher is present. As another approach, students can assess the participation and cooperation of their peers. These peer evaluations can be used for the students' own development and shared among peers but not with the teacher, or they can be incorporated by the teacher in the grade for the group project. Students can also be asked to assess their own participation in the group.

Self-Assessment

Self-assessment is the ability of students to assess their own clinical competencies and identify where further learning is needed. Self-evaluation begins with the first clinical course and develops throughout the nursing program, continuing into professional practice. Through self-evaluation, students examine their clinical performance and identify both strengths and areas for improvement. Using students' own assessments, teachers can develop plans to assist students in gaining the knowledge and skills they need to meet the outcomes of the course. It is important for teachers to establish a positive climate for learning in the course, or students will not be likely to share an honest self-evaluation with them.

In addition to developing a supportive learning environment, the teacher should hold planned conferences with each student to review performance. In these conferences, the teacher can:

- Give specific feedback on performance
- Obtain the student's perceptions of his or her competencies
- Identify strengths and areas for learning from the teacher's and student's perspectives
- Plan with the student learning activities for improving performance, which is critical if the student is not passing the clinical course
- Enhance communication between teacher and student.

Self-evaluation is appropriate only for formative evaluation and should never be graded.

CLINICAL EVALUATION IN DISTANCE EDUCATION

Nursing programs use different strategies for offering the clinical component of distance education courses. Often preceptors in the local area guide student learning in the clinical setting and evaluate performance. If cohorts of students are available in an area, adjunct or part-time faculty members might be hired to teach a small group of students in the clinical setting. In other programs, students independently complete clinical learning activities to gain the clinical knowledge and competencies of a course. Regardless of how the clinical component is structured, the course syllabus, competencies to be developed, rating forms, guidelines for clinical practice, and other materials associated with the clinical course need to be available to whomever is providing the instruction and evaluating student learning. Course management systems facilitate communication among students, preceptors, course faculty, and others involved in the students' clinical activities.

The clinical evaluation methods presented in this chapter can be used for distance education. The critical decision for the teacher is to identify which clinical competencies and skills, if any, need to be observed and the performance rated, because that decision suggests different evaluation methods than if the focus of the evaluation is on the cognitive outcomes of the clinical course. In programs in which preceptors or adjunct faculty members are available on site, any of the clinical evaluation methods presented in this chapter can be used as long as they are congruent with the outcomes and competencies. There should be consistency, though, in how the evaluation is done across preceptors and clinical settings.

Strategies should be implemented in the course for preceptors and other educators involved in the performance evaluation to discuss as a group the competencies to be rated, what each competency means, and the performance of those competencies at different levels on the rating scale. This is a critical activity to ensure reliability across preceptors and other evaluators. Preceptor development activities of this type should be done before the course begins and at least once during the course to ensure that evaluators are using the tool as intended and are consistent across students and clinical settings.

Even in clinical courses involving preceptors, faculty members may decide to evaluate clinical skills themselves by reviewing digital recordings of performance or observing students through videoconferencing and other technology. Digitally recording performance is valuable as a strategy for summative evaluation, to assess competencies at the end of a clinical course or another designated point in time, and for review by students for self-assessment and by faculty members to give feedback.

Simulations and standardized patients are other strategies useful in assessing clinical performance in distance education. Performance with standardized patients can be recorded, and students can submit their patient histories and other written documentation that would commonly be done in practice in that situation. Students can also complete case analyses related to the standardized patient encounter for assessing their knowledge base and rationale for their decisions.

Simulations, analyses of cases, case presentations, written assignments, and other strategies presented in this chapter can be used for clinical evaluation in distance education courses. Similar to clinical evaluation in general, a combination of approaches is more effective than one method alone.

GRADING CLINICAL PRACTICE

Grading systems for clinical practice are often two-dimensional, such as pass–fail, satisfactory–unsatisfactory, and met or did not meet the clinical objectives. Some nursing programs add a third category, honors, to acknowledge performance that exceeds the level required. Other grading systems are multidimensional—for example, using letter grades A through F; integers 1 through 5; and percentages. With any of these grading systems, it is not always easy to summarize the multiple types of evaluation data collected about the student's performance into a symbol representing a grade. This is true even in a pass–fail system; it may be difficult to arrive at a judgment to pass or fail based on the evaluation data and the circumstances associated with the student's clinical and simulated practice.

Regardless of the grading system for clinical practice, there are two criteria to be met: (1) the evaluation methods for collecting data about student performance should reflect the clinical competencies and outcomes for which a grade will be assigned, and (2) students must understand how their clinical practice will be evaluated and graded. In planning the course, the teacher needs to decide which of the evaluation methods should be incorporated in the clinical grade. Some of these methods are for summative evaluation, thereby providing a source of information for including in the clinical grade. Other methods, though, are used in clinical practice for feedback only and are not incorporated in the grade.

Categories for grading clinical practice such as pass–fail and satisfactory–unsatisfactory have advantages over a system with multiple levels, although there are some disadvantages as well. Pass–fail places greater emphasis on giving feedback to the learner, because only two categories of performance need to be determined. With a pass–fail grading system, faculty members may be more inclined to provide continual feedback to learners, because they do not have to ultimately differentiate performance according to four or five levels of proficiency such as with a multidimensional system. Performance that exceeds the requirements and expectations, though, is not reflected in the grade for clinical practice unless a third category is included—honors–pass–fail. Pass–fail is used most frequently in nursing programs (Oermann et al., 2009).

A pass–fail system requires only two types of judgment about clinical performance. Do the evaluation data indicate that the student has demonstrated satisfactory performance of the competencies to indicate a pass? Or do the data suggest that the performance of those competencies is not at a satisfactory level? Deciding whether the learner has passed or failed is often easier for the teacher than using the same evaluation information for deciding on multiple levels of performance. A letter system for grading clinical practice, however, acknowledges the different levels of clinical proficiency students may have demonstrated in their clinical practice.

A disadvantage of pass–fail for grading clinical practice is the inability to include a clinical grade into the course grade. One strategy is to separate nursing courses into two components for grading: one for theory and the second for clinical practice (designated as pass–fail), even though the course is considered a whole. Typically, guidelines for the course indicate that the students must pass the clinical component to pass the course. A second mechanism is to offer two separate courses with the clinical course graded on a pass–fail basis.

Methods for Assigning the Clinical Grade

Once the grading system is determined, there are varied ways of using it to arrive at the clinical grade. The grade can be assigned based on the competencies or outcomes achieved by the student. To use this method, the faculty should consider designating some of the competencies or outcomes as critical for achievement in the course. For example, an A might be assigned if all of the clinical competencies or outcomes were met; a B might be assigned if all of the competencies designated by the faculty as critical behaviors and at least half of the others were met.

For pass–fail grading, the faculty can indicate that all of the competencies or outcomes must be met to pass the course or can designate critical behaviors required for passing the course. For both of these grading systems, the clinical evaluation methods provide the data for determining whether the student's performance reflects achievement of the competencies. These evaluation methods may or may not be graded separately as part of the course grade.

Another way of arriving at the clinical grade is to base it on the evaluation methods. In this system, the clinical evaluation methods become the source of data for the grade. For example,

Paper on analysis of clinical practice issue	10%
Analysis of clinical cases	5%
Conference presentation	10%
Community resource paper	10%
Portfolio	25%
Rating scale (of performance)	40%

In this illustration, the clinical grade is computed according to the evaluation methods. Observation of performance, and the rating on the clinical evaluation tool, is only a portion of the clinical grade. An advantage of this approach is that it incorporates into the grade the summative evaluation methods completed by students.

If pass–fail is used for grading clinical practice, the grade might be computed as follows:

Paper on analysis of clinical practice issue	10%
Analysis of clinical cases	5%
Conference presentation	10%
Community resource paper	10%
Portfolio	25%
Clinical examination, simulations	40%
Rating scale (of performance)	Pass required

This discussion of grading clinical practice suggests a variety of appropriate mechanisms. The teacher must make it clear to students and others how the evaluation and grading will be carried out in clinical practice, through simulations, and in other settings.

FAILING CLINICAL PRACTICE

Teachers will be faced with determining when students have not met the outcomes of the clinical practicum—that is, when students have not demonstrated sufficient competence to pass the clinical course. There are principles that should be followed in evaluating and grading clinical practice, which are critical if a student fails a clinical course or has the potential for failing it. These principles are discussed below.

Communicate Evaluation and Grading Methods in Writing

The evaluation methods used in a clinical course; how each will be graded, if at all; and how the clinical grade will be assigned should be in writing and communicated to the students. The teacher's practices in evaluating and grading clinical performance must reflect this written information. In courses with preceptors, it is critical that preceptors and others involved in teaching and assessing student performance understand the outcomes of the course, the evaluation methods, how to observe and rate performance, and responsibilities when students are not performing adequately. Preceptors are reluctant to assign failing grades to students whose competence is questionable (Heaslip & Scammell, 2012).

There is a need for faculty development, especially for new and part-time teachers. The decision whether to assign a pass or fail grade to a nursing student is difficult, and some nursing faculty members feel insecure about making that decision (DeBrew & Lewallen, 2013; Larocque & Luhanga, 2013). As part of this development, teachers should explore their own beliefs and values about grading clinical performance, the meaning of grades, and their views of what constitutes satisfactory performance (Scanlan & Care, 2008).

Identify Effect of Failing Clinical Practicum on Course Grade

If failing clinical practice, whether in a pass–fail or a letter system, means failing the nursing course, this should be stated clearly in the course syllabus and policies. By stating it in the syllabus, which all students receive, they have it in writing before clinical learning activities begin. A sample policy statement for pass–fail clinical grading is:

> The clinical component of NUR XXX is evaluated with a pass or fail. A failing grade in the clinical component results in failure of the course, even if the theory grade is 75% or higher.

In a letter grade system, the policy should include the letter grade representing a failure in clinical practice—for example, below a C grade. A sample policy statement is:

> Students must pass the clinical component of NUR XXX with the grade of C or higher. A grade lower than a C in the clinical component of the course results in failure of the course, even if the theory grade is 75% or higher.

Ask Students to Sign Rating Forms and Evaluation Summaries

Students should sign any written clinical evaluation documents—rating forms (of clinical practicum, clinical examinations, and performance in simulations), notes and any other narrative comments about the student's performance, and summaries of conferences in which performance was discussed. Their signatures do not mean they agree with the ratings or comments, only that they have read them. Students should have an opportunity to write in their own comments. These materials are important, because they document the student's performance and indicate that the teacher provided feedback and shared concerns about that performance. This is critical in situations in which students may be failing the clinical course because of performance problems.

Identify Performance Problems Early and Develop Learning Plans

Students need continuous feedback on their clinical performance. Observations made by the teacher, the preceptor, and others and evaluation data from other sources should be shared with the student. Together they should discuss the data. Students may have different perceptions of their performance and, in some cases, may provide new information that influences the teacher's judgment about clinical competencies.

When the teacher or preceptor identifies performance problems and clinical deficiencies that may affect passing the course, conferences should be held with the student to discuss these areas of concern and develop a plan for remediation. It is critical that these conferences focus on problems in performance combined with specific learning activities for addressing them. The conferences should not be the teacher telling the student everything that is wrong with clinical performance; the student needs an opportunity to respond to the teacher's concerns and identify how to address them.

One of the goals of the conference is to develop a plan with learning activities for the student to correct deficiencies and develop competencies further. The plan should indicate that (1) completing the remedial learning activities does not guarantee that the student will pass the course, (2) one satisfactory performance of the competencies will not constitute a pass clinical grade (the improvement must be sustained), and (3) the student must demonstrate satisfactory performance of the competencies by the end of the course. A template is provided in Exhibit 15.7 that can be used to develop a learning plan for students. It is important to remember that students have until the end of the course to improve their performance unless they are unsafe in the clinical setting. In that case, the student may be removed from the clinical course depending on the policies of the nursing program, which every teacher and student should understand.

Any discussions with students at risk of failing clinical practice should focus on the student's inability to meet the clinical objectives and perform the specified competencies, not on the teacher's perceptions of the student's intelligence and overall ability. In addition, opinions about the student's ability in general should not be discussed with others.

Conferences should be held in private, and a summary of the discussion should be prepared. The summary should include the date and time of the conference, who participated, areas of concern about clinical performance, and the learning plan with a time frame for completion. The summary should be signed by the teacher, the student, and other participants.

Exhibit 15.7

TEMPLATE OF A LEARNING PLAN

1. Identify the knowledge and areas of performance to be improved in clinical practice (specify the related outcomes or competencies).

2. For each of the areas to be improved, identify learning activities to be completed by the student with due dates.

3. List relevant resources to guide student learning and practice.

4. Plan and specify the process to be used for evaluating progress and performance. Include dates for achieving outcomes and developing competencies, and set up specific meeting times for feedback on progress.

Faculty members should review related policies of the nursing education program, because they might specify other requirements.

Identify Support Services

Students who are at risk of failing clinical practice may have other problems affecting their performance. Teachers should refer students to counseling and other support services and not attempt to provide these resources themselves. Attempting to counsel the student and help the student cope with other problems may bias the teacher and influence judgment of the student's clinical performance.

Document Performance

As the clinical course progresses, the teacher should give feedback to the student about performance and continue to guide learning. It is important to document the observations made, other types of evaluation data collected, and the learning activities completed by the student. The documentation should be shared routinely with students, discussions about performance should be summarized, and students should sign these summaries to confirm that they read them.

The teacher cannot observe and document the performance of only the student at risk of failing the course. There should be a minimum number of observations and documentation of other students in the clinical group, or the student failing the course might believe that he or she was treated differently than others in the group. One strategy is to plan the number of observations of performance to be made for each student in the clinical group to avoid focusing only on the student with performance problems. However, teachers may observe students who are believed to be at risk for failure more closely and document their observations and conferences with those students more thoroughly and frequently than is necessary for the majority of students. When observations result in feedback to students that can be used to improve performance, at-risk students do not usually object to this extra attention.

Follow Policy on Unsafe Clinical Performance

There should be a policy in the nursing program about actions to be taken if a student is unsafe in clinical practice. Students who are not meeting the outcomes of the course or have problems performing some of the competencies can continue in the clinical course as long as they demonstrate safe care. This is because the outcomes and clinical competencies are identified for achievement at the end of the course, not during it.

If the student demonstrates performance that is potentially unsafe, however, the teacher can remove the student from the clinical setting, following the policy and procedures of the nursing education program. Specific learning activities outside of the clinical setting need to be offered for students to develop the knowledge and skills they lack; practice with simulators is valuable in these situations. A learning plan should be prepared and implemented as described earlier.

Follow Policy for Failure of a Clinical Course

In all instances, the teacher must follow the policies of the nursing program. If the student fails the clinical course, the student must be notified of the failure and its consequences as indicated in these policies. In some nursing programs, students are allowed to repeat only one clinical course, and there may be other requirements to be met. If the student will be dismissed from the program because of the failure, the student must be informed of this in writing. Generally, there is a specific time frame for each step in the process, which must be adhered to by the faculty, administrators, and students.

SUMMARY

Through clinical evaluation, a teacher arrives at judgments about students' performance in clinical practice. The teacher's observations of performance should focus on the outcomes to be met or competencies to be developed in the clinical course. These provide the framework for learning in clinical practice and the basis for evaluating performance. Although such a framework is essential in clinical evaluation, teachers also need to examine their own beliefs about the evaluation process and purposes it serves in nursing. Clarifying one's own values, beliefs, attitudes, and biases that may affect evaluation is an important first step.

Many clinical evaluation methods are available for assessing student competencies in clinical practice. The teacher should choose evaluation methods that provide information on how well students are performing the clinical competencies. The teacher also decides whether the evaluation method is intended for formative or summative evaluation. Some of the methods designed for clinical evaluation are strictly to provide feedback to students on areas for improvement and are not graded. Other methods, such as rating forms and certain written assignments, may be used for summative purposes.

The predominant method for clinical evaluation is in observing the performance of students in clinical practice. Although observation is widely used, there are threats to its validity and reliability. Observations of students may be influenced by the teacher's or preceptor's values, attitudes, and biases. In observing clinical performance, there are many aspects of that performance on which the teacher may focus attention. Every observation reflects only a sampling of the learner's performance during a clinical learning activity. Such issues point to the need for a series of observations before drawing conclusions about performance. There are several ways of recording observations of students, including anecdotal notes, checklists, and rating scales.

Other methods for clinical evaluation are simulations, standardized patients, OSCEs, written assignments, portfolios, conferences, group projects, and self-evaluation. Some methods are appropriate only for formative evaluation and providing feedback to students. Other methods can be used for both formative and summative evaluation (i.e., graded).

Important guidelines for grading clinical practice and working with students who are at risk for failing a clinical course were discussed in the chapter. These guidelines give direction to teachers in establishing sound grading practices and following them when working with students in clinical practice.

Exhibit 15.8

CNE EXAMINATION TEST BLUEPRINT CORE COMPETENCIES

3. **Use Assessment and Evaluation Strategies**

   A. Provide input for the development of nursing program standards and policies regarding
      2. progression

   B. Enforce nursing program standards related to
      1. admission
      2. progression

(continued)

C. Use a variety of strategies to assess and evaluate learning in these domains
   1. cognitive
   2. psychomotor
   3. affective
D. Incorporate current research in assessment and evaluation practices
E. Analyze available resources for learner assessment and evaluation
F. Create assessment instruments to evaluate outcomes
G. Use assessment instruments to evaluate outcomes
H. Implement evaluation strategies that are appropriate to the learner and learning outcomes
I. Analyze assessment and evaluation data
J. Use assessment and evaluation data to enhance the teaching-learning process
K. Advise learners regarding assessment and evaluation criteria
L. Provide timely, constructive, and thoughtful feedback to learners

NOTE

This chapter was adapted from *Evaluation and Testing in Nursing Education*, 4th ed. (Chapters 13, 14, and 17), by M. H. Oermann and K. B. Gaberson, 2014, New York, NY: Springer Publishing. Copyright ©2014 by Springer Publishing. Adapted with permission.

REFERENCES

Boland, D. L. (2009). Developing curriculum frameworks, outcomes, and competencies. In D. M. Billings & J. A. Halstead (Eds.), *Teaching in nursing: A guide for faculty* (3rd ed., pp. 137–153). St. Louis, MO: Saunders.

Bonnel, W. (2008). Improving feedback to students in online courses. *Nursing Education Perspectives, 29*, 290–294.

Bourke, M. P., & Ihrke, B. A. (2009). The evaluation process: An overview. In D. M. Billings & J. Halstead (Eds.), *Teaching in nursing* (3rd ed., pp. 391–408). St. Louis, MO: Saunders Elsevier.

Chickering, A. W., & Gamson, Z. F. (1987). Seven principles for good practice in undergraduate education. *AAHE Bulletin, 39*(7), 3–7.

Clynes, M. P., & Raftery, S. E. (2008). Feedback: An essential element of student learning in clinical practice. *Nurse Education in Practice, 8*, 405–411.

DeBrew, J. K., & Lewallen, L. P. (2013). To pass or to fail? Understanding the factors considered by faculty in the clinical evaluation of nursing students. *Nurse Education Today.* doi:10.1016/j.nedt.2013.05.014

Di Leonardi Case, B., & Oermann, M. H. (2010). Clinical teaching and evaluation. In L. Caputi (Ed.), *Teaching nursing: The art and science* (2nd ed., pp. 82–141). Glen Ellyn, IL: College of DuPage.

Gigante, J., Dell, M., & Sharkey, A. (2011). Getting beyond "Good job": How to give effective feedback. *Pediatrics, 127*, 205–207.

Hall, M. A. (2013). An expanded look at evaluating clinical performance: Faculty use of anecdotal notes in the U.S. and Canada. *Nurse Education in Practice, 13*, 271–276. doi: 10.1016/j.nepr.2013.02.001

Hawkins, R. E., & Boulet, J. R. (2008). Direct observation: Standardized patients. In E. S. Holmboe & R. E. Hawkins (Eds.), *Practical guide to the evaluation of clinical competencies* (pp. 102–118). Philadelphia, PA: Mosby.

Heaslip, V., & Scammell, J. M. E. (2012). Failing underperforming students: The role of grading in practice assessment. *Nurse Education in Practice, 12*, 95–100.

Larocque, S., & Luhanga, F. L. (2013). Exploring the issue of failure to fail in a nursing program. *International Journal of Nursing Education Scholarship, 10*, 1–8. doi: 10.1515/ijnes-2012-0037

McWilliam, P. L., & Botwinski, C. A. (2012). Identifying strengths and weaknesses in the utilization of Objective Structured Clinical Examination (OSCE) in a nursing program. *Nursing Education Perspectives, 33*, 35–39.

Nitko, A. J., & Brookhart, S. M. (2011). *Educational assessment of students* (6th ed.). Upper Saddle River, NJ: Pearson Education.

Oermann, M. H. (2008). Clinical evaluation. In B. Penn (Ed.), *Mastering the teaching role: A guide for nurse educators* (pp. 299–313). Philadelphia, PA: F. A. Davis.

Oermann, M. H., Yarbrough, S. S., Ard, N., Saewert, K. J., & Charasika, M. (2009). Clinical evaluation and grading practices in schools of nursing: National Survey Findings Part II. *Nursing Education Perspectives, 30*, 274–279.

Quality and Safety Education for Nurses. (2013). *Competencies*. Retrieved from http://qsen.org/competencies/

Scanlan, J. M., & Care, W. D. (2008). Issues with grading and grade inflation in nursing education. In M. H. Oermann, (Ed.), *Annual review of nursing education* (Vol. 6, pp. 173–188). New York, NY: Springer Publishing.

Appendix: Certified Nurse Educator (CNE™) Examination Detailed Test Blueprint*

1. Facilitate Learning—22%

A. Implement a variety of teaching strategies appropriate to:

    1. content

    2. setting (i.e., clinical versus classroom)

    3. learner needs

    4. learning style

    5. desired learner outcomes

    6. method of delivery (e.g., face-to-face, remote, simulation)

B. Use teaching strategies based on:

    1. educational theory

    2. evidence-based practices related to education

C. Modify teaching strategies and learning experiences based on consideration of learners':

    1. cultural background

    2. past clinical experiences

    3. past educational and life experiences

    4. generational groups (i.e., age)

D. Use information technologies to support the teaching-learning process

* Reprinted with permission of the National League for Nursing (NLN). © Copyright 2012. All rights reserved. The test blueprint is subject to revision, and the most current version can be obtained in the CNE Candidate Handbook, which can be obtained on the NLN website.

E. Practice skilled oral and written (including electronic) communication that reflects an awareness of self and relationships with learners (e.g., evaluation, mentorship, and supervision)

F. Communicate effectively orally and in writing with an ability to convey ideas in a variety of contexts

G. Model reflective thinking practices, including critical thinking

H. Create opportunities for learners to develop their own critical thinking skills

I. Create a positive learning environment that fosters a free exchange of ideas

J. Show enthusiasm for teaching, learning, and the nursing profession that inspires and motivates students

K. Demonstrate personal attributes that facilitate learning (e.g., caring, confidence, patience, integrity, respect, and flexibility)

L. Respond effectively to unexpected events that affect instruction

M. Develop collegial working relationships with clinical agency personnel to promote positive learning environments

N. Use knowledge of evidence-based practice to instruct learners

O. Demonstrate ability to teach clinical skills

P. Act as a role model in practice settings

Q. Foster a safe learning environment

2. **Facilitate Learner Development and Socialization—14%**

A. Identify individual learning styles and unique learning needs of learners with these characteristics:
   1. culturally diverse (including international);
   2. English as an additional language
   3. traditional *vs.* non-traditional (i.e., recent high school graduates vs. those in school later)
   4. at-risk (e.g., educationally disadvantaged, learning and/or physically challenged, social, and economic issues)
   5. previous nursing education

B. Provide resources for diverse learners to meet their individual learning needs

C. Advise learners in ways that help them meet their professional goals

D. Create learning environments that facilitate learners' self-reflection, personal goal setting, and socialization to the role of the nurse

E. Foster the development of learners in these areas:
1. cognitive domain
2. psychomotor domain
3. affective domain

F. Assist learners to engage in thoughtful and constructive self and peer evaluation

G. Encourage professional development of learners

3. Use Assessment and Evaluation Strategies—17%

A. Provide input for the development of nursing program standards and policies regarding:
1. admission
2. progression
3. graduation

B. Enforce nursing program standards related to
1. admission
2. progression
3. graduation

C. Use a variety of strategies to assess and evaluate learning in these domains:
1. cognitive
2. psychomotor
3. affective

D. Incorporate current research in assessment and evaluation practices

E. Analyze available resources for learner assessment and evaluation

F. Create assessment instruments to evaluate outcomes

G. Use assessment instruments to evaluate outcomes

H. Implement evaluation strategies that are appropriate to the learner and learning outcomes

I. Analyze assessment and evaluation data

J. Use assessment and evaluation data to enhance the teaching-learning process

K. Advise learners regarding assessment and evaluation criteria

L. Provide timely, constructive, and thoughtful feedback to learners

4. **Participate in Curriculum Design and Evaluation of Program Outcomes—19%**

   A. Demonstrate knowledge of curriculum development including:
   1. identifying program outcomes
   2. developing competency statements
   3. writing course objectives
   4. selecting appropriate learning activities
   5. selecting appropriate clinical experiences
   6. selecting appropriate evaluation strategies

   B. Actively participate in the design of the curriculum to reflect:
   1. institutional philosophy and mission
   2. current nursing and health care trends
   3. community and societal needs
   4. nursing principles, standards, theory, and research
   5. educational principles, theory, and research
   6. use of technology

   C. Lead the development of curriculum design

   D. Lead the development of course design

   E. Analyze results of program evaluation

   F. Revise the curriculum based on evaluation of:
   1. program outcomes
   2. learner needs
   3. societal and health care trends
   4. stakeholder feedback (e.g., from learners, agency personnel, accrediting agencies, advisory boards)

   G. Implement curricular revisions using appropriate change theories and strategies

   H. Collaborate with community and clinical partners to support educational goals

   I. Design program assessment plans that promote continuous quality improvement

J. Implement the program assessment plan

K. Evaluate the program assessment plan

5. **Pursue Systematic Self-Evaluation and Improvement in the Academic Nurse Educator Role—9%**

   A. Engage in activities that promote one's socialization to the role

   B. Maintain membership in professional organizations

   C. Participate actively in professional organizations through committee work and/or leadership roles

   D. Demonstrate a commitment to lifelong learning

   E. Participate in professional development opportunities that increase one's effectiveness in the role

   F. Manage the teaching, scholarship, and service demands as influenced by the requirements of the institutional setting

   G. Use feedback gained from self, peer, learner, and administrative evaluation to improve role effectiveness

   H. Practice according to legal and ethical standards relevant to higher education and nursing education

   I. Mentor and support faculty colleagues in the role of an academic nurse educator

   J. Engage in self-reflection to improve teaching practices

6. **Engage in Scholarship, Service, and Leadership—21%**

   A. Function as a Change Agent and Leader
      1. Model cultural sensitivity when advocating for change
      2. Evaluate organizational effectiveness in nursing education
      3. Enhance the visibility of nursing and its contributions by providing leadership in the:
         a. nursing program
         b. parent institution
         c. local community
         d. state or region

    4. Participate in interdisciplinary efforts to address health care and educational needs:

      a. within the institution

      b. locally

      c. regionally

    5. Implement strategies for change within the:

      a. nursing program

      b. institution

      c. local community

    6. Develop leadership skills in others to shape and implement change

    7. Adapt to changes created by external factors

    8. Create a culture for change within the:

      a. nursing program

      b. institution

    9. Advocate for nursing, nursing education, and higher education in the political arena

B. Engage in Scholarship of Teaching

    1. Exhibit a spirit of inquiry about teaching and learning, student development, and evaluation methods

    2. Use evidence-based resources to improve and support teaching

    3. Participate in research activities related to nursing education

    4. Share teaching expertise with colleagues and others

    5. Demonstrate integrity as a scholar

C. Function Effectively within the Institutional Environment and the Academic Community

    1. Identify how social, economic, political, and institutional forces influence nursing and higher education

    2. Make decisions based on knowledge of historical and current trends and issues in higher education

    3. Integrate the values of respect, collegiality, professionalism, and caring to build an organizational climate that fosters the development of learners and colleagues

    4. Consider the goals of the nursing program and the mission of the parent institution when proposing change or managing issues

    5. Participate on institutional and departmental committees

Index

AACN. *See* American Association of Colleges of Nursing
academic deficiencies, 136
academic dishonesty, 33, 130–133
academic integrity policy, 132–133
academic-service partnerships, 57
academic standards, 134, 136
accommodations, 129, 134
accreditation
  agency, 56, 76
  of nursing education programs, 76
ACIP. *See* Advisory Committee on Immunization Practices
acute care units, as clinical learning sites, 39, 40, 62
adult learning theory, 191
advance practice nurses (APNs), 102, 115, 190
Advisory Committee on Immunization Practices (ACIP), 74
affective domain outcomes, 30
affective preparation for clinical learning activities, 85–86
Affordable Care Act (2010), 41
agencies, clinical. *See also* clinical learning settings
  accreditation of, 76
  acute care, 39, 40, 62
  contracts with, 56
  licensure, 76

  orientation to, 86–87
  preparation of, 57–59, 78–81
  requirements of, 74
Agency for Health care Research (AHRQ), 228
altering a document, 130
American Association of Colleges of Nursing (AACN), 23, 41
American Association of Colleges of Nursing QSEN Education Consortium, 25
American Association of Critical Care Nurses Synergy Model for Patient Care, 5
American Nurses Association (ANA)
  Code of Ethics for Nurses, 30
  Principles for Social Networking and the Nurse, 128
Americans with Disabilities Act of 1990, 133
ANA. *See* American Nurses Association
anecdotal notes, 142, 143
  clinical performance and, 332
anxiety, 53, 85
AORN. *See* Association of periOperative Registered Nurses
appeals of academic decisions, 131, 137, 138

electronic health records (EHRs), 28, 211, 220, 224
End-of-Life Nursing Education Consortium (ELNEC), 47
errors
  concealing, 131
  correcting, 259
  preventing, 33, 70
  with rating scales, 343–344
espoused curriculum, 13, 14
ethical issues, 125–133, 144, 145
  academic dishonesty, 130–133
  competent teaching, 130
  learners in service setting, 125–126
  student–faculty relationships, 127–128
  students' privacy rights, 129
ethical values, 30, 35
evaluation, 10, 105, 117
  of clinical competence, 53
  in distance education, 52, 53
  of media and multimedia, 175–176
  preceptors, 286, 287
  of presentations, 263
  role of staff members in, 80–81
  of simulations, 203–209, 211
  student, of guided observation activity, 163–164
  technology, 233
  of textbooks, 219
  written assignments, 311–317
  written communication of, 355–356
evidence-based practice papers, 305–307
experience. *See* clinical experience
experiential learning theory, 191
extended care facilities, 45–47

Facebook, 127
faculty, 90, 106
  clinical competence of, 76–77
  clinical setting familiarity, 77
  development, 182
  preparation, 76
failure, 356–360
Fair Credit Reporting Act, 75

fairness, 127–128, 324–325
false representation, 131
Family Education Rights and Privacy Act (FERPA), 75, 129
feedback
  in clinical evaluation, 325–326
  principles of providing, 326–327
  in simulations, 204–209
feelings, examining, 298
feminism, 5
fieldwork, 159
formative clinical evaluation, 105, 117, 323–324
The Future of Nursing (Institute of Medicine), 41

game-based learning, 228–231
grading
  academic dishonesty and, 130–133
  assignments, 313–317
  versus clinical evaluation, 322
  clinical practice, 353–355
  group projects, 349–351
  methods for assigning, 354–355
  pass–fail, 353–354
grand rounds, 237, 250–252
  clinical judgment and, 239
  cognitive skill development and, 237–239
  critical thinking and, 238–239
  problem solving and, 238
grievance process, 135–138
group discussions. *See* discussions
group projects, 349–351
group writing, 309
guided observation, 159–164
guided reflection, 199–203
guidelines
  for community-based learning, 61–62
  for discussions, 257–260
  multimedia, 181–182
  for preceptors, 280
  for rating scales, 346
  safety, 61–62

Lightning Source UK Ltd.
Milton Keynes UK
UKOW05f0100230916

283576UK00001B/204/P